Oxygen Variations

Oxygen Variations

Editors

Costantino Balestra
Fabio Virgili
Simona Mrakic-Sposta

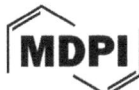

Basel • Beijing • Wuhan • Barcelona • Belgrade • Novi Sad • Cluj • Manchester

Editors
Costantino Balestra
Environmental, Occupational,
Aging Physiology Laboratory
Haute Ecole
Bruxelles-Brabant (HE2B)
Brussels
Belgium

Fabio Virgili
National Institute for
Bio-Structures and
Bio-Systems—I.N.B.B.
Interuniversitary Consortium
Rome
Italy

Simona Mrakic-Sposta
Institute of Clinical
Physiology
National Research
Council (CNR)
Milan
Italy

Editorial Office
MDPI
St. Alban-Anlage 66
4052 Basel, Switzerland

This is a reprint of articles from the Special Issue published online in the open access journal *International Journal of Molecular Sciences* (ISSN 1422-0067) (available at: www.mdpi.com/journal/ijms/special_issues/Oxygen_Variations).

For citation purposes, cite each article independently as indicated on the article page online and as indicated below:

Lastname, A.A.; Lastname, B.B. Article Title. *Journal Name* **Year**, *Volume Number*, Page Range.

ISBN 978-3-0365-8892-6 (Hbk)
ISBN 978-3-0365-8893-3 (PDF)
doi.org/10.3390/books978-3-0365-8893-3

© 2023 by the authors. Articles in this book are Open Access and distributed under the Creative Commons Attribution (CC BY) license. The book as a whole is distributed by MDPI under the terms and conditions of the Creative Commons Attribution-NonCommercial-NoDerivs (CC BY-NC-ND) license.

Contents

About the Editors vii

Preface ix

Costantino Balestra, Simona Mrakic-Sposta and Fabio Virgili
Oxygen Variations—Insights into Hypoxia, Hyperoxia and Hyperbaric Hyperoxia—Is the Dose the Clue?
Reprinted from: *Int. J. Mol. Sci.* **2023**, 24, 13472, doi:10.3390/ijms241713472 1

Costantino Balestra, Awadhesh K. Arya, Clément Leveque, Fabio Virgili, Peter Germonpré, Kate Lambrechts, et al.
Varying Oxygen Partial Pressure Elicits Blood-Borne Microparticles Expressing Different Cell-Specific Proteins—Toward a Targeted Use of Oxygen?
Reprinted from: *Int. J. Mol. Sci.* **2022**, 23, 7888, doi:10.3390/ijms23147888 9

Michele Salvagno, Giacomo Coppalini, Fabio Silvio Taccone, Giacomo Strapazzon, Simona Mrakic-Sposta, Monica Rocco, et al.
The Normobaric Oxygen Paradox—Hyperoxic Hypoxic Paradox: A Novel Expedient Strategy in Hematopoiesis Clinical Issues
Reprinted from: *Int. J. Mol. Sci.* **2023**, 24, 82, doi:10.3390/ijms24010082 25

Liang-Ti Huang and Chung-Ming Chen
Kidney Injuries and Evolution of Chronic Kidney Diseases Due to Neonatal Hyperoxia Exposure Based on Animal Studies
Reprinted from: *Int. J. Mol. Sci.* **2022**, 23, 8492, doi:10.3390/ijms23158492 41

Clément Leveque, Simona Mrakic-Sposta, Pierre Lafère, Alessandra Vezzoli, Peter Germonpré, Alexandre Beer, et al.
Oxidative Stress Response's Kinetics after 60 Minutes at Different (30% or 100%) Normobaric Hyperoxia Exposures
Reprinted from: *Int. J. Mol. Sci.* **2023**, 24, 664, doi:10.3390/ijms24010664 55

Simona Mrakic-Sposta, Maristella Gussoni, Mauro Marzorati, Simone Porcelli, Gerardo Bosco, Costantino Balestra, et al.
The "ON-OFF" Switching Response of Reactive Oxygen Species in Acute Normobaric Hypoxia: Preliminary Outcome
Reprinted from: *Int. J. Mol. Sci.* **2023**, 24, 4012, doi:10.3390/ijms24044012 69

Clément Leveque, Simona Mrakic Sposta, Sigrid Theunissen, Peter Germonpré, Kate Lambrechts, Alessandra Vezzoli, et al.
Oxidative Stress Response Kinetics after 60 Minutes at Different Levels (10% or 15%) of Normobaric Hypoxia Exposure
Reprinted from: *Int. J. Mol. Sci.* **2023**, 24, 10188, doi:10.3390/ijms241210188 81

Qianqian Shao, Jia Liu, Gaifen Li, Yakun Gu, Mengyuan Guo, Yuying Guan, et al.
Proteomic Analysis Reveals That Mitochondria Dominate the Hippocampal Hypoxic Response in Mice
Reprinted from: *Int. J. Mol. Sci.* **2022**, 23, 14094, doi:10.3390/ijms232214094 95

Clément Leveque, Simona Mrakic Sposta, Sigrid Theunissen, Peter Germonpré, Kate Lambrechts, Alessandra Vezzoli, et al.
Oxidative Stress Response Kinetics after 60 Minutes at Different (1.4 ATA and 2.5 ATA) Hyperbaric Hyperoxia Exposures
Reprinted from: *Int. J. Mol. Sci.* **2023**, 24, 12361, doi:10.3390/ijms241512361 113

Rada Jeremic, Sanja Pekovic, Irena Lavrnja, Ivana Bjelobaba, Marina Djelic, Sanja Dacic and Predrag Brkic
Hyperbaric Oxygenation Prevents Loss of Immature Neurons in the Adult Hippocampal Dentate Gyrus Following Brain Injury
Reprinted from: *Int. J. Mol. Sci.* **2023**, *24*, 4261, doi:10.3390/ijms24054261 . . . . **127**

Awadhesh K. Arya, Costantino Balestra, Veena M. Bhopale, Laura J. Tuominen, Anne Räisänen-Sokolowski, Emmanuel Dugrenot, et al.
Elevations of Extracellular Vesicles and Inflammatory Biomarkers in Closed Circuit SCUBA Divers
Reprinted from: *Int. J. Mol. Sci.* **2023**, *24*, 5969, doi:10.3390/ijms24065969 . . . . **147**

About the Editors

Costantino Balestra

Costantino Balestra completed his Master's degree in 1986, then started his PhD and research in neurophysiology, successfully defending his thesis on the physiology of human fatigue in 1995. He produced an annexed thesis on the Doppler analysis of venous gas emboli in disabled scuba divers. This initiated his investigations into diving and other environmental physiology issues. He now teaches physiology, biostatistics, research methodology and biomechanics, as well as other subjects. Since 2000, Tino has been the Director of the Environmental, Occupational and Ageing Physiology Laboratory and a full time professor at the Haute Ecole Bruxelles-Brabant (Brussels)—Pôle Universitaire Bruxelles-Wallonie and Universite Libre de Bruxelles (ULB). He is also part of the anatomy and morphology research unit of VUB (Vrije Universiteit Brussels), based on 15 years previous experience teaching anatomy and physiology. He lectures in the pathophysiology of diving on several internationally recognized courses. He is the Vice President of DAN Europe for research and education and a past President of the European Underwater and Baromedical Society, and the VP of the Underwater and Hyperbaric Medical Society (UHMS) and VP of the Belgian Society for Diving and Hyperbaric Medicine. Tino has co-authored five books, including one entitled "Patent Foramen Ovale and the Diver" (in English), one entitled "Science of Diving" (in English), and another on communication skills (in French); he is also the author or co-author of over 150 scientific publications and has contributed sections to several books on physiology and human field research.

Fabio Virgili

Fabio Virgili graduated in Biology from the University of Rome with a first class honors, and completed his PhD on "Cellular and Tissue Pathology" at the University of Modena and Reggio Emilia, Italy. He has been a visiting scientist at the Rowett Research Institute of Aberdeen (UK), at the Department of Pathology of the University of Modena (Italy), and at the Department of Molecular and Cellular Biology of the University of California, Berkeley (USA. He is a Senior Scientist at the Research Centre for Food and Nutrition of the National Council for Agricultural Research and Economics in (CREA-AN). He was appointed Professor of Biochemistry in the Faculty of Sciences of the University of Roma-Tre, Rome, and participates in the board of teachers for different Master and PhD courses held by several Italian universities. His research addresses the effect of molecules of nutritional interest on the transcriptional control of gene expression and on the effect of the presence of specific genetic variants and epigenetic modifications on the risk of degenerative diseases having a nutritional component. Fabio Virgili has coordinated several research studies funded by the Italian Ministry of Research, the Italian Ministry for Agricultural and Nutritional Policies and the EU. He has authored more than 90 peer-reviewed scientific papers and book chapters.

Simona Mrakic-Sposta

Simona Mrakic-Sposta graduated in Neurophysiopathology and Biotechnology from the University of Milan, and completed her Ph.D. in Molecular Medicine. She is currently a researcher at the Institute of Clinical Physiology for the Italian National Council of Research (IFC-CNR). Since 2017, she has been a part-time Professor of "Human Anatomy and Histology", formerly in Milan and now in Rome (UNIROMA5). In 2017, she qualified as an Associate Professor. She is currently the Secretary of the Italian Society of Mountain Medicine (SIMeM), a position that she has held since October 2017. In 2016, she won the prize for Best Oral communication at the Italian Society of Mountain Medicine (SIMeM), and in 2022, won the prize for Best Poster and Oral communication at the Italian Society of Underwater Medicine (SIMSI). Her research interests include oxidative stress and inflammation studies in physiological and pathological conditions and/or during/after dietary supplementation, as well as specific long-term diets. Part of her research has focused, in particular, on the physiological adaptation of the whole body to extreme environmental conditions (i.e., high altitudes, hypobaric and normobaric hypoxia, hyperoxia), with or without adaptation to exercise. Furthermore, her research has addressed the following research topics: muscle atrophy, aging processes, and neurodegeneration; the measurement of oxidative damage biomarkers using enzymatic-immuno and fluorescent-assays; the detection of direct free radicals using Electron Paramagnetic Resonance (EPR); the assessment of the production of Reactive Oxygen Species (ROS) and antioxidant capacity in biological samples (blood, saliva, urine, cells, and tissues: in vivo and in vitro via human and animals) using the EPR technique; and studies of the role of myoglobin in human muscle. She is also the author or co-author of over 100 scientific publications.

Preface

For many years, diving and hyperbaric medicine has strived to increase our understanding of the effects of environmental stressors on human pathophysiology. It has demonstrated the importance of oxygen and has taught us not to fear this oxidative molecule, the name of which is derived from the ancient Greek meaning the "acid generator" or Oxy-Gene; indeed, at that time, it was believed that all acids were derived from oxygen.

Oxygen levels in the atmosphere have not always been stable, and enormous changes in its content have induced many adaptive reactions. The Great Oxidative Event (GOE) took place around 2.3–2.5 million years ago and the following great change took place with the GOE, which occurred approximately 0.8 million years ago. After these "catastrophic" changes, the oxygen level altered drastically, reaching 35% and being around 25–28% in the carboniferous era.

Amazingly enough, all the known anti-oxidative protections that we continue to employ were present then and able to survive such tremendous changes. We still utilize a well-known "protective" effect produced by hyperoxic vasoconstriction.

Despite the extensive number of years that medical science has employed oxygen, we have not totally mastered its use. Hypoxia (normobaric or hypobaric), normobaric hyperoxia and hyperbaric hyperoxia refer to the various "levels" of oxygen that humans are submitted to, either in the medical field or during sports activities such as scuba diving or mountaineering. In chronic situations such as living at high altitudes, we submit our bodies to prolonged hypoxia. One such example of a human settlement at extreme altitudes is the town of La Rinconada in Peru (around 4500–5500 m, approximately 11% of inspired oxygen). In physiological situations, hypoxemia is frequently observed in the absence of hypoxia in athletes who experience very high maximum oxygen consumption during maximal exercise (Dempsey effect); in this case, we find an extremely high pulmonary blood flow associated with a reduced capillary transit time, which does not allow the blood to complete sufficient oxygen loading.

Prolonged hyperoxia is more difficult to achieve than prolonged hypoxia, but is possible, for instance, if people live below sea level, such as near to The Dead Sea in Israel.

This Special Issue aims to provide an overview of the various approaches and physiological mechanisms or reactions to oxygen variations, and will be of great interest to scholars, physicians, researchers, sportsmen, coaches, and biologists, or, indeed, anyone interested on oxygen.

Costantino Balestra, Fabio Virgili, and Simona Mrakic-Sposta
Editors

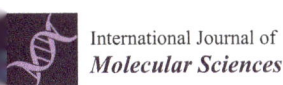

Editorial

Oxygen Variations—Insights into Hypoxia, Hyperoxia and Hyperbaric Hyperoxia—Is the Dose the Clue?

Costantino Balestra [1,2,3,4,*], Simona Mrakic-Sposta [5] and Fabio Virgili [6]

1. Environmental, Occupational, Aging (Integrative) Physiology Laboratory, Haute Ecole Bruxelles-Brabant (HE2B), 1160 Brussels, Belgium
2. Anatomical Research and Clinical Studies, Vrije Universiteit Brussels (VUB), 1090 Brussels, Belgium
3. DAN Europe Research Division (Roseto-Brussels), 1160 Brussels, Belgium
4. Physical Activity Teaching Unit, Motor Sciences Department, Université Libre de Bruxelles (ULB), 1050 Brussels, Belgium
5. Institute of Clinical Physiology, National Research Council (CNR), 20162 Milan, Italy; simona.mrakicsposta@cnr.it
6. Interuniversitary Consortium "National Institute for Bio-Structures and Bio-Systems"—I.N.B.B., 00136 Rome, Italy; fvirgili@outlook.com
* Correspondence: cbalestra@he2b.be

Molecular oxygen (O_2) is one of the four most important elements on Earth (alongside carbon, nitrogen and hydrogen); aerobic organisms depend on it to release energy from carbon-based molecules. The concentration of oxygen in the atmosphere is ~20.93–20.95% (209–460 ppm), but this has fluctuated markedly throughout geological history. It stabilized within a habitable range, between ~15% and 35%, which has been maintained from the Cambrian period 540 million years ago until today [1].

The history of the use and the study of oxygen is of great interest, yet we firmly believe that it has not yet reached a final point.

Nowadays, the therapeutic use of oxygen is not only limited to restoring hypoxia, but several newly developed approaches use oxygen not only as a "restoring agent" [2] but also as a potent stimulus [3]. Salvagno et al. based their review on the paradoxical response of the intermittent shift between hyperoxic–normoxic exposure, which was shown to enhance erythropoietin production and raise hemoglobin levels with numerous different potential applications in many fields of therapy as a new strategy for surgical preconditioning aimed at frail patients and prevention of postoperative anemia. They summarize the physiological processes behind the proposed "normobaric oxygen paradox", focusing on the latest scientific evidence and the potential applications for this strategy [4,5].

The Renaissance physician Paracelsus noted that "Nothing is without poison—the poison is in the dose". The contemporary interpretation of this statement is that dose and effect move together in a predictably linear fashion, and therefore, lower exposures to a hazardous compound will always generate lower risks. The new data presented in this Special Issue open new perspectives and explore the "linearity" of cellular responses to oxygen doses [1,6–8].

Balestra et al. [9] focused on the production of cellular microparticles after one hour of different levels of oxygen exposure in healthy subjects. They analyzed six different oxygen breathing concentrations from hypoxia to hyperbaric hyperoxia (See Figure 1).

Microparticles (MPs) expressing proteins specific to different cells were analyzed, including platelets (CD41), neutrophils (CD66b), endothelial cells (CD146), and microglia (TMEM). Phalloidin binding and thrombospondin-1 (TSP), which are related to neutrophil and platelet activation, were also analyzed. The responses were found to be different and sometimes contrasting. Significant elevations were identified for MPs expressing CD41, CD66b, TMEM, and phalloidin binding in all conditions apart from 1.4 ATA, which elicited significant decreases. Few changes were found for CD146 and TSP [10–13].

Citation: Balestra, C.; Mrakic-Sposta, S.; Virgili, F. Oxygen Variations—Insights into Hypoxia, Hyperoxia and Hyperbaric Hyperoxia—Is the Dose the Clue?. *Int. J. Mol. Sci.* **2023**, *24*, 13472. https://doi.org/10.3390/ijms241713472

Received: 23 August 2023
Accepted: 29 August 2023
Published: 30 August 2023

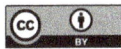

Copyright: © 2023 by the authors. Licensee MDPI, Basel, Switzerland. This article is an open access article distributed under the terms and conditions of the Creative Commons Attribution (CC BY) license (https://creativecommons.org/licenses/by/4.0/).

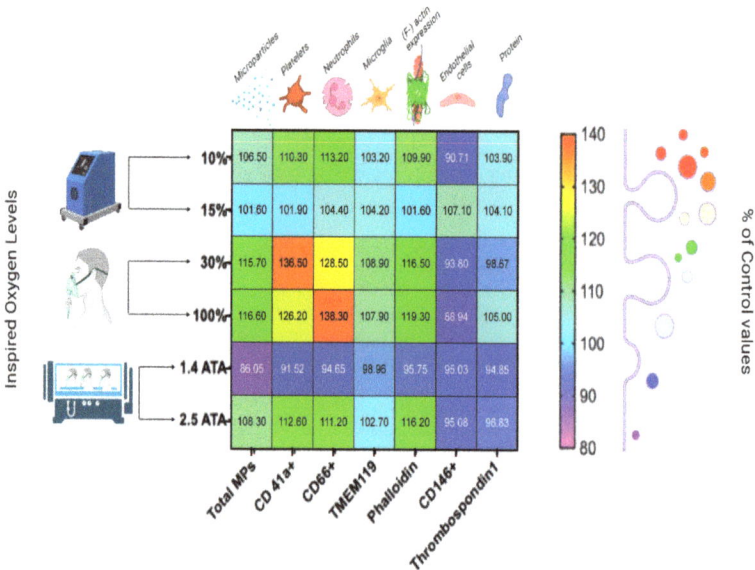

Figure 1. Percentual variations in microparticles (MPs) after 60 min of oxygen breathing. Levels of oxygen are shown on the ordinate, and total MPs and MP sub-types are shown on the abscissa. Blood sampling occurred 120 min after exposures (in a total of 48 subjects). Results are expressed in the heat map as mean percentage change (modified from [9]).

Such results challenge the "paracelsian" view on oxygen. Previous studies have already shown the different magnitudes and speeds of reactions after oxygen exposure of cellular HIF-1 α at various levels. Fratantonio et al. [14] described the activation time trend of oxygen-sensitive transcription factors in human peripheral blood mononuclear cells (PBMCs) obtained from healthy subjects after one hour of exposure to mild (MH), high (HH), and very high (VHH) hyperoxia, corresponding to 30%, 100%, and 140% O_2, respectively. They confirmed that MH is perceived as a hypoxic stress, characterized by the activation of HIF-1 α and nuclear factor (erythroid-derived 2)-like 2 (NRF2), but not of the Nuclear Factor kappa-light-chain-enhancer of activated B cells (NF-kB). Conversely, HH is associated with a progressive increase in oxidative stress leading to NRF2 and NF-kB activation, accompanied by the synthesis of glutathione (GSH). After VHH, HIF-1 α activation is totally absent and oxidative stress response, accompanied by NF-kB activation, is prevalent. Intracellular GSH and Matrix metallopeptidase 9 (MMP-9) plasma levels parallel the transcription factors' activation patterns and remain elevated throughout the observation time (24 h). This confirms that, in vivo, the return to normoxia after MH is sensed as a hypoxic trigger characterized by HIF-1 α activation. On the contrary, HH and VHH induce a shift toward an oxidative stress response, characterized by NRF2 and NF-kB activation in the first 24 h post-exposure.

1. Hypoxic Oxygen levels

To reach hypoxic oxygen levels, two different modalities are possible: one is dependent on a higher percentage of nitrogen in the inhaled mixture at atmospheric pressure (normobaric hypoxia or dilution hypoxia), while the other modality requires a reduced atmospheric pressure to reach lesser oxygen molecules per volume of breathed air (hypobaric hypoxia, such as that found during altitude stay or in a hypobaric chamber) [15].

Leveque et al. [16] compared the metabolic responses of normobaric hypoxic breathing for 1 h to inspired fractions of 10% and 15% oxygen in healthy humans (roughly mimicking altitudes of 6000 and 2400 m) [17]. Blood samples were taken before, and at 30 min, 2 h, 8 h,

24 h, and 48 h after exposure. The level of oxidative stress was evaluated by considering reactive oxygen species (ROS), nitric oxide metabolites (NOx), lipid peroxidation, and immune inflammation by interleukin-6 (IL-6) and neopterin, while antioxidant systems were observed in terms of the total antioxidant capacity (TAC) and urates. Hypoxia abruptly and rapidly increased ROS, while TAC showed a U-shape pattern, with a nadir between 30 min and 2 h. The regulation of ROS and NOx could be explained by the antioxidant action of uric acid and creatinine. The kinetics of ROS allowed for the stimulation of the immune system, as shown by increases in neopterin [18], IL-6, and NOx. This study provides insights into the mechanisms through which acute hypoxia affects various bodily functions and how the body sets up the protective mechanisms to maintain redox homeostasis in response to oxidative stress.

Another approach to acute hypoxia (12.5% of inspired fraction) was proposed by Mrakic-Sposta et al. [19]. Exposure to acute normobaric hypoxia elicited reactive oxygen species (ROS) accumulation [20], whose production kinetics and oxidative damage were investigated [21,22]. Subjects were monitored while breathing a hypoxic mixture (0.125 FiO_2 in air, mimicking about 4100 m) and during recovery with room air. ROS production was assessed using Electron Paramagnetic Resonance in capillary blood. Total antioxidant capacity, lipid peroxidation (TBARS and 8-iso-PFG2alpha) [23,24], protein oxidation (PC), and DNA oxidation (8-OH-dG) were measured in plasma and/or urine [23,25]. The ROS production rate was monitored (5, 15, 30, 60, 120, 240, and 300 min). A production peak (+50%) was reached at 4 h. The on-transient kinetics, exponentially fitted (t(1/2) = 30 min r(2) = 0.995), were ascribable to the low O_2 tension transition and the mirror-like related SpO(2) decrease: 15 min: -12%; 60 min: -18%. The exposure did not seem to affect the prooxidant/antioxidant balance. Significant increases in PC (+88%) and 8-OH-dG (+67%) at 4 h in TBARS (+33%) one hour after hypoxia offset were also observed. General malaise was described by most of the subjects. Under acute NH, ROS production and oxidative damage resulted in time and SpO_2-dependent reversible phenomena.

In an animal model (mice), Shao et al. [26] studied the impact of hypoxia (a total of 30 mice were randomly divided into three groups (10 mice in each): control (CON) and chronic hypoxia (continuously with 13% O_2 for 1 and 3 days (H1D and H3D), respectively) on advanced brain function (learning and memory skills in particular), and the effects of hypoxic stress on hippocampal function were assessed. Specifically, the effects of the dysfunction of mitochondrial oxidative phosphorylation using global proteomics. The authors found that hypoxic stress impaired cognitive and motor abilities, whereas it caused no substantial changes in the brain morphology or structure of mice. Bioinformatics analysis reported that hypoxia affected the expression of 516 proteins, of which 71.1% were upregulated and 28.5% were downregulated. The mitochondrial function was altered and manifested as a decrease in NADH dehydrogenase (ubiquinone) 1 alpha subcomplex 4 expression, accompanied by increased reactive oxygen species generation, resulting in further neuronal injury.

Their results may provide some new insights into how hypoxic stress alters hippocampal function via the dysfunction of mitochondrial oxidative phosphorylation [27].

2. Normobaric Hyperoxic Oxygen levels

In clinical practice, preventing or counteracting hypoxia is achieved providing normobaric oxygen. Even though hyperoxia may seem harmless, it can have detrimental effects even at modest levels if administered for prolonged periods, especially in critically ill patients [28].

One example is preterm babies, since their postnatal exposure to factors such as high oxygen concentrations may likely adversely influence postnatal growth and ongoing organ development [29–32]. The renal consequences of preterm births have attracted increasing attention and include a high risk of chronic kidney disease. The third trimester of pregnancy is the most active period of fetal nephrogenesis, during which more than 60% of nephrons are formed. Preterm birth (within <37 gestational weeks) interrupts the development and maturation of the kidneys during the critical growth period since neonates born preterm have an immature antioxidant defense system [33] and present an imbalance between the oxidant and the antioxidant system, leading to an increased level of oxygen free radicals, with subsequent increased risk of oxidative damage to organs.

Hyperoxia during the neonatal period impairs renal tubular development. Human and animal studies have demonstrated that neonatal hyperoxia increases oxidative stress and induces glomerular and tubular injuries, which are manifested as renal corpuscle enlargement, renal tubular necrosis, interstitial inflammation, and kidney fibrosis during the perinatal period [34–36].

Huang et al. [37] showed a global approach in their manuscript (see their Figure 1); they analyzed several animal studies (murine) of preterm birth interrupting the development and maturation of the kidneys during the critical growth period. They found that kidneys can exhibit structural defects and functional impairment due to hyperoxia. Furthermore, hyperoxia during nephrogenesis impairs renal tubular development and induces glomerular and tubular injuries, which manifest as renal corpuscle enlargement, renal tubular necrosis, interstitial inflammation, and kidney fibrosis. Preterm birth along with hyperoxia exposure induces a pathological predisposition to chronic kidney disease. Hyperoxia-induced kidney injuries are influenced by several molecular factors, including hypoxia-inducible factor-1 alpha and interleukin-6/Smad2/transforming growth factor-beta and Wnt/beta-catenin signaling pathways; these are key to cell proliferation, tissue inflammation, and cell membrane repair. Hyperoxia-induced oxidative stress is characterized by the attenuation or the induction of multiple molecular factors associated with kidney damage. This review focuses on the molecular pathways involved in the pathogenesis of hyperoxia-induced kidney injuries.

In terms of human studies on hyperoxia, Leveque et al. [38] compared two 60 min hyperoxic exposures on healthy humans. Since the effects of oxygen over time and at different partial pressures remain poorly understood, they measured the metabolic responses of a normobaric oxygen intake for 1 h to mild (30%) and high (100%) inspired fractions. Blood samples were taken before the intake, and at 30 min, 2 h, 8 h, 24 h, and 48 h after the single oxygen exposure. The level of oxidation was evaluated by the rate of reactive oxygen species (ROS) and the levels of isoprostane. Antioxidant reactions were observed by total antioxidant capacity (TAC), superoxide dismutase (SOD), and catalase (CAT). The inflammatory response was measured using interleukins-6 (IL-6), neopterin, creatinine, and urates. Oxidation markers increased from 30 min on to reach a peak at 8 h. From 8 h post-exposure, the markers of inflammation increased more significantly in the 100% condition than in the 30% condition. This study suggests a biphasic response over time characterized by an initial "permissive oxidation" followed by increased inflammation and the antioxidant protection system seems to not be the leading actor. The authors concluded that the kinetics of enzymatic reactions need to be better studied to establish therapeutic, training, or rehabilitation protocols for a more targeted use of oxygen.

3. Hyperbaric Hyperoxic Oxygen levels

To reach oxygen levels above 100%, a hyperbaric environment is needed; increasing the surrounding pressure is achieved in a hyperbaric chamber and is usually achieved for therapeutic reasons. Hyperbaric oxygen therapy (HBOT) is a therapeutic approach based on breathing pure oxygen (O_2) in an augmented atmospheric pressure [39,40].

Two directions are found in the field of immature (or premature) organisms; on the one hand, as previously reported, some adverse normobaric hyperoxic effects may occur, but on the other hand, several sessions of hyperbaric oxygen treatment have been reported to be beneficial [29,41,42].

In a murine model, Jeremic et al. [43] showed evidence suggesting that hyperbaric oxygenation may affect the activity of adult neural stem cells (NSCs) [44–46]. Since the role of NSCs in recovery from brain injury is still unclear, the purpose of this study was to investigate the effects of sensorimotor cortex ablation (SCA) and HBO treatment (HBOT) on the processes of neurogenesis in the adult dentate gyrus (DG), a region of the hippocampus that is the site of adult neurogenesis. Ten-week-old Wistar rats were divided into groups:

Control (C, intact animals), Sham control (S, animals that underwent the surgical procedure without opening the skull), SCA (animals in whom the right sensorimotor cortex was removed via suction ablation), and SCA + HBO (operated animals that passed HBOT). HBOT protocol: pressure applied at 2.5 absolute atmospheres for 60 min, once daily for 10 days. Using immunohistochemistry and double immunofluorescence labeling, it was shown that SCA causes significant loss of neurons in the DG. Newborn neurons in the subgranular zone (SGZ), inner third, and partially mid-third of the granule cell layer are predominantly affected by SCA. HBOT decreases the SCA-caused loss of immature neurons, prevents reduction of dendritic arborization, and increases the proliferation of progenitor cells.

A protective effect of HBO can be considered by reducing the vulnerability of immature neurons in the adult DG to SCA injury.

The only other way to increase oxygen partial pressure above one atmosphere is to breathe underwater while diving. A particular diving procedure using closed-circuit rebreathers (CCR) allows a constant PO_2 to be set that will be kept stable during the whole dive regardless of depth variations (with concomitant ambient pressure changes). Arya et al. [47] measured blood-borne extracellular vesicles and inflammatory mediators in divers using closed-circuit rebreathing apparatus and custom-mixed gases to diminish some diving risks. "Deep" divers (n = 8) dove once to mean (±SD) 102.5 ± 1.2 m of sea water (msw) for 167.3 ± 11.5 min. "Shallow" divers (n = 6) dove three times on day 1 and then repeatedly over 7 days to 16.4 ± 3.7 msw for 49.9 ± 11.9 min. There were statistically significant elevations of microparticles (MPs) in deep divers (day 1) and shallow divers at day 7 that expressed proteins specific to microglia, neutrophils, platelets and endothelial cells, as well as thrombospondin (TSP)-1 and filamentous (F-) actin. Intra-MP IL-1β increased by 7.5-fold ($p < 0.001$) after day 1 and 41-fold ($p = 0.003$) at day 7. Intra-MP nitric oxide synthase-2 (NOS2) increased 17-fold ($p < 0.001$) after day 1 and 19-fold ($p = 0.002$) at day 7. Plasma gelsolin (pGSN) level decreased by 73% ($p < 0.001$) in deep divers (day 1) and 37% in shallow divers by day 7. Plasma samples containing exosomes and other lipophilic particles increased from 186 to 490% among the divers but contained no IL-1β or NOS2.

The authors concluded that diving triggers inflammatory events even when controlling for hyperoxia and many are not proportional to the depth of diving.

In terms of the therapeutic side of hyperbaric oxygen, it is strange that, despite having been used for years, the exact kinetics of the reactive oxygen species between different levels of hyperbaric oxygen exposure are still not clearly evidenced and, without much scientific evidence, it is common practice to apply HBOT sessions every 24 h [48]. The need for several sessions to reach a relevant effect is likewise commonly accepted, however, the optimal hyperbaric oxygen levels and the time needed between each session to optimize cellular responses—such as Hypoxia-inducible factor (HIF-1α) or nuclear factor kappa β (NF-Kβ), erythroid related factor 2 (NRF2), cellular vesicles, and microparticles, such as Caspase 3 [5,9,14]—are still debated and stand solely on observational clinical outcomes.

Leveque et al. [49] studied the metabolic responses of hyperbaric hyperoxia exposures for 1 h at 1.4 and 2.5 ATA.

Fourteen healthy non-smoking subjects volunteered for the study. Blood samples were taken before, and at 30 min, 2 h, 24 h, and 48 h after 1 h hyperbaric hyperoxic exposure. The level of oxidation was evaluated by the rate of ROS production, nitric oxide metabolites (NOx), and the levels of isoprostane. Antioxidant reactions were assessed through measuring superoxide dismutase (SOD), catalase (CAT), cysteinylglycine, and glutathione (GSH). The inflammatory response was measured using interleukine-6, neopterin, and creatinine. A short (60 min) period of mild (1.4 ATA) and high (2.5 ATA) hyperbaric hyperoxia led to a similar significant increase in the production of ROS and antioxidant reactions. Immunomodulation and inflammatory responses, on the contrary, responded proportionally to the hyperbaric oxygen dose. Further research is warranted on the dose and the inter-dose recovery time to optimize the potential therapeutic benefits of this promising intervention.

These encouraging but also challenging results lead us to question if some oxygen levels formerly considered as 'HBOT sham' [50,51] may be of therapeutic interest [9,51,52].

Oxygen and its variations are certainly the most powerful cellular triggers that can be found in nature.

Returning to Philippus Theophrastus Aureolus Bombast von Hohenheim (Paracelsus), he was known to have quite a hot temper and be "bombastic". Nevertheless, he was very respectful of previous scholars, such as Aulus Cornelius Celsus (who wrote "De Medicina"); he respected deep knowledge, which is likely why the name "Paracelsus" was appropriate to him, since he considered himself not equal to Celsus.

Oxygen can be considered bombastic sometimes, but is also as indispensable; deeper knowledge on its biology is vital in the present day, and the simple "dose is the poison" approach is not appropriate for such a metabolically active molecule [41].

To better describe this concept, we constructed Figure 2 after three manuscripts from Leveque et al. [16,38,49] to illustrate how relative changes of reactive oxygen species are not directly dependent on the dose up to 48 h following 60 min of exposure.

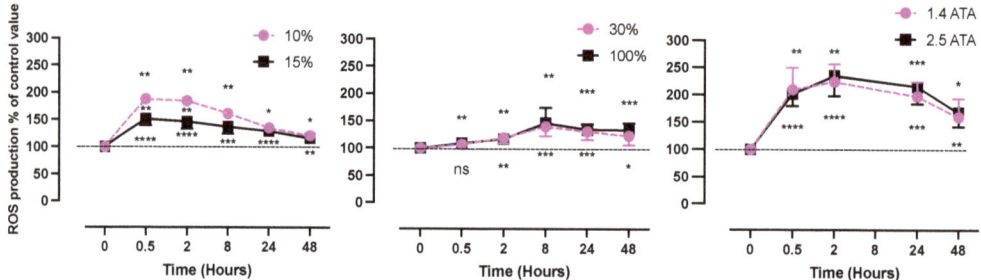

Figure 2. Percentual variations in ROS production after 60 min of oxygen breathing. Levels of oxygen are shown in the figure legend (48 subjects in total). Results are expressed as mean percentage change of control values (modified from [16,38,49]) (*: $p < 0.05$, **: $p < 0.01$, ***: $p < 0.001$, ****: $p < 0.0001$; RM-ANOVA and Dunnet's post hoc test).

As can be seen from Figure 2, no real difference in ROS production is present during hyperoxia for as long as 48 h between two rather different doses of oxygen on the hypoxic side; on the contrary, some acute differences even in slightly different doses can be seen (in the first few hours after exposure). The dose seems to not be the only clue!

This editorial, drawing a general picture of the Special Issue it accompanies, clearly shows how much new material can aid understanding of the underlying mechanisms elicited by oxygen exposures.

Oxygen biology is still a very fruitful research field, and we strongly believe that "oxygen variations" will, in the coming years, be a promising and proficuous field to explore.

Conflicts of Interest: The authors declare no conflict of interest.

References

1. Brugniaux, J.V.; Coombs, G.B.; Barak, O.F.; Dujic, Z.; Sekhon, M.S.; Ainslie, P.N. Highs and lows of hyperoxia: Physiological, performance, and clinical aspects. *Am. J. Physiol. Regul. Integr. Comp. Physiol.* **2018**, *315*, R1–R27. [CrossRef] [PubMed]
2. Samaja, M.; Chiumello, D. Oxygen administration during general anaesthesia for surgery. *BMJ* **2022**, *379*, o2823. [CrossRef]
3. Hadanny, A.; Efrati, S. The Hyperoxic-Hypoxic Paradox. *Biomolecules* **2020**, *10*, 958. [CrossRef]
4. Salvagno, M.; Coppalini, G.; Taccone, F.S.; Strapazzon, G.; Mrakic-Sposta, S.; Rocco, M.; Khalife, M.; Balestra, C. The Normobaric Oxygen Paradox-Hyperoxic Hypoxic Paradox: A Novel Expedient Strategy in Hematopoiesis Clinical Issues. *Int. J. Mol. Sci.* **2022**, *24*, 82. [CrossRef] [PubMed]
5. Cimino, F.; Balestra, C.; Germonpre, P.; De Bels, D.; Tillmans, F.; Saija, A.; Speciale, A.; Virgili, F. Pulsed high oxygen induces a hypoxic-like response in Human Umbilical Endothelial Cells (HUVECs) and in humans. *J. Appl. Physiol.* **2012**, *113*, 1684–1689. [CrossRef]

6. Arieli, R.; Yalov, A.; Goldenshluger, A. Modeling pulmonary and CNS O_2 toxicity and estimation of parameters for humans. *J. Appl. Physiol.* **2002**, *92*, 248–256. [CrossRef]
7. Samaja, M.; Ottolenghi, S. The Oxygen Cascade from Atmosphere to Mitochondria as a Tool to Understand the (Mal)adaptation to Hypoxia. *Int. J. Mol. Sci.* **2023**, *24*, 3670. [CrossRef] [PubMed]
8. Mancardi, D.; Ottolenghi, S.; Attanasio, U.; Tocchetti, C.G.; Paroni, R.; Pagliaro, P.; Samaja, M. Janus, or the Inevitable Battle Between Too Much and Too Little Oxygen. *Antioxid. Redox Signal.* **2022**, *37*, 972–989. [CrossRef] [PubMed]
9. Balestra, C.; Arya, A.K.; Leveque, C.; Virgili, F.; Germonpre, P.; Lambrechts, K.; Lafere, P.; Thom, S.R. Varying Oxygen Partial Pressure Elicits Blood-Borne Microparticles Expressing Different Cell-Specific Proteins-Toward a Targeted Use of Oxygen? *Int. J. Mol. Sci.* **2022**, *23*, 7888. [CrossRef]
10. Thom, S.R.; Bhopale, V.M.; Arya, A.K.; Ruhela, D.; Bhat, A.R.; Mitra, N.; Hoffstad, O.; Malay, D.S.; Mirza, Z.K.; Lantis, J.C.; et al. Blood-Borne Microparticles Are an Inflammatory Stimulus in Type 2 Diabetes Mellitus. *Immunohorizons* **2023**, *7*, 71–80. [CrossRef]
11. Bhopale, V.M.; Ruhela, D.; Brett, K.D.; Nugent, N.Z.; Fraser, N.K.; Levinson, S.L.; DiNubile, M.J.; Thom, S.R. Plasma gelsolin modulates the production and fate of IL-1β-containing microparticles following high-pressure exposure and decompression. *J. Appl. Physiol.* **2021**, *130*, 1604–1613. [CrossRef] [PubMed]
12. Thom, S.R.; Bhopale, V.M.; Yu, K.; Huang, W.; Kane, M.A.; Margolis, D.J. Neutrophil microparticle production and inflammasome activation by hyperglycemia due to cytoskeletal instability. *J. Biol. Chem.* **2017**, *292*, 18312–18324. [CrossRef] [PubMed]
13. Thom, S.R.; Hampton, M.; Troiano, M.A.; Mirza, Z.; Malay, D.S.; Shannon, S.; Jennato, N.B.; Donohue, C.M.; Hoffstad, O.; Woltereck, D.; et al. Measurements of CD34+/CD45-dim Stem Cells Predict Healing of Diabetic Neuropathic Wounds. *Diabetes* **2016**, *65*, 486–497. [CrossRef] [PubMed]
14. Fratantonio, D.; Virgili, F.; Zucchi, A.; Lambrechts, K.; Latronico, T.; Lafere, P.; Germonpre, P.; Balestra, C. Increasing Oxygen Partial Pressures Induce a Distinct Transcriptional Response in Human PBMC: A Pilot Study on the "Normobaric Oxygen Paradox". *Int. J. Mol. Sci.* **2021**, *22*, 458. [CrossRef] [PubMed]
15. Camacho-Cardenosa, A.; Burtscher, J.; Burtscher, M.; Camacho-Cardenosa, M. Editorial: Hypoxia as a therapeutic tool in search of healthy aging. *Front. Physiol.* **2023**, *13*, 1112129. [CrossRef]
16. Leveque, C.; Mrakic Sposta, S.; Theunissen, S.; Germonpré, P.; Lambrechts, K.; Vezzoli, A.; Gussoni, M.; Levenez, M.; Lafère, P.; Guerrero, F.; et al. Oxidative Stress Response Kinetics after 60 Minutes at Different Levels (10% or 15%) of Normobaric Hypoxia Exposure. *Int. J. Mol. Sci.* **2023**, *24*, 10188. [CrossRef]
17. Peacock, A.J. ABC of oxygen: Oxygen at high altitude. *BMJ* **1998**, *317*, 1063–1066. [CrossRef]
18. Bavunoglu, I.; Genc, H.; Konukoglu, D.; Cicekci, H.; Sozer, V.; Gelisgen, R.; Uzun, H. Oxidative stress parameters and inflammatory and immune mediators as markers of the severity of sepsis. *J. Infect. Dev. Ctries.* **2016**, *10*, 1045–1052. [CrossRef]
19. Mrakic-Sposta, S.; Gussoni, M.; Marzorati, M.; Porcelli, S.; Bosco, G.; Balestra, C.; Montorsi, M.; Lafortuna, C.; Vezzoli, A. The "ON-OFF" Switching Response of Reactive Oxygen Species in Acute Normobaric Hypoxia: Preliminary Outcome. *Int. J. Mol. Sci.* **2023**, *24*, 4012. [CrossRef]
20. Sies, H.; Jones, D.P. Reactive oxygen species (ROS) as pleiotropic physiological signalling agents. *Nat. Rev. Mol. Cell Biol.* **2020**, *21*, 363–383. [CrossRef]
21. Mathew, T.; Sarada, S.K.S. Intonation of Nrf2 and Hif1-α pathway by curcumin prophylaxis: A potential strategy to augment survival signaling under hypoxia. *Respir. Physiol. Neurobiol.* **2018**, *258*, 12–24. [CrossRef] [PubMed]
22. Joanny, P.; Steinberg, J.; Robach, P.; Richalet, J.P.; Gortan, C.; Gardette, B.; Jammes, Y. Operation Everest III (Comex'97): The effect of simulated sever hypobaric hypoxia on lipid peroxidation and antioxidant defence systems in human blood at rest and after maximal exercise. *Resuscitation* **2001**, *49*, 307–314. [CrossRef] [PubMed]
23. Schmidt, M.C.; Askew, E.W.; Roberts, D.E.; Prior, R.L.; Ensign, W.Y., Jr.; Hesslink, R.E., Jr. Oxidative stress in humans training in a cold, moderate altitude environment and their response to a phytochemical antioxidant supplement. *Wilderness Environ. Med.* **2002**, *13*, 94–105. [CrossRef] [PubMed]
24. Araneda, O.F.; García, C.; Lagos, N.; Quiroga, G.; Cajigal, J.; Salazar, M.P.; Behn, C. Lung oxidative stress as related to exercise and altitude. Lipid peroxidation evidence in exhaled breath condensate: A possible predictor of acute mountain sickness. *Eur. J. Appl. Physiol.* **2005**, *95*, 383–390. [CrossRef]
25. Møller, P.; Loft, S.; Lundby, C.; Olsen, N.V. Acute hypoxia and hypoxic exercise induce DNA strand breaks and oxidative DNA damage in humans. *FASEB J.* **2001**, *15*, 1181–1186. [CrossRef] [PubMed]
26. Shao, Q.; Liu, J.; Li, G.; Gu, Y.; Guo, M.; Guan, Y.; Tian, Z.; Ma, W.; Wang, C.; Ji, X. Proteomic Analysis Reveals That Mitochondria Dominate the Hippocampal Hypoxic Response in Mice. *Int. J. Mol. Sci.* **2022**, *23*, 14094. [CrossRef]
27. Li, A.L.; Lian, L.; Chen, X.N.; Cai, W.H.; Fan, X.B.; Fan, Y.J.; Li, T.T.; Xie, Y.Y.; Zhang, J.P. The role of mitochondria in myocardial damage caused by energy metabolism disorders: From mechanisms to therapeutics. *Free Radic. Biol. Med.* **2023**, *208*, 236–251. [CrossRef]
28. Baude, J.; Cooper, J.S. Hyperbaric Contraindicated Chemotherapeutic Agents. In *StatPearls*; StatPearls Publishing LLC.: Treasure Island, FL, USA, 2023.
29. Yehiam, S.Z.; Simkin, S.K.; Al-Taie, R.; Wong, M.; Battin, M.; Dai, S. Incomplete peripheral retinal vascularisation in retinopathy of prematurity: Is it the consequence of changing oxygen saturation? *Front. Pediatr.* **2023**, *11*, 1203068. [CrossRef]
30. Shetty, S.; Tolentino, D.; Kulkarni, A.; Duffy, D.; Greenough, A. Comparison of Outcomes of Less Invasive Surfactant Administration in Prematurely Born Infants in the Delivery Suite and the Neonatal Unit. *Am. J. Perinatol.* **2023**. [CrossRef]

31. Kim, E.S.; Calkins, K.L.; Chu, A. Retinopathy of Prematurity: The Role of Nutrition. *Pediatr. Ann.* **2023**, *52*, e303–e308. [CrossRef]
32. Dormishian, A.; Schott, A.; Aguilar, A.C.; Jimenez, V.; Bancalari, E.; Tolosa, J.; Claure, N. Etiology and Mechanism of Intermittent Hypoxemia Episodes in Spontaneously Breathing Extremely Premature Infants. *J. Pediatr.* **2023**, *262*, 113623. [CrossRef] [PubMed]
33. Georgeson, G.D.; Szony, B.J.; Streitman, K.; Varga, I.S.; Kovács, A.; Kovács, L.; László, A. Antioxidant enzyme activities are decreased in preterm infants and in neonates born via caesarean section. *Eur. J. Obstet. Gynecol. Reprod. Biol.* **2002**, *103*, 136–139. [CrossRef] [PubMed]
34. Chu, Y.T.; Chen, B.H.; Chen, H.H.; Lee, J.C.; Kuo, T.J.; Chiu, H.C.; Lu, W.H. Hypoxia-Induced Kidney Injury in Newborn Rats. *Toxics* **2023**, *11*, 260. [CrossRef] [PubMed]
35. Perrone, S.; Mussap, M.; Longini, M.; Fanos, V.; Bellieni, C.V.; Proietti, F.; Cataldi, L.; Buonocore, G. Oxidative kidney damage in preterm newborns during perinatal period. *Clin. Biochem.* **2007**, *40*, 656–660. [CrossRef]
36. Torbati, D.; Tan, G.H.; Smith, S.; Frazier, K.S.; Gelvez, J.; Fakioglu, H.; Totapally, B.R. Multiple-organ effect of normobaric hyperoxia in neonatal rats. *J. Crit. Care* **2006**, *21*, 85–93; discussion 93–84. [CrossRef]
37. Huang, L.-T.; Chen, C.-M. Kidney Injuries and Evolution of Chronic Kidney Diseases Due to Neonatal Hyperoxia Exposure Based on Animal Studies. *Int. J. Mol. Sci.* **2022**, *23*, 8492. [CrossRef]
38. Leveque, C.; Mrakic-Sposta, S.; Lafere, P.; Vezzoli, A.; Germonpre, P.; Beer, A.; Mievis, S.; Virgili, F.; Lambrechts, K.; Theunissen, S.; et al. Oxidative Stress Response's Kinetics after 60 Minutes at Different (30% or 100%) Normobaric Hyperoxia Exposures. *Int. J. Mol. Sci.* **2022**, *24*, 664. [CrossRef]
39. Vinkel, J.; Arenkiel, B.; Hyldegaard, O. The Mechanisms of Action of Hyperbaric Oxygen in Restoring Host Homeostasis during Sepsis. *Biomolecules* **2023**, *13*, 1228. [CrossRef]
40. Gottfried, I.; Schottlender, N.; Ashery, U. Hyperbaric Oxygen Treatment-From Mechanisms to Cognitive Improvement. *Biomolecules* **2021**, *11*, 1520. [CrossRef]
41. Robba, C.; Battaglini, D.; Cinotti, R.; Asehnoune, K.; Stevens, R.; Taccone, F.S.; Badenes, R.; Pelosi, P. Individualized Thresholds of Hypoxemia and Hyperoxemia and their Effect on Outcome in Acute Brain Injured Patients: A Secondary Analysis of the ENIO Study. In *Neurocritical Care*; Springer: Berlin/Heidelberg, Germany, 2023. [CrossRef]
42. Yılmaz, A.; Kaya, N.; Meriç, R.; Bayramli, Z.; Öroğlu, B.; Celkan, T.T.; Vural, M.; Perk, Y. Use of hyperbaric oxygen therapy of purpura fulminans in an extremely low birth weight preterm: A case report. *J. Neonatal. Perinatal. Med.* **2023**, *16*, 339–342. [CrossRef]
43. Jeremic, R.; Pekovic, S.; Lavrnja, I.; Bjelobaba, I.; Djelic, M.; Dacic, S.; Brkic, P. Hyperbaric Oxygenation Prevents Loss of Immature Neurons in the Adult Hippocampal Dentate Gyrus Following Brain Injury. *Int. J. Mol. Sci.* **2023**, *24*, 4261. [PubMed]
44. Lavrnja, I.; Parabucki, A.; Brkic, P.; Jovanovic, T.; Dacic, S.; Savic, D.; Pantic, I.; Stojiljkovic, M.; Pekovic, S. Repetitive hyperbaric oxygenation attenuates reactive astrogliosis and suppresses expression of inflammatory mediators in the rat model of brain injury. *Mediat. Inflamm.* **2015**, *2015*, 498405. [CrossRef]
45. Parabucki, A.B.; Bozić, I.D.; Bjelobaba, I.M.; Lavrnja, I.C.; Brkić, P.D.; Jovanović, T.S.; Savić, D.Z.; Stojiljković, M.B.; Peković, S.M. Hyperbaric oxygenation alters temporal expression pattern of superoxide dismutase 2 after cortical stab injury in rats. *Croat. Med. J.* **2012**, *53*, 586–597. [CrossRef] [PubMed]
46. Brkic, P.; Stojiljkovic, M.; Jovanovic, T.; Dacic, S.; Lavrnja, I.; Savic, D.; Parabucki, A.; Bjelobaba, I.; Rakic, L.; Pekovic, S. Hyperbaric oxygenation improves locomotor ability by enhancing neuroplastic responses after cortical ablation in rats. *Brain Inj.* **2012**, *26*, 1273–1284. [CrossRef]
47. Arya, A.K.; Balestra, C.; Bhopale, V.M.; Tuominen, L.J.; Raisanen-Sokolowski, A.; Dugrenot, E.; L'Her, E.; Bhat, A.R.; Thom, S.R. Elevations of Extracellular Vesicles and Inflammatory Biomarkers in Closed Circuit SCUBA Divers. *Int. J. Mol. Sci.* **2023**, *24*, 5969. [CrossRef] [PubMed]
48. De Wolde, S.D.; Hulskes, R.H.; de Jonge, S.W.; Hollmann, M.W.; van Hulst, R.A.; Weenink, R.P.; Kox, M. The Effect of Hyperbaric Oxygen Therapy on Markers of Oxidative Stress and the Immune Response in Healthy Volunteers. *Front. Physiol.* **2022**, *13*, 826163. [CrossRef]
49. Leveque, C.; Mrakic Sposta, S.; Theunissen, S.; Germonpré, P.; Lambrechts, K.; Vezzoli, A.; Bosco, G.; Lévénez, M.; Lafère, P.; Guerrero, F.; et al. Oxidative Stress Response Kinetics after 60 Minutes at Different (1.4 ATA and 2.5 ATA) Hyperbaric Hyperoxia Exposures. *Int. J. Mol. Sci.* **2023**, *24*, 12361. [CrossRef]
50. Louge, P.; Pignel, R.; Serratrice, J.; Stirnemann, J. Validation of sham treatment in hyperbaric medicine: A randomised trial. *Diving Hyperb. Med.* **2023**, *53*, 51–54. [CrossRef]
51. Mozayeni, B.R.; Duncan, W.; Zant, E.; Love, T.L.; Beckman, R.L.; Stoller, K.P. The National Brain Injury Rescue and Rehabilitation Study—A multicenter observational study of hyperbaric oxygen for mild traumatic brain injury with post-concussive symptoms. *Med. Gas Res.* **2019**, *9*, 1–12. [CrossRef]
52. MacLaughlin, K.J.; Barton, G.P.; Braun, R.K.; MacLaughlin, J.E.; Lamers, J.J.; Marcou, M.D.; Eldridge, M.W. Hyperbaric air mobilizes stem cells in humans; a new perspective on the hormetic dose curve. *Front. Neurol.* **2023**, *14*, 1192793. [CrossRef]

Disclaimer/Publisher's Note: The statements, opinions and data contained in all publications are solely those of the individual author(s) and contributor(s) and not of MDPI and/or the editor(s). MDPI and/or the editor(s) disclaim responsibility for any injury to people or property resulting from any ideas, methods, instructions or products referred to in the content.

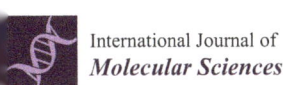

Article

Varying Oxygen Partial Pressure Elicits Blood-Borne Microparticles Expressing Different Cell-Specific Proteins—Toward a Targeted Use of Oxygen?

Costantino Balestra [1,2,3,4,*], Awadhesh K. Arya [5], Clément Leveque [1], Fabio Virgili [6], Peter Germonpré [1,3,7], Kate Lambrechts [1], Pierre Lafère [1,3] and Stephen R. Thom [5]

1. Environmental, Occupational, Aging (Integrative) Physiology Laboratory, Haute Ecole Bruxelles-Brabant (HE2B), 1180 Brussels, Belgium; clement.leveque.kinepro@gmail.com (C.L.); pgermonpre@gmail.com (P.G.); klambrechts@he2b.be (K.L.); plafere@he2b.be (P.L.)
2. Anatomical Research and Clinical Studies, Vrije Universiteit Brussels (VUB), 1090 Brussels, Belgium
3. DAN Europe Research Division (Roseto-Brussels), 1160 Brussels, Belgium
4. Motor Sciences Department, Physical Activity Teaching Unit, Université Libre de Bruxelles (ULB), 1050 Brussels, Belgium
5. Department of Emergency Medicine, University of Maryland School of Medicine, Baltimore, MD 21201, USA; aarya@som.umaryland.edu (A.K.A.); sthom@som.umaryland.edu (S.R.T.)
6. Council for Agricultural Research and Economic-Food and Nutrition Research Centre (C.R.E.A.-AN), 00187 Rome, Italy; fabio.virgili@crea.gov.it
7. Hyperbaric Centre, Queen Astrid Military Hospital, 1120 Brussels, Belgium
* Correspondence: costantinobalestra@gmail.com

Abstract: Oxygen is a powerful trigger for cellular reactions, but there are few comparative investigations assessing the effects over a large range of partial pressures. We investigated a metabolic response to single exposures to either normobaric (10%, 15%, 30%, 100%) or hyperbaric (1.4 ATA, 2.5 ATA) oxygen. Forty-eight healthy subjects (32 males/16 females; age: 43.7 ± 13.4 years, height: 172.7 ± 10.07 cm; weight 68.4 ± 15.7 kg) were randomly assigned, and blood samples were taken before and 2 h after each exposure. Microparticles (MPs) expressing proteins specific to different cells were analyzed, including platelets (CD41), neutrophils (CD66b), endothelial cells (CD146), and microglia (TMEM). Phalloidin binding and thrombospondin-1 (TSP), which are related to neutrophil and platelet activation, respectively, were also analyzed. The responses were found to be different and sometimes opposite. Significant elevations were identified for MPs expressing CD41, CD66b, TMEM, and phalloidin binding in all conditions but for 1.4 ATA, which elicited significant decreases. Few changes were found for CD146 and TSP. Regarding OPB, further investigation is needed to fully understand the future applications of such findings.

Keywords: hypoxia; hyperoxia; hyperbaric oxygen; cellular reactions; decompression sickness; diving; altitude; normobaric oxygen paradox; hyperoxic-hypoxic paradox

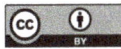

1. Introduction

Oxygen (O_2), which belongs to the WHO list of essential medicines, has long been recognized as a common treatment for both acute and chronic diseases, and is widely applied from pre-hospital emergency medical services to home oxygen therapy [1]. Its main therapeutic objective is to correct tissue or cellular hypoxia [2]. However, pure O_2 breathing is not only devoted to patients needing oxygen support. Indeed, other therapeutic uses of oxygen need to be considered. In those therapies, oxygen is considered as a drug capable of inducing a targeted clinical response, such as Hyperbaric Oxygen Therapy (HBOT) [3,4] or in therapies using the "Normobaric Oxygen Paradox" or the "Hyperoxic-Hypoxic Paradox" [5–8]. Moreover, O_2 breathing goes beyond mere therapeutic use. Breathing an O_2 mixture at different concentrations, either hypoxic or hyperoxic, has been used for sport training [9], cardiovascular conditioning [10,11], or before extreme environmental exposure, such as SCUBA diving [12,13], military high-altitude free fall [14,15], or space flight [16,17], to avoid the occurrence of decompression sickness (DCS).

DCS arises when tissues become supersaturated with metabolically inert gases. On decompression, Nitrogen (N_2) or similar gases diffuse from sites of high concentration as a function of both the pressure gradient and blood flow, which can induce vascular gas emboli (VGE), a key element in the development of DCS. Indeed, the amount of VGE is statistically related to the risk of DCS [18]. Conversely, the absence of detectable VGE is correlated with a very low probability of DCS in both hyperbaric [19] or hypobaric [20] settings, hence the development of pre-conditioning strategies that aim to reduce VGE production. Oxygen pre-breathing (OPB), a standard approach to remove dissolved N_2 from tissues in anticipation of exposures to sub-normal pressures associated with high-altitude aviation and extra-vehicular transits while in space, is one of those strategies [21]. OPB has been associated with a decreased incidence of DCS, especially when combined with moderate exercise [22]. However, although DCS risk is lowered, OPB does not seem to alter the time when VGE is first detected in decompressed research subjects, except in small animal research where the metabolic rate is different [18,23,24]. This is interpreted as indicating that the number of bubble nucleation sites, so-called micronuclei, present at baseline is not clearly influenced by varying the O_2 concentration, but N_2 mobilization or 'wash-out' decreases bubble formation except for a limited population of such nuclei [18]. There are also alternative strategies that appear to diminish bubble micronuclei [25]. These issues highlight the complexity of the physio-pathological mechanisms related to DCS.

The literature has identified several contributing factors to pressure exposures and DCS, such as vascular dysfunction, oxidative stress, and blood-borne microparticles (MPs) [26,27], which have been considered potential targets for pre-conditioning interventions. MPs are of particular interest since a growing body of data suggest that they are a potential bubble nucleation site and play a role in DCS pathophysiology [27–31]. MPs are 0.1–1 µm vesicles generated by an outward budding of the plasma membrane in a process that results in the surface expression of phosphatidylserine. As with most types of extracellular vesicles, MPs are found in all body fluids and increase in association with most human disease and injuries [32]. They are generated by virtually all cells, can be beneficial or exacerbate pathology, and exert effects due to the content of nucleic acids, inflammatory mediators, and enzymes or organelles that generate free radicals [33–36].

Oxidative stress is also considered among the issues related to DCS, especially with OPB in mind. It is known to occur with diving and documented as the upregulation of antioxidant genes and elevation of plasma and intracellular antioxidant enzyme levels [37–42]. High-pressure exposures also increase the number of MPs in human divers, marine mammals, and small animals used in models of DCS [27–30,43–47]. Studies with isolated human and murine neutrophils demonstrate that MP production is an oxidative stress response [48].

Since OPB protocols were developed based on pragmatic factors and the limitations of resources—such as those present during space flight—with only a view toward N_2 removal, the aim of this investigation was to evaluate the impact of varying concentrations of O_2 on the number of blood-borne MPs in a group of human research subjects. We considered that examining MP responses may offer more objective criteria for choices of O_2 partial pressure.

However, when it comes to analyzing the biological responses to oxygen level variation, the trade-off between hypoxia and hyperoxia is not obvious. Large deviations from normoxia generally lead to increased oxidative stress, while the slight modulation of oxygen levels can enhance the antioxidant defenses [1,49]. We therefore investigated extremes, from 0.1 ATA (Summit of Kilimanjaro (5791 m)) to 2.5 ATA (therapeutic hyperbaric oxygen sessions), and several intermediate oxygen levels relevant to high-altitude exposure (2400 to 2700 m) or O_2 levels used during closed circuit rebreather (CCR) diving—either in recreational, technical, or military diving (0.15, 0.30, 1.0, and 1.4 ATA) [12,50,51].

2. Results

2.1. Microparticles Elicited after One Hour of Different Oxygen Exposures

Research subjects had blood samples obtained prior to and at two hours after a one-hour exposure to various O_2 partial pressures. MPs were identified based on size and surface expression of annexin V (a protein that binds to phosphatidylserine at the particle surface).

Figure 1 illustrates the changes in the number of blood-borne MPs. Elevations were found across the range of hypo- to hyperoxic exposures, with significant elevations following 10%, 30%, 100%, and 2.5 ATA. Breathing 15% oxygen elicited no change, while 1.4 ATA is the only O_2 level showing a significant decrease in MP production.

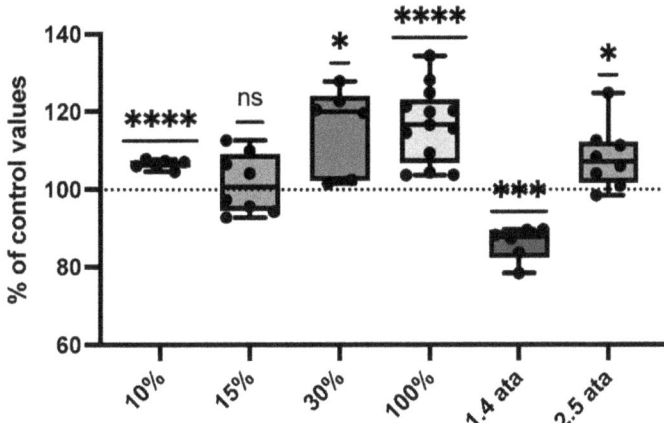

Figure 1. Total microparticle response following different oxygen levels. Box and Whisker plots indicating median, 1st quartile, 3rd quartile, interquartile range, min., and max. in comparison to baseline (before oxygen exposure), which was set at 100%. (One-sample t test: **** $p < 0.0001$, *** $p < 0.001$, * $p < 0.05$, ns = non-significant).

2.2. Microparticles Expressing Proteins from Platelets, Neutrophils, Endothelial Cells, and Microglia after One Hour of Different Oxygen Exposures

The expression of antigens on the MPs surface were probed to evaluate cells generating MPs and several cells' signaling proteins.

Thus, we assessed the percent of MPs expressing proteins specific to platelets (CD41)—see Figure 2, neutrophils (CD66b)—see Figure 3, endothelial cells (CD146)—see Figure 4, and microglia (TMEM119)—see Figure 5.

The response pattern of MPs expressing platelet-specific CD41 after different oxidative stressors shows an ambivalent trend that approaches a sinusoidal pattern following PO_2 increase. Every oxygen level increases CD41+ expression except 15% (ns) and an opposite reaction (a decrease) is elicited for 1.4-ATA exposure.

Neutrophil responses linked to inflammatory reactions show an interesting response pattern. Normobaric hyperoxia exposures share the same trend—mainly an increase of CD66b+. This is also the case for the 10% hypoxic stimulus, however with a smaller magnitude. Interestingly, the 1.4-ATA exposure again elicited an opposite reaction, suggesting a sort of "inhibitory" action.

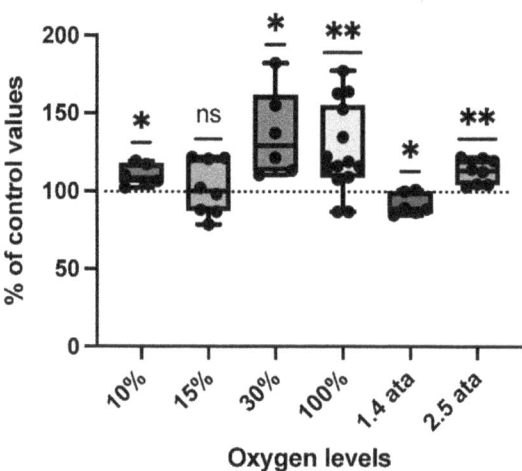

Figure 2. CD41+ response following different oxygen levels exposure. Box and Whisker plots indicating median, 1st quartile, 3rd quartile, interquartile range, min., and max. in comparison to baseline (before oxygen exposure), which was set at 100%. (One-sample t test: ** $p < 0.01$, * $p < 0.05$, ns = non-significant).

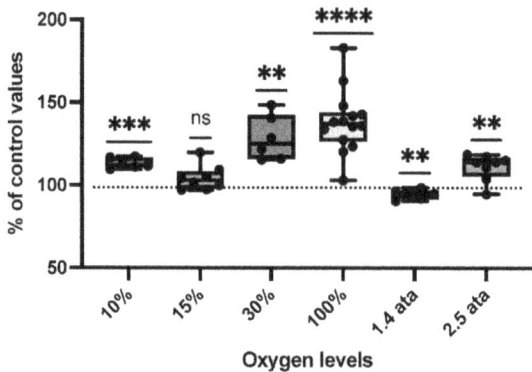

Figure 3. CD66b+ response following different oxygen levels exposure. Box and Whisker plots indicating median, 1st quartile, 3rd quartile, interquartile range, min., and max. in comparison to baseline (before oxygen exposure), which was set at 100%. (One-sample t test: **** $p < 0.0001$, *** $p < 0.001$, ** $p < 0.01$, ns = non-significant).

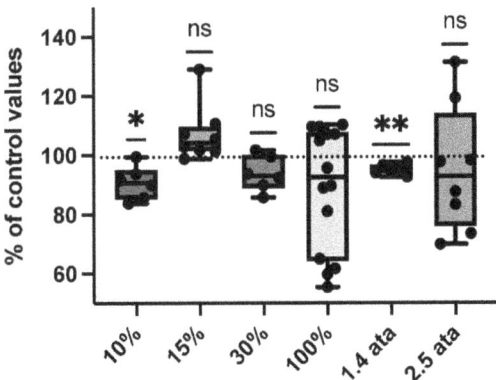

Figure 4. CD146+ response following different oxygen levels exposure. Box and Whisker plots indicating median, 1st quartile, 3rd quartile, interquartile range, min., and max. in comparison to baseline (before oxygen exposure), which was set at 100%. (One-sample t test: ** $p < 0.01$, * $p < 0.05$, ns = non-significant).

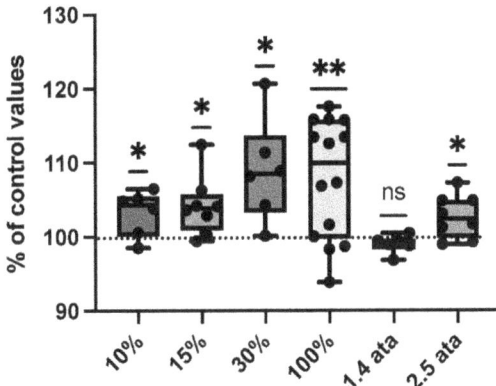

Figure 5. TMEM119+ response following different oxygen levels exposure. Box and Whisker plots indicating median, 1st quartile, 3rd quartile, interquartile range, min., and max. in comparison to baseline (before oxygen exposure), which was set at 100%. (One-sample t test: ** $p < 0.01$, * $p < 0.05$, ns = non-significant).

CD146+ is a protein expressed by endothelial cells, which are known to react to oxidative stress but also to increased hydrostatic pressure [52]. It is interesting to note that hypoxic breathing gives a scattered response, although not reaching statistical significance—except for 10% and 1.4-ATA exposures, which elicited a significant reduction.

Microglia-derived responses (TMEM119+) show a global increase, except for 1.4 ATA; another example of varied reactions elicited by this specific PO_2.

2.3. Microparticles Expressing Proteins from Cell Activation after One Hour of Different Oxygen Exposures

MPs expressing thrombospondin-1 (TSP) (see Figure 6) and those binding phalloidin (See Figure 7) were also evaluated, seeking evidence for particles arising from cell activation. Phalloidin binding, a manifestation of membrane surface filamentous (F-) actin expression, occurs on particles released by activated neutrophils and possibly other cells, and TSP can be released by activated platelets and astrocytes [53–55].

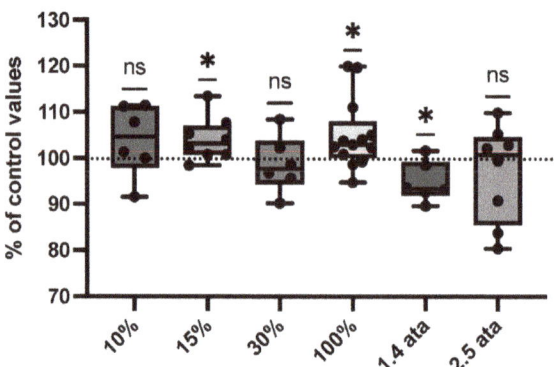

Figure 6. Thrombospondin-1 response following different oxygen levels exposure. Box and Whisker plots indicating median, 1st quartile, 3rd quartile, interquartile range, min., and max. in comparison to baseline (before oxygen exposure), which was set at 100%. (One-sample t test: * $p < 0.05$, ns = non-significant).

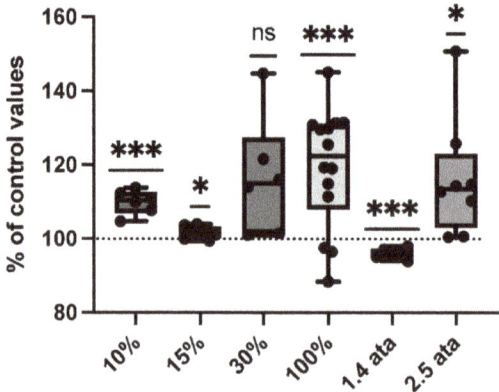

Figure 7. Phalloidin response following different oxygen levels exposure. Box and Whisker plots indicating median, 1st quartile, 3rd quartile, interquartile range, min., and max. in comparison to baseline (before oxygen exposure), which was set at 100%. (One-sample t test: *** $p < 0.001$, * $p < 0.05$, ns = non-significant).

Cellular reactions from platelets and astrocytes may demonstrate a neurovascular reaction of the body to cope with oxidative stress. Again, all oxygen levels react with an increment or without significant change, except for the 1.4 ATA, which shows a limited but significant decrease.

Cellular reactions eliciting filamentous actin liberation are extremely variable, but clearly demonstrate a membrane stress, and again the only reduction is found after 1.4-ATA exposure.

2.4. Percentual and Absolute Changes of Microparticles Expressing Proteins after One Hour of Different Oxygen Exposures

Significant elevations across many exposures were identified for CD41, CD66b, TMEM119, and phalloidin binding, whereas few changes were found for CD146 and TSP.

The magnitude and direction of changes among all MP sub-types are illustrated as a heat map in Figure 8, while absolute values are presented in Table 1. It should be noted that when adding each % change in MPs, as shown in Table 1, the sum exceeds 100%. This is a common finding that is thought to indicate that MPs collide and share antigens [27,56].

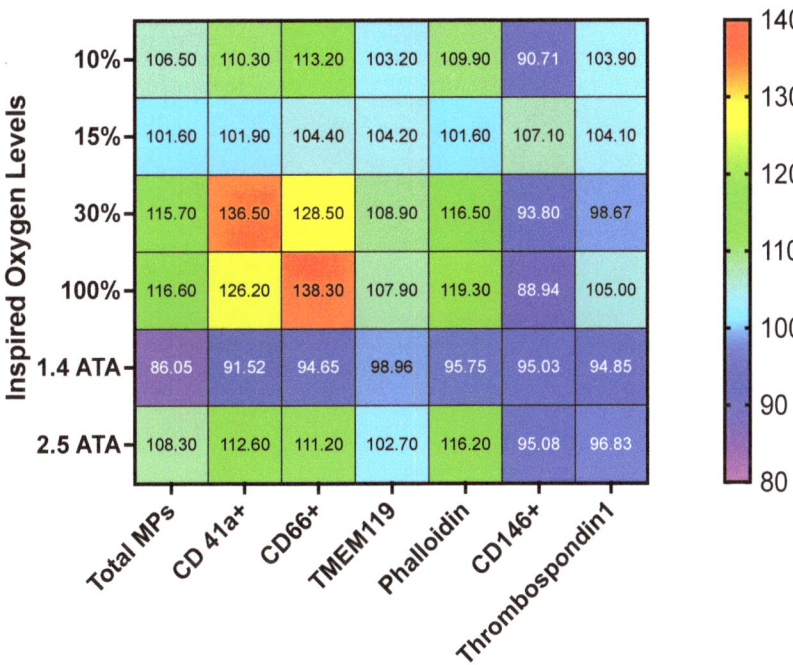

Figure 8. Percentual variations in MPs after 60 min of oxygen breathing. Levels of oxygen are shown on the ordinate, and Total MPs and MP sub-types are shown on the abscissa. Blood sampling occurred 120 min after exposures (in total 48 subjects participated to the experiment). Results are expressed in the heat map as mean percentage change.

Table 1. Absolute values for microparticle-derived responses (MPs/µL). Results are given in mean ± SD. (Paired t-test: **** $p < 0.0001$, *** $p < 0.001$, ** $p < 0.01$, * $p < 0.05$).

Exposition	Baseline	After 120 min	p Value	n
Extreme Hypoxia 10% (0.1 ATA)	MPs/µL	Mps/µL	Paired t Test	
Total MPs	2241 ± 77.5	2388 ± 101.4	<0.0001 ****	6
Thrombospondin 1	12 ± 0.9338	12.44 ± 0.9422	0.2862	6
TMEM119	26.97 ± 0.4024	27.84 ± 0.8396	0.0480 *	6
CD 146+	33.11 ± 2.934	30.31 ± 2.329	0.0260 *	6
CD 41a+	4.5 ± 0.1117	4.962 ± 0.2962	0.0125 *	6
CD 66b+	13.56 ± 1.006	15.33 ± 0.9346	<0.0001 ****	6
Phalloidin	14.24 ± 0.6746	15.66 ± 0.9320	0.0007 ***	6
Moderate Hypoxia 15% (0.15 ATA)				
Total MPs	2085 ± 79.27	2114 ± 80.54	0.6174	8
Thrombospondin 1	18.28 ± 0.6066	19.03 ± 0.9983	0.0473 *	8
TMEM119	33.96 ± 0.4660	35.36 ± 1.141	0.0234 *	8
CD 146+	33.94 ± 0.5551	36.32 ± 2.880	0.0156 *	8
CD 41a+	10.60 ± 1.136	10.64 ± 1.008	0.9582	8
CD 66b+	22.26 ± 0.5924	23.20 ± 1.216	0.1563	8
Phalloidin	20.60 ± 0.2195	20.93 ± 0.1674	0.0315 *	8
Moderate Hyperoxia 30% (0.3 ATA)				
Total MPs	1838 ± 123.2	2116 ± 68.66	0.0159 *	6
Thrombospondin 1	17.86 ± 1.4	17.55 ± 0.8321	0.0473 *	6
TMEM119	30.98 ± 2.081	33.60 ± 0.3714	0.0203 *	6
CD 146+	33.13 ± 2.933	30.94 ± 1.841	0.0472 *	6
CD 41a+	8.227 ± 0.7471	11.06 ± 1.192	0.0149 *	6
CD 66b+	17 ± 1.849	21.64 ± 0.5708	0.001 ***	6
Phalloidin	17.91 ± 2.438	20.54 ± 0.2030	0.0356 *	6
Hyperoxia 100% (1 ATA)				
Total MPs	1786 ± 118.0	2072 ± 56.29	<0.0001 ****	14
Thrombospondin 1	17.16 ± 0.5448	18.01 ± 1.218	0.0266 *	14
TMEM119	30.80 ± 1.993	33.10 ± 0.5293	0.0031 **	14
CD 146+	42.38 ± 12.31	35.32 ± 4.333	0.0785	14
CD 41a+	7.751 ± 0.9495	9.552 ± 1.086	0.0035 **	14
CD 66b+	14.85 ± 1.662	20.30 ± 1.723	<0.0001 ****	14
Phalloidin	16.74 ± 2.008	19.65 ± 0.7498	0.0023 **	14
Hyperbaric Hyperoxia 1.4 ATA				
Total MPs	2766.69 ± 80.74	2381.7 ± 156.3	0.0004 ***	6
Thrombospondin 1	11.82 ± 0.26	11.21 ± 0.4	0.0354 *	6
TMEM119	31.27 ± 0.35	30.94 ± 0.36	0.087	6
CD 146+	22.62 ± 0.3	21.5 ± 0.32	0.0011 **	6
CD 41a+	6.56 ± 0.40	5.6 ± 0.22	0.0336 **	6
CD 66b+	17.65 ± 0.18	16.7 ± 0.4	0.0077 **	6
Phalloidin	16.86 +/− 0.22	16.15 +/− 0.09	0.001 ***	6
Hyperbaric Hyperoxia 2.5 ATA				
Total MPs	1846 ± 128.8	1989 ± 44.05	0.0206 *	8
Thrombospondin 1	17.08 ± 2.048	16.37 ± 0.865	0.6406	8
TMEM119	32.13 ± 0.445	32.98 ± 0.5293	0.0347 *	8
CD 146+	39.47 ± 4.985	36.88 ± 6.047	0.3828	8
CD 41a+	8.114 ± 0.6390	9.109 ± 0.5885	0.0078 **	8
CD 66b+	17.64 ± 0.8149	19.59 ± 1.327	0.0057 **	8
Phalloidin	16.80 ± 1.893	19.22 ± 0.4839	0.0149 *	8

3. Discussion

DCS is mostly known as an occupational risk for SCUBA divers or caisson workers (chamber hyperbaric technician, tunnellers), but also concerns space flight and extra-vehicular activity involving decompression from 1 ATA to 0.3 ATA in space-suit use [57], or altitude exposure up to 8000 m with an estimated probability of 0.2% [58] to 15–20% [59], respectively. Given its potential deleterious outcome, it must be prevented, especially in the occupational setting.

As mentioned earlier, OPB is one possible strategy. Unfortunately, available protocols are varied and complex, involving intervals of exercise while breathing O_2 at partial pressures from 1 to 0.3 ATA for over more than 24 h [60]. The rationale behind the protocol is denitrogenating the astronaut to prevent the supersaturation of inert gas and subsequent DCS.

However, this hypothesis does not provide a full explanation for phenomena like the variability between bubblers and non-bubblers, the bi-phasic mechanism of VGE expansion, increased VGE formation with depth, potential endothelial injury, or the presence of MPs [57,61].

While the role of MPs in decompression stress is not clear, they seem to play a major role as VGE precursors or as a mediator of inflammation [62]. To the best of our knowledge, this is the first study describing blood-borne MP responses to different PO_2. Although net changes are a balance between production/liberation to the blood stream and sequestration/removal, we interpret differences in the patterns among the MP subsets elicited as reflecting the propensity for production because alternative cell types have different O_2 tolerances and there is little evidence for the selective uptake of circulating MPs [32].

The first interesting results from our data are that the complex pattern of changes in MP numbers approximate a sinusoidal curve with nodes of nominal change in total number at 15% O_2 and 1.4 ATA. This is consistent with the oxygen-sensing mechanism within the body. In case of hypoxia, hypoxia-inducible factors (HIFs) activate the transcription of numerous target genes that mediate both adaptive and maladaptive responses, including erythropoiesis, angiogenesis, metabolic reprogramming, or cardiovascular disease [1], while hyperoxia involves the production of ROS, which initiate signaling via the modulation of many molecules, such as NF-E2, Nrf2, or NF-kB [63]. At the same time, hyperoxia elicits an antioxidant scavenging adaptive response that can mimic the effect of hypoxia. Indeed, a sudden and sustained decrease in tissue oxygen tension, even in the absence of hypoxia (e.g., after hyperoxic oxygen breathing), acts as a trigger for HIF liberation and subsequent transcription [64,65].

Secondly, we anticipated that some changes in specific MP numbers are due to oxidative stress at the extremes of hypoxia and hyperoxia, as demonstrated by the elevations in plasma TSP levels [54]. However, the trade-off between both conditions is not obvious. Neutrophil MP generation was most prominent at 30% and 100%. Similarly, an intimate balance exists between the redox state and platelet activation, which may be reflected by MPs expressing CD41 [66]. On this particular point, previous work on hip replacement surgery, and randomized Oxygen administration one hour per day compared to one hour of air, showed a significant reduction of transfusions in the oxygen group, and also an increase of reticulocytes, both outcomes possibly resulting on the one hand due to CD41 increase and better bleeding reduction [67], and on the other hand, due to the normobaric oxygen paradox [6].

The same observation may apply to TMEM119, a fixed macrophage-like leukocyte resident within the central nervous system (CNS) [68]. All these features are consistent with a pro-inflammatory response related to oxygen breathing but does not concern the 1.4-ATA exposure that exhibits an inhibitory rather than an activation pattern. One possible explanation pertains to F-actin instability that occurs at high O_2 partial pressures, thereby leading to the impairment of MP formation [69]. Alternatively, since phalloidin-binding MPs seem to play a role in tissue damage associated with DCS and can be generated by leukocytes [53,54], this can be interpreted as demonstrating membrane stress that is not found after 1.4-ATA exposure.

Despite the limitations to our study, including the observational, non-randomized trial design, hidden processes because of unmeasured confounders and the small sample sizes that may have altered the resulting patterns, these results question the unique profile of 1.4-ATA exposure. This is a reasonable interpretation since the end-points were objective and the participating research subjects served as their own control. Therefore, a clearer understanding of hyperoxia-induced signal transduction pathways is crucial to facilitate the design of successful therapeutic strategies as well as prevention strategies, such as OPB.

Indeed, this investigation poses numerous questions as to the impact of O_2 partial pressure on MPs. Regarding OPB, the production of MPs is maximal when breathing 100% oxygen, which could constitute a risk. However, it must be put into perspective. De-nitrogenation is a clear benefit while the kinetics of the production and elimination of MPs are unknown, with multiple O_2 partial pressures being used during OPB. The results from this investigation also highlight questions such as the presumed innocuity of sham procedures in HBOT research [5].

Therefore, elucidating the mechanisms for changes and subsequent applications will require substantial future effort. Further experiments will also need to investigate the specific compensatory reactive adaptations at longer periods of pulsed hyperoxia.

4. Materials and Methods

4.1. Experimental Protocol

After written informed consent, 48 healthy non-smoking subjects (32 males and 16 females) volunteered for this study. None of them had a history of previous cardiac abnormalities or were under any cardio or vaso-active medication. The sample age was 43.7 ± 13.4 years old; height was 172.7 ± 10.07 cm; and weight was 68.4 ± 15.7 kg.

All experimental procedures were conducted in accordance with the Declaration of Helsinki [70] and approved by the Ethics Committee approval from the Bio-Ethical Committee for Research and Higher Education, Brussels (N° B200-2020-088).

Participants were prospectively randomized into 6 groups of 6–14 persons each (Figure 9).

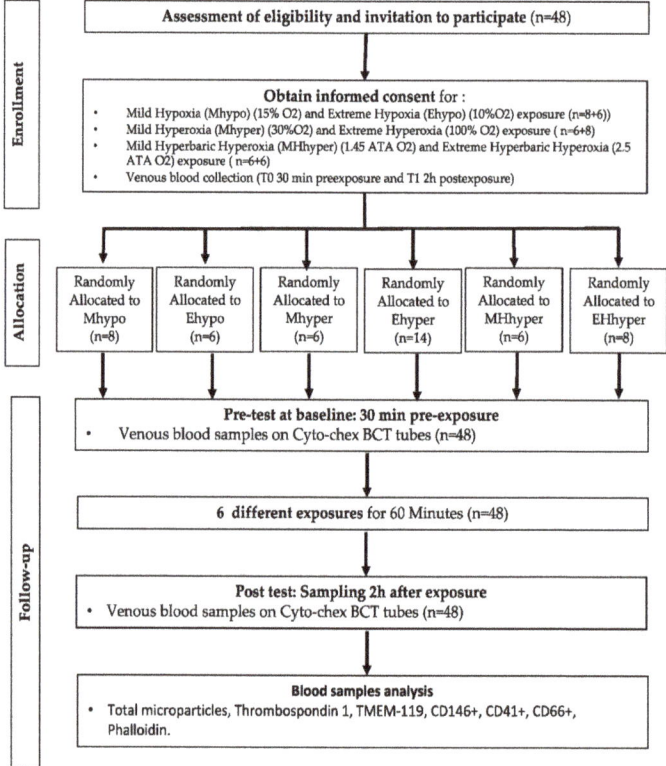

Figure 9. Experimental flowchart.

Subjects breathed different oxygen levels for a total duration of 60 min delivered by an oro-facial mask (non-rebreather mask) with a reservoir for the 10%, 15%, 30%, and 100% exposures, or a dedicated mask adapted to the hyperbaric environment (1.4 and 2.5 ATA) (Adult Silicone Mask–Laerdael, Laerdal Benelux, Vilvoorde, Belgium) were proposed.

The hypoxic gas supplies (10% and 15%) were achieved using a hypoxia generator and calibrated to reach the chosen level of oxygen (HYP 123, Hypoxico–Hypoxico Europe GmbH, Bickenbach, Germany). Normobaric hyperoxia was delivered using generated free-flow oxygen or medical oxygen tanks. Every exposure flow was calibrated by means of an oxymeter (Solo-O_2 Divesoft, Halkova, Czech Republic) in the mask used by the subject to ascertain that the desired oxygen level was reached. Hyperbaric exposures were performed at the Hyperbaric Centre, Queen Astrid Military Hospital, 1120 Brussels, Belgium.

4.2. Blood Sampling and Laboratory Procedure

Blood samples were obtained before and 120 min after the different oxygen breathing sessions, the chosen time windows were achieved according to our previous work showing a clear variation in MP numbers 120-min post-exposure [71]. Blood (~5 mL) was drawn into Cyto-Chex BCT test tubes that contain a proprietary preservative (Streck, Inc., Omaha, NE, USA). Samples were sent by express mail to the University of Maryland (Dr. Thom) laboratory where all analyses were performed by following published techniques described in previous publications [54,72,73]. In brief, blood was centrifuged for 5 min at $1500\times g$, the supernatant was added to 12.5 mmol/L EDTA to impede MP aggregation, and then centrifuged at $15,000\times g$ for 30 min. Aliquots of the $15,000\times g$ supernatant were stained with antibodies for MP analysis by flow cytometry. Total MPs and sub-types were assayed in an 8-color, triple laser MACSQuant (Miltenyi Biotec Corp., Auburn, CA, USA) flow cytometer with the manufacturers' acquisition software using standard methods, including a "fluorescence minus one control test" [73]. This analysis provides a way to define the boundary between positive and negative particles in an unbiased manner by defining the maximum fluorescence expected for a given subset after outlining the area in a two-dimensional scatter diagram when a fluorophore-tagged antibody is omitted from the stain set. This analysis allows a simple decision as to where to place the upper boundary for non-staining particles in a fluorescence channel. We define MPs as annexin V-positive particles with diameters from 0.3 to 1 µm. All supplies, reagents, and manufacturer sources have been described in previous publications [46,47].

4.3. Statistical Analysis

The normality of the data was verified by means of the Shapiro–Wilk test. Since a Gaussian distribution could be verified, crude data were analyzed by means of a paired t-test. When compared to air-breathing control values with the baseline measures set as 100%, changes were calculated for each exposure protocol and analyzed with a one-sample t test to allow an appreciation of the magnitude of change rather than the absolute values. All statistical tests were performed using a standard computer statistical package, GraphPad Prism version 9.00 for Mac (GraphPad Software, San Diego CA, USA). A threshold of $p < 0.05$ was considered statistically significant. All Table 1 data are presented as mean $\pm$ standard deviation (SD) and the figures are presented as box and whisker plots of median and quartiles.

Author Contributions: All authors listed have made a substantial, direct and intellectual contribution to the work, and approved it for publication: Conceptualization: C.B., P.L., P.G., C.L., S.R.T., K.L. and F.V.; Investigation: P.L., C.L., S.R.T., C.B., K.L., P.G. and A.K.A.; Writing: S.R.T., K.L., C.B., P.G., P.L., A.K.A. and C.L.; Funding: C.B., F.V., K.L. and S.R.T.; Data Analysis: S.R.T., C.B., P.L., A.K.A. and P.G. All authors have read and agreed to the published version of the manuscript.

Funding: This work was supported in part by grants from the National Institutes for Health (NINDS) R01-NS122855 and the US Office of Naval Research N00014-20-1-2641 and by the DELTO2X Project funded by WBE (Wallonia-Brussels-Education) Belgium to the Environmental, Occupational, Aging (Integrative) Physiology Laboratory, Haute Ecole Bruxelles-Brabant (HE2B), Belgium. The sponsors had no role in the design and conduct of the study; collection, management, analysis, and interpretation of the data; preparation, review, or approval of the manuscript; and the decision to submit the manuscript for publication.

Institutional Review Board Statement: Ethics Committee approval from the Bio-Ethical Committee for Research and Higher Education, Brussels (N° B 200-2020-088).

Informed Consent Statement: Informed consent was obtained from all subjects involved in the study.

Data Availability Statement: Data are available at request from the authors.

Acknowledgments: Authors are grateful to all volunteer participants specially to students of the Haute Ecole Bruxelles-Brabant, Motor Sciences Department (Physiotherapy).

Conflicts of Interest: The authors declare no conflict of interest.

Abbreviations

MPs	Blood Borne Microparticles
OPB	Oxygen Pre-Breathing
VGE	Vascular Gas Emboli
DCS	Decompression Sickness
NF-kB	Nuclear Factor kappa-light-chain-enhancer of activated B cells
NRF2	Nuclear Factor Erythroid 2 Related–Factor 2
PO_2	Oxygen Partial Pressure
TSP	Thrombospondin 1
NF-E2	Nuclear Factor, Erythroid 2
HIFs	Hypoxia Inducible Factors

References

1. Nakane, M. Biological effects of the oxygen molecule in critically ill patients. *J. Intensive Care* **2020**, *8*, 95. [CrossRef] [PubMed]
2. Girault, C.; Boyer, D.; Jolly, G.; Carpentier, D.; Béduneau, G.; Frat, J.P. Operating principles, physiological effects and practical issues of high-flow nasal oxygen therapy. *Rev. Mal. Respir.* **2022**, *39*, 455–468. [CrossRef] [PubMed]
3. De Wolde, S.D.; Hulskes, R.H.; Weenink, R.P.; Hollmann, M.W.; Van Hulst, R.A. The Effects of Hyperbaric Oxygenation on Oxidative Stress, Inflammation and Angiogenesis. *Biomolecules* **2021**, *11*, 1210. [CrossRef] [PubMed]
4. Mathieu, D.; Marroni, A.; Kot, J. Tenth European Consensus Conference on Hyperbaric Medicine: Recommendations for accepted and non-accepted clinical indications and practice of hyperbaric oxygen treatment. *Diving Hyperb. Med.* **2017**, *47*, 24–32. [CrossRef] [PubMed]
5. Hadanny, A.; Efrati, S. The Hyperoxic-Hypoxic Paradox. *Biomolecules* **2020**, *10*, 958. [CrossRef]
6. Lafere, P.; Schubert, T.; De Bels, D.; Germonpre, P.; Balestra, C. Can the normobaric oxygen paradox (NOP) increase reticulocyte count after traumatic hip surgery? *J. Clin. Anesth.* **2013**, *25*, 129–134. [CrossRef]
7. De Bels, D.; Corazza, F.; Germonpre, P.; Balestra, C. The normobaric oxygen paradox: A novel way to administer oxygen as an adjuvant treatment for cancer? *Med. Hypotheses* **2011**, *76*, 467–470. [CrossRef]
8. Burk, R. Oxygen breathing may be a cheaper and safer alternative to exogenous erythropoietin (EPO). *Med. Hypotheses* **2007**, *69*, 1200–1204. [CrossRef]
9. Balestra, C.; Lambrechts, K.; Mrakic-Sposta, S.; Vezzoli, A.; Levenez, M.; Germonpre, P.; Virgili, F.; Bosco, G.; Lafere, P. Hypoxic and Hyperoxic Breathing as a Complement to Low-Intensity Physical Exercise Programs: A Proof-of-Principle Study. *Int. J. Mol. Sci.* **2021**, *22*, 9600. [CrossRef]
10. Bestavashvili, A.; Glazachev, O.; Bestavashvili, A.; Suvorov, A.; Zhang, Y.; Zhang, X.; Rozhkov, A.; Kuznetsova, N.; Pavlov, C.; Glushenkov, D.; et al. Intermittent Hypoxic-Hyperoxic Exposures Effects in Patients with Metabolic Syndrome: Correction of Cardiovascular and Metabolic Profile. *Biomedicines* **2022**, *10*, 566. [CrossRef]
11. Matta, A.; Nader, V.; Lebrin, M.; Gross, F.; Prats, A.C.; Cussac, D.; Galinier, M.; Roncalli, J. Pre-Conditioning Methods and Novel Approaches with Mesenchymal Stem Cells Therapy in Cardiovascular Disease. *Cells* **2022**, *11*, 1620. [CrossRef] [PubMed]
12. Lafère, P.; Lambrechts, K.; Germonpré, P.; Balestra, A.; Germonpré, F.L.; Marroni, A.; Cialoni, D.; Bosco, G.; Balestra, C. Heart Rate Variability During a Standard Dive: A Role for Inspired Oxygen Pressure? *Front. Physiol.* **2021**, *12*, 635132. [CrossRef] [PubMed]

13. Balestra, C.; Theunissen, S.; Papadopoulou, V.; Le Mener, C.; Germonpré, P.; Guerrero, F.; Lafère, P. Pre-dive Whole-Body Vibration Better Reduces Decompression-Induced Vascular Gas Emboli than Oxygenation or a Combination of Both. *Front. Physiol.* **2016**, *7*, 586. [CrossRef]
14. Webb, J.T.; Pilmanis, A.A. Fifty years of decompression sickness research at Brooks AFB, TX: 1960–2010. *Aviat. Space Environ. Med.* **2011**, *82*, A1–A25. [CrossRef] [PubMed]
15. Sannigrahi, P.; Sushree, S.K.; Agarwal, A. Aeromedical Concerns and Lessons Learned during Oxygen Jump at Dolma Sampa. *IJASM Indian J. Aerosp. Med.* **2018**, *62*, 16–20.
16. Kluis, L.; Diaz-Artiles, A. Revisiting decompression sickness risk and mobility in the context of the SmartSuit, a hybrid planetary spacesuit. *NPJ Microgravity* **2021**, *7*, 46. [CrossRef] [PubMed]
17. Wessel, J.H., 3rd; Schaefer, C.M.; Thompson, M.S.; Norcross, J.R.; Bekdash, O.S. Retrospective Evaluation of Clinical Symptoms Due to Mild Hypobaric Hypoxia Exposure in Microgravity. *Aerosp. Med. Hum. Perform.* **2018**, *89*, 792–797. [CrossRef]
18. Imbert, J.P.; Egi, S.M.; Germonpre, P.; Balestra, C. Static Metabolic Bubbles as Precursors of Vascular Gas Emboli During Divers' Decompression: A Hypothesis Explaining Bubbling Variability. *Front. Physiol.* **2019**, *10*, 807. [CrossRef]
19. Mollerlokken, A.; Gaustad, S.E.; Havnes, M.B.; Gutvik, C.R.; Hjelde, A.; Wisloff, U.; Brubakk, A.O. Venous gas embolism as a predictive tool for improving CNS decompression safety. *Eur. J. Appl. Physiol.* **2012**, *112*, 401–409. [CrossRef]
20. Ånell, R.; Grönkvist, M.; Gennser, M.; Eiken, O. High-altitude decompression strain can be reduced by an early excursion to moderate altitude while breathing oxygen. *Eur. J. Appl. Physiol.* **2021**, *121*, 3225–3232. [CrossRef]
21. Webb, J.T.; Pilmanis, A.A. Breathing 100% oxygen compared with 50% oxygen: 50% nitrogen reduces altitude-induced venous gas emboli. *Aviat. Space Environ. Med.* **1993**, *64*, 808–812. [PubMed]
22. Webb, J.T.; Fischer, M.D.; Heaps, C.L.; Pilmanis, A.A. Exercise-enhanced preoxygenation increases protection from decompression sickness. *Aviat. Space Environ. Med.* **1996**, *67*, 618–624. [PubMed]
23. Arieli, R.; Boaron, E.; Abramovich, A. Combined effect of denucleation and denitrogenation on the risk of decompression sickness in rats. *J. Appl. Physiol.* **2009**, *106*, 1453–1458. [CrossRef] [PubMed]
24. Arieli, Y.; Katsenelson, K.; Arieli, R. Bubble reduction after decompression in the prawn Palaemon elegans by pretreatment with hyperbaric oxygen. *Undersea Hyperb. Med.* **2007**, *34*, 369–378. [PubMed]
25. Lambrechts, K.; Germonpre, P.; Vandenheede, J.; Delorme, M.; Lafere, P.; Balestra, C. Mini Trampoline, a New and Promising Way of SCUBA Diving Preconditioning to Reduce Vascular Gas Emboli? *Int. J. Environ. Res. Public Health* **2022**, *19*, 5410. [CrossRef]
26. Thom, S.R.; Bennett, M.; Banham, N.D.; Chin, W.; Blake, D.F.; Rosen, A.; Pollock, N.W.; Madden, D.; Barak, O.; Marroni, A.; et al. Association of microparticles and neutrophil activation with decompression sickness. *J. Appl. Physiol.* **2015**, *119*, 427–434. [CrossRef]
27. Thom, S.R.; Yang, M.; Bhopale, V.M.; Huang, S.; Milovanova, T.N. Microparticles initiate decompression-induced neutrophil activation and subsequent vascular injuries. *J. Appl. Physiol.* **2011**, *110*, 340–351. [CrossRef]
28. Vince, R.V.; McNaughton, L.R.; Taylor, L.; Midgley, A.W.; Laden, G.; Madden, L.A. Release of VCAM-1 associated endothelial microparticles following simulated SCUBA dives. *Eur. J. Appl. Physiol.* **2009**, *105*, 507–513. [CrossRef]
29. Thom, S.R.; Bhopale, V.M.; Yu, K.; Yang, M. Provocative decompression causes diffuse vascular injury in mice mediated by microparticles containing interleukin-1beta. *J. Appl. Physiol.* **2018**, *125*, 1339–1348. [CrossRef]
30. Brett, K.D.; Nugent, N.Z.; Fraser, N.K.; Bhopale, V.M.; Yang, M.; Thom, S.R. Microparticle and interleukin-1beta production with human simulated compressed air diving. *Sci. Rep.* **2019**, *9*, 13320. [CrossRef]
31. Pontier, J.M.; Gempp, E.; Ignatescu, M. Blood platelet-derived microparticles release and bubble formation after an open-sea air dive. *Appl. Physiol. Nutr. Metab.* **2012**, *37*, 888–892. [CrossRef] [PubMed]
32. Meldolesi, J. Exosomes and Ectosomes in Intercellular Communication. *Curr. Biol.* **2018**, *28*, R435–R444. [CrossRef] [PubMed]
33. Cabral, J.; Ryan, A.E.; Griffin, M.D.; Ritter, T. Extracellular vesicles as modulators of wound healing. *Adv. Drug. Deliv. Rev.* **2018**, *129*, 394–406. [CrossRef] [PubMed]
34. Mause, S.F.; Weber, C. Microparticles: Protagonists of a novel communication network for intercellular information exchange. *Circ. Res.* **2010**, *107*, 1047–1057. [CrossRef]
35. Slater, T.W.; Finkielsztein, A.; Mascarenhas, L.A.; Mehl, L.C.; Butin-Israeli, V.; Sumagin, R. Neutrophil Microparticles Deliver Active Myeloperoxidase to Injured Mucosa To Inhibit Epithelial Wound Healing. *J. Immunol.* **2017**, *198*, 2886–2897. [CrossRef]
36. Thom, S.R.; Yang, M.; Bhopale, V.M.; Milovanova, T.N.; Bogush, M.; Buerk, D.G. Intramicroparticle nitrogen dioxide is a bubble nucleation site leading to decompression-induced neutrophil activation and vascular injury. *J. Appl. Physiol.* **2013**, *114*, 550–558. [CrossRef]
37. Eftedal, I.; Ljubkovic, M.; Flatberg, A.; Jorgensen, A.; Brubakk, A.O.; Dujic, Z. Acute and potentially persistent effects of scuba diving on the blood transcriptome of experienced divers. *Physiol. Genom.* **2013**, *45*, 965–972. [CrossRef]
38. Ferrer, M.D.; Sureda, A.; Batle, J.M.; Tauler, P.; Tur, J.A.; Pons, A. Scuba diving enhances endogenous antioxidant defenses in lymphocytes and neutrophils. *Free Radic. Res.* **2007**, *41*, 274–281. [CrossRef]
39. Morabito, C.; Bosco, G.; Pilla, R.; Corona, C.; Mancinelli, R.; Yang, Z.; Camporesi, E.M.; Fano, G.; Mariggio, M.A. Effect of pre-breathing oxygen at different depth on oxidative status and calcium concentration in lymphocytes of scuba divers. *Acta Physiol. Oxf.* **2011**, *202*, 69–78. [CrossRef]

40. Sureda, A.; Batle, J.M.; Capo, X.; Martorell, M.; Cordova, A.; Tur, J.A.; Pons, A. Scuba diving induces nitric oxide synthesis and the expression of inflammatory and regulatory genes of the immune response in neutrophils. *Physiol. Genom.* **2014**, *46*, 647–654. [CrossRef]
41. Sureda, A.; Batle, J.M.; Ferrer, M.D.; Mestre-Alfaro, A.; Tur, J.A.; Pons, A. Scuba diving activates vascular antioxidant system. *Int. J. Sports Med.* **2012**, *33*, 531–536. [CrossRef] [PubMed]
42. Sureda, A.; Ferrer, M.D.; Batle, J.M.; Tauler, P.; Tur, J.A.; Pons, A. Scuba diving increases erythrocyte and plasma antioxidant defenses and spares NO without oxidative damage. *Med. Sci. Sports Exerc.* **2009**, *41*, 1271–1276. [CrossRef] [PubMed]
43. Madden, D.; Thom, S.R.; Milovanova, T.N.; Yang, M.; Bhopale, V.M.; Ljubkovic, M.; Dujic, Z. Exercise before scuba diving ameliorates decompression-induced neutrophil activation. *Med. Sci. Sports Exerc.* **2014**, *46*, 1928–1935. [CrossRef]
44. Madden, D.; Thom, S.R.; Yang, M.; Bhopale, V.M.; Ljubkovic, M.; Dujic, Z. High intensity cycling before SCUBA diving reduces post-decompression microparticle production and neutrophil activation. *Eur. J. Appl. Physiol.* **2014**, *114*, 1955–1961. [CrossRef] [PubMed]
45. Madden, L.A.; Chrismas, B.C.; Mellor, D.; Vince, R.V.; Midgley, A.W.; McNaughton, L.R.; Atkin, S.L.; Laden, G. Endothelial function and stress response after simulated dives to 18 msw breathing air or oxygen. *Aviat. Space Environ. Med.* **2010**, *81*, 41–45. [CrossRef] [PubMed]
46. Thom, S.R.; Milovanova, T.N.; Bogush, M.; Bhopale, V.M.; Yang, M.; Bushmann, K.; Pollock, N.W.; Ljubkovic, M.; Denoble, P.; Dujic, Z. Microparticle production, neutrophil activation, and intravascular bubbles following open-water SCUBA diving. *J. Appl. Physiol.* **2012**, *112*, 1268–1278. [CrossRef]
47. Thom, S.R.; Milovanova, T.N.; Bogush, M.; Yang, M.; Bhopale, V.M.; Pollock, N.W.; Ljubkovic, M.; Denoble, P.; Madden, D.; Lozo, M.; et al. Bubbles, microparticles, and neutrophil activation: Changes with exercise level and breathing gas during open-water SCUBA diving. *J. Appl. Physiol.* **2013**, *114*, 1396–1405. [CrossRef]
48. Thom, S.R.; Bhopale, V.M.; Yang, M. Neutrophils generate microparticles during exposure to inert gases due to cytoskeletal oxidative stress. *J. Biol. Chem.* **2014**, *289*, 18831–18845. [CrossRef]
49. Fu, Q.; Duan, R.; Sun, Y.; Li, Q. Hyperbaric oxygen therapy for healthy aging: From mechanisms to therapeutics. *Redox Biol.* **2022**, *53*, 102352. [CrossRef]
50. Balestra, C.; Guerrero, F.; Theunissen, S.; Germonpre, P.; Lafere, P. Physiology of repeated mixed gas 100-m wreck dives using a closed-circuit rebreather: A field bubble study. *Eur. J. Appl. Physiol.* **2022**, *122*, 515–522. [CrossRef]
51. Dugrenot, E.; Balestra, C.; Gouin, E.; L'Her, E.; Guerrero, F. Physiological effects of mixed-gas deep sea dives using a closed-circuit rebreather: A field pilot study. *Eur. J. Appl. Physiol.* **2021**, *121*, 3323–3331. [CrossRef] [PubMed]
52. Wang, Q.; Guerrero, F.; Lambrechts, K.; Mazur, A.; Buzzacott, P.; Belhomme, M.; Theron, M. Simulated air dives induce superoxide, nitric oxide, peroxynitrite, and Ca^{2+} alterations in endothelial cells. *J. Physiol. Biochem.* **2020**, *76*, 61–72. [CrossRef] [PubMed]
53. Bhopale, V.M.; Ruhela, D.; Brett, K.D.; Nugent, N.Z.; Fraser, N.K.; Levinson, S.L.; DiNubile, M.J.; Thom, S.R. Plasma gelsolin modulates the production and fate of IL-1beta-containing microparticles following high-pressure exposure and decompression. *J. Appl. Physiol.* **2021**, *130*, 1604–1613. [CrossRef] [PubMed]
54. Chen, J.K.; Zhan, Y.J.; Yang, C.S.; Tzeng, S.F. Oxidative stress-induced attenuation of thrombospondin-1 expression in primary rat astrocytes. *J. Cell. Biochem.* **2011**, *112*, 59–70. [CrossRef]
55. Novelli, E.M.; Kato, G.J.; Ragni, M.V.; Zhang, Y.; Hildesheim, M.E.; Nouraie, M.; Barge, S.; Meyer, M.P.; Hassett, A.C.; Gordeuk, V.R.; et al. Plasma thrombospondin-1 is increased during acute sickle cell vaso-occlusive events and associated with acute chest syndrome, hydroxyurea therapy, and lower hemolytic rates. *Am. J. Hematol.* **2012**, *87*, 326–330. [CrossRef]
56. Yang, M.; Kosterin, P.; Salzberg, B.M.; Milovanova, T.N.; Bhopale, V.M.; Thom, S.R. Microparticles generated by decompression stress cause central nervous system injury manifested as neurohypophysial terminal action potential broadening. *J. Appl. Physiol.* **2013**, *115*, 1481–1486. [CrossRef]
57. Foster, P.P.; Pollock, N.W.; Conkin, J.; Dervay, J.P.; Caillot, N.; Chhikara, R.S.; Vann, R.D.; Butler, B.D.; Gernhardt, M.L. Protective mechanisms in hypobaric decompression. *Aviat. Space Environ. Med.* **2013**, *84*, 212–225. [CrossRef]
58. Eckmann, D.M.; Zhang, J.; Lampe, J.; Ayyaswamy, P.S. Gas embolism and surfactant-based intervention: Implications for long-duration space-based activity. *Ann. N. Y. Acad. Sci.* **2006**, *1077*, 256–269. [CrossRef]
59. Molenat, F.; Boussuges, A. Operation Everest III (Comex'97): Altitude-induced decompression sickness during a hypobaric chamber experiment: Necessity for circulating venous gas emboli monitoring for the investigators. *Chest* **2002**, *121*, 173–177. [CrossRef]
60. Ross, J.; Duncan, M. Prebreathe protocol for extravehicular activity: Technical consultation report. *NASA Eng. Saf. Cent. Tech. Consult. Rep. Doc.* **2008**, RP-05-91, 1–169.
61. Arieli, R. Nanobubbles Form at Active Hydrophobic Spots on the Luminal Aspect of Blood Vessels: Consequences for Decompression Illness in Diving and Possible Implications for Autoimmune Disease-An Overview. *Front. Physiol.* **2017**, *8*, 591. [CrossRef] [PubMed]
62. Magri, K.; Eftedal, I.; Petroni Magri, V.; Matity, L.; Azzopardi, C.P.; Muscat, S.; Pace, N.P. Acute Effects on the Human Peripheral Blood Transcriptome of Decompression Sickness Secondary to Scuba Diving. *Front. Physiol.* **2021**, *12*, 660402. [CrossRef] [PubMed]
63. Fratantonio, D.; Virgili, F.; Zucchi, A.; Lambrechts, K.; Latronico, T.; Lafère, P.; Germonpré, P.; Balestra, C. Increasing Oxygen Partial Pressures Induce a Distinct Transcriptional Response in Human PBMC: A Pilot Study on the "Normobaric Oxygen Paradox". *Int. J. Mol. Sci.* **2021**, *22*, 458. [CrossRef] [PubMed]

64. Balestra, C.; Germonpré, P.; Poortmans, J.R.; Marroni, A. Serum erythropoietin levels in healthy humans after a short period of normobaric and hyperbaric oxygen breathing: The "normobaric oxygen paradox". *J. Appl. Physiol.* **2006**, *100*, 512–518. [CrossRef] [PubMed]
65. Cimino, F.; Balestra, C.; Germonpré, P.; De Bels, D.; Tillmans, F.; Saija, A.; Speciale, A.; Virgili, F. Pulsed high oxygen induces a hypoxic-like response in human umbilical endothelial cells and in humans. *J. Appl. Physiol.* **2012**, *113*, 1684–1689. [CrossRef]
66. Masselli, E.; Pozzi, G.; Vaccarezza, M.; Mirandola, P.; Galli, D.; Vitale, M.; Carubbi, C.; Gobbi, G. ROS in Platelet Biology: Functional Aspects and Methodological Insights. *Int. J. Mol. Sci.* **2020**, *21*, 866. [CrossRef]
67. Ferraris, V.A. Microparticles: The good, the bad, and the ugly. *J. Thorac. Cardiovasc. Surg.* **2015**, *149*, 312–313. [CrossRef]
68. Bennett, M.L.; Bennett, F.C.; Liddelow, S.A.; Barres, B.A. New tools for studying microglia in the mouse and human CNS. *Proc. Natl. Acad. Sci. USA* **2016**, *113*, E1738–E1746. [CrossRef]
69. Thom, S.R.; Bhopale, V.M.; Yang, M. Microparticle-induced vascular injury in mice following decompression is inhibited by hyperbaric oxygen: Effects on microparticles and interleukin-1beta. *J. Appl. Physiol.* **2019**, *126*, 1006–1014. [CrossRef]
70. World Medical, A. World Medical Association Declaration of Helsinki: Ethical principles for medical research involving human subjects. *JAMA* **2013**, *310*, 2191–2194. [CrossRef]
71. Thom, S.R.; Bhopale, V.M.; Yu, K.; Huang, W.; Kane, M.A.; Margolis, D.J. Neutrophil microparticle production and inflammasome activation by hyperglycemia due to cytoskeletal instability. *J. Biol. Chem.* **2017**, *292*, 18312–18324. [CrossRef] [PubMed]
72. Thom, S.R.; Hampton, M.; Troiano, M.A.; Mirza, Z.; Malay, D.S.; Shannon, S.; Jennato, N.B.; Donohue, C.M.; Hoffstad, O.; Woltereck, D.; et al. Measurements of CD34+/CD45-dim Stem Cells Predict Healing of Diabetic Neuropathic Wounds. *Diabetes* **2016**, *65*, 486–497. [CrossRef] [PubMed]
73. Tung, J.W.; Parks, D.R.; Moore, W.A.; Herzenberg, L.A.; Herzenberg, L.A. New approaches to fluorescence compensation and visualization of FACS data. *Clin. Immunol.* **2004**, *110*, 277–283. [CrossRef] [PubMed]

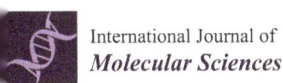

Review

The Normobaric Oxygen Paradox—Hyperoxic Hypoxic Paradox: A Novel Expedient Strategy in Hematopoiesis Clinical Issues

Michele Salvagno [1,†], Giacomo Coppalini [1,†], Fabio Silvio Taccone [1], Giacomo Strapazzon [2], Simona Mrakic-Sposta [3], Monica Rocco [4], Maher Khalife [5] and Costantino Balestra [6,7,8,9,*]

1. Department of Intensive Care, Hôpital Universitaire de Bruxelles (HUB), 1070 Brussels, Belgium
2. Institute of Mountain Emergency Medicine, Eurac Research, 39100 Bolzano, Italy
3. Institute of Clinical Physiology—National Research Council (CNR-IFC), 20162 Milano, Italy
4. Dipartimento di Scienze Medico Chirurgiche e Medicina Traslazionale, Sapienza University of Rome, 00189 Rome, Italy
5. Department of Anesthesiology, Institut Jules Bordet, Université Libre de Bruxelles (ULB), 1070 Brussels, Belgium
6. Environmental, Occupational, Aging (Integrative) Physiology Laboratory, Haute Ecole Bruxelles-Brabant (HE2B), 1050 Brussels, Belgium
7. Anatomical Research and Clinical Studies, Vrije Universiteit Brussels (VUB), 1090 Brussels, Belgium
8. DAN Europe Research Division (Roseto-Brussels), 1020 Brussels, Belgium
9. Physical Activity Teaching Unit, Motor Sciences Department, Université Libre de Bruxelles (ULB), 1050 Brussels, Belgium

* Correspondence: costantino.balestra@ulb.be
† These authors contributed equally to this work.

Abstract: Hypoxia, even at non-lethal levels, is one of the most stressful events for all aerobic organisms as it significantly affects a wide spectrum of physiological functions and energy production. Aerobic organisms activate countless molecular responses directed to respond at cellular, tissue, organ, and whole-body levels to cope with oxygen shortage allowing survival, including enhanced neo-angiogenesis and systemic oxygen delivery. The benefits of hypoxia may be evoked without its detrimental consequences by exploiting the so-called normobaric oxygen paradox. The intermittent shift between hyperoxic-normoxic exposure, in addition to being safe and feasible, has been shown to enhance erythropoietin production and raise hemoglobin levels with numerous different potential applications in many fields of therapy as a new strategy for surgical preconditioning aimed at frail patients and prevention of postoperative anemia. This narrative review summarizes the physiological processes behind the proposed normobaric oxygen paradox, focusing on the latest scientific evidence and the potential applications for this strategy. Future possibilities for hyperoxic-normoxic exposure therapy include implementation as a synergistic strategy to improve a patient's pre-surgical condition, a stimulating treatment in critically ill patients, preconditioning of athletes during physical preparation, and, in combination with surgery and conventional chemotherapy, to improve patients' outcomes and quality of life.

Keywords: hypoxia; hyperoxia; HIF-1α; oxygen biology; human; stimulus; cancer; intensive care; rehabilitation; human performance; preconditioning; pre-habilitation

1. Introduction

Oxygen is essential to support cellular biology and most vital cell reactions. Hypoxemia is a condition where below-normal levels of oxygen are dissolved in the blood and may result in poor oxygen delivery to peripheral tissues and organs, causing a supply/demand discrepancy called hypoxia [1]. If this state persists, tissues may develop hypoxemic stress, leading to organ dysfunction and permanent functional impairment [2]. To prevent this kind of damage, hypoxia is a key inducer of cellular gene expression, promoting many processes (aimed at improving oxygen delivery), such as angiogenesis,

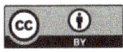

stem cell proliferation and differentiation, but also cellular protection and repair, or cell death. Most of this gene expression is guided by the activity of transcription factors called Hypoxia Inducible Factors (HIF) [3].

To prevent or counteract hypoxia, oxygen, which is considered as inexpensive and safe, is one of the most widely used treatments in clinical settings, especially in the intensive care unit (ICU) [4]. However, hyperoxemia is not constantly assessed. In fact, hypoxemia is usually monitored using peripheral oxygen saturation (SpO_2), which cannot detect whether the oxygen level is too high. Oxygen administration is therefore not often titrated to achieve normoxia. Consequently, many patients in the ICU may be exposed to episodes of hyperoxemia (high PaO_2), generally considered more acceptable by clinicians than hypoxia.

Even though hyperoxia may seem harmless, it can have detrimental effects even at modest levels if prolonged, especially in critically ill patients. In fact, hyperoxia is associated with increased mortality [5], and other possible adverse effects, such as reduced mucociliary clearance and atelectasis [6], pulmonary vascular vasoconstriction [7], which may further limit oxygen delivery and cause direct tissue damage [8], and neurotoxicity [9]. Nevertheless, administration of high partial pressure of oxygen is sometimes necessary for specific treatments such as hyperbaric oxygen therapy [10] and pre-oxygenation maneuvers to prevent hypoxia (during procedures such as bronchoscopy or oro/nasotracheal intubation where brief moments of apnea cannot be avoided) [11].

There is currently a move toward not only targeting normoxia but using intermittent hyperoxic stimuli with cyclical exposure to hyperoxygenation [12]. An intermittent hyperoxic stimulus is defined as an elevated oxygen concentration supplied for a limited period, followed by a return to a lower oxygen concentration, repeated for several days or even several times per day [12,13]. The decrease from a hyperoxic level has been shown to act paradoxically because the cells respond to it as they would respond to a hypoxic state [14,15]. It appears that fluctuations in oxygen concentration are translated by cells as a lack of oxygen and can trigger the hypoxic stress response even when there is no persistent hypoxia. This phenomenon happens especially with small and cyclical variations in partial oxygen pressure [16–18] and is linked with increased production of erythropoietin (EPO) in humans [15,19].

This review will discuss the main studies related to this "normobaric oxygen paradox" and its mechanism with a specific concern for clinical issues in hematopoietic physiology.

2. Hypoxia

2.1. Biological Cellular Response: Hypoxia Inducible Factors (HIFs)

Hypoxia generates a natural and multi-aspect response inside the organism through the involvement of various systems (e.g., hematopoietic, metabolic, respiratory, cardiovascular) and biological processes with specific cellular reactions and temporal regulation, all aimed at maintaining adequate tissue oxygenation [20,21].

The hypoxic stress inside cells activates a family of transcriptional factors called Hypoxia Inducible Factors (HIF-1α, HIF-2α, HIF-3α) [3,22]. First discovered at the Johns Hopkins University by Semenza, Kaelin and Ratcliffe more than 30 years ago [23], Semenza and colleagues isolated and purified HIF-1, confirming the presence of two subunits: HIF-1α and HIF-1β [24,25]. Later, it was shown that there is a family of HIFs: the subunit α could be one among HIF-1α, HIF-2α and HIF-3α; the β subunit is represented by one protein (HIF-1β). HIF-1α is widely expressed in all body tissues, while HIF-2α and HIF-3α are only detected in a few specific tissues [3,26,27]. HIFs modulate the response to hypoxia by prompting the expression of hundreds of genes that are involved in metabolism regulation, angiogenesis, cell growth/death, cell proliferation and division, glycolysis, microbial infection, tumor genesis and metastasis, oxygen consumption, erythrocyte production, mitochondrial metabolism, immune and inflammatory response [28–30]. HIFs can be considered one of the main regulators of O_2 detection, driving cellular adaptation to a specific oxygen level.

2.2. HIF Regulation

In the presence of oxygen, prolyl hydroxylase domain (PHD) proteins which contain oxygen-sensing hydroxylases, continuously hydroxylase specific residuals on the α subunit of HIF (Figure 1) [31].

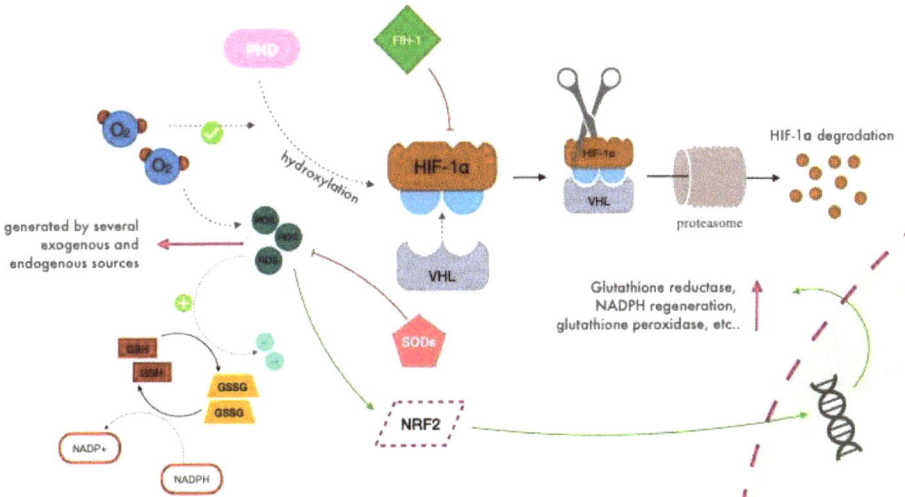

Figure 1. Simplified schematic representation of HIF activity during normoxia.

When HIF-1α is hydroxylated, it becomes a viable target for von Hippel–Lindau (VHL) protein, which activates its ubiquitin ligase system, leading to the proteasomal degradation of HIF-α [32,33]. Moreover, VHL acts as a repressor of HIF-1α by binding the inhibitory domain, as does FIH-1 (Factor Inhibiting HIF-1), which interacts with both HIF-1α and VHL via independent binding sites [34].

By contrast, in hypoxic conditions, HIF-1α is stabilized, driving its translocation to the nucleus, its dimerization with HIF-1β, and its binding to hypoxia response elements (HREs) sequence on DNA, thus regulating the transcription of around 400 genes, including the gene for EPO [29,35,36].

As a counterpart of HIF transcriptional activity, the nuclear factor erythroid 2-related factor 2 (NRF2) has a central role, coordinating the activation of a vast array of cytoprotective genes. In response to different activating stimuli following disturbances of the cellular redox status, NRF2 is stabilized, and it translocates to the nucleus where it binds to antioxidant response elements (AREs) in the promoter regions of genes encoding for antioxidant, cytoprotective proteins including glutathione synthesis, as well as glutathione reductase and enzymes involved in NADPH regeneration, xenobiotic detoxification and heme metabolism [37,38].

Despite the importance of these other actors in the cellular redox status control, this review will focus on HIF activity redirecting the readers to more specialized publications for more in-depth analysis.

2.3. Reactive Oxygen Species (ROS)

In this complex mechanism, mitochondria have a central role, representing the core of cellular respiration. Here, oxygen reacts with glucose to produce ATP (adenosine triphosphate), which serves as energy for the body [39]. In particular, oxygen molecules sit at the end of the electron transport chain, necessary for ATP production, as electron acceptors. During this process, a minimum amount of reactive oxygen species (ROS) is produced. These represent a group of highly reactive molecules characterized by unpaired electrons derived from oxygen reduction, which can quickly react with other cellular molecules [40,41].

The detrimental effects of the reactive species of oxygen are counteracted through the activation of NRF2, which tightly regulates an antioxidant response through the encoding of several genes, as forementioned. Thus, ROS are kept under control by scavengers, such as superoxide dismutases (SODs, a group of metalloproteins, which catalyzes the reduction of superoxide anions to hydrogen peroxide) and glutathione (GSH, a substrate of glutathione reductase that reduces hydroperoxides to the corresponding alcohol, oxidizing itself to the oxidized disulfide form, GSSG) [42–44].

Nowadays, ROS are no longer considered just as harmful, rather are they are believed to play a role as mediators in physiological signaling, linked to the regulation of the HIF system [45,46]. HIF, NRF2, ROS, scavengers, and other regulators appear to be tightly linked, highlighting the importance of cellular control of oxygen levels, which still needs to be fully understood.

Not every molecule and biological reaction involved in the fascinating process of cellular response to hypoxia have been cited here (there are indeed many other participants including peroxiredoxin reductase/oxygenases and catalase, to name just a few), both for the sake of simplicity and because out of the focus of our review which is not to provide a full biological molecular description (thoroughly described elsewhere [38,47,48]) but to summarize new experimental evidence of practical application of the normobaric oxygen paradox and illustrate the perspective of its desirable future clinical applications.

Hypoxic Inducible Factor 1 (HIF-1) is a heterodimer composed of 2 subunits: HIF-1α in the cytosol (HIF-1α is widely expressed in all body tissues, whereas HIF-2α and HIF-3α are only detected in a few specific tissues), and HIF-β in the nucleus. During normoxia prolyl hydroxylase domain (PHD) proteins which contain oxygen-sensing hydroxylases, continuously hydroxylase specific residues on the α subunit of HIF (blue circles). When HIF-1α is hydroxylated, it becomes a viable target for von Hippel–Lindau (VHL) protein, which activates its ubiquitin ligase system, leading to the proteasomal degradation of HIF-1α. Moreover, VHL acts as a direct repressor of HIF-1α by binding the inhibitory domain, as does FIH-1 (factor inhibiting HIF-1). Reactive species of oxygen (ROS) are kept under control by scavengers such as superoxide dismutases (SODs) and glutathione. The latter acts as a scavenger of H_2O_2, oxidizing from GSH to GSSG thanks to the activity of glutathione peroxidase. The reduction in GSH is led by glutathione reductase, which consumes NADPH. Moreover, in response to different activating stimuli following disturbances of the cellular redox status, NRF2 is stabilized, and it translocates to the nucleus where it binds to antioxidant response elements in the promoter regions of genes encoding for antioxidant, cytoprotective proteins including glutathione synthesis and reduction, as well as enzymes involved in NADPH regeneration.

3. The Normobaric Oxygen Paradox

3.1. Background

It has been proposed that relative changes in oxygen availability, rather than an absolute hypoxic or hyperoxic value, play an essential role in the transcriptional effects of HIF [49]. The *normobaric oxygen paradox* (NOP, also called *hyperoxic-hypoxic paradox* when considered in other than normobaric pressure) postulates that a period of hyperoxemia (obtained with normobaric or hyperbaric oxygen inhalation) followed by a return to normoxia would be interpreted by our cells as an oxygen shortage, thus potentially triggering a HIF-1α regulated gene synthesis cascade, including synthesis of EPO.

This paradox was proposed for the first time in 2006 by Balestra et al. [15]. In that study, the authors found that intermittent hyperoxia/normoxia exposure induced EPO synthesis. The authors reported that hyperbaric oxygen (HBO) was an essential depressor of serum EPO levels up to 24 h after hyperbaric treatment. In 2012, Cimino and colleagues reported that reducing the O_2 concentration from hyperoxic to normoxic levels could stimulate HIF-1α expression in human umbilical endothelial cells [14]. They also showed an increase in hemoglobin concentration in healthy volunteers ($n = 24$) when exposed to 30 min cycles of hypoxia (FiO$_2$ 0.15) and hyperoxia (FiO$_2$ 1.0) every other day for 10 days (5 sessions). These studies confirmed the hypothesis that a hyperoxic stimulus may re-create the benefits of a hypoxic-like response (through the production or non-inhibition of HIF-1α) without inducing potentially harmful hypoxic status.

3.2. The Proposed Mechanism

In a recent review, Hadanny and Efrati [33] redescribed the same explanation for the normobaric oxygen paradox but focused on hyperbaric oxygen exposure. However, intermittent Hyperbaric or Normobaric oxygen exposures will elicit the same reactions. The general process proposed (Figure 2) lies in the fundamental cellular mechanism of adaptation to hypoxia, namely on the O$_2$ availability of free radicals. The ratio of ROS to scavenging capacity is the key to understanding the process. The different steps of this phenomenon can be summarized as follows:

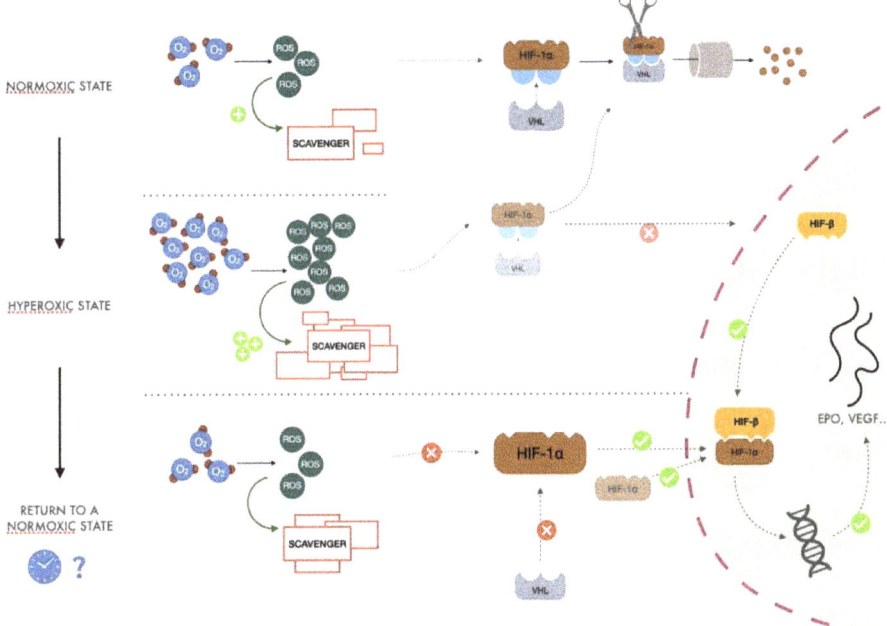

Figure 2. A simplified description of the proposed normobaric oxygen paradox.

(1) After exposure to hyperoxia, the increased presence of ROS causes an increase in activity of the glutathione synthetase enzyme. This increase in scavenger molecules keeps the oxidative conditions of the cells under control, thus preventing the potential harm caused by reactive species to DNA and other pivotal cellular processes.

(2) When returning to normoxia, normalization of oxygen levels and therefore of ROS is rapidly established, but activity of the scavenger power of the cells remains high for a longer period, exceeding the amount of ROS normally produced in the presence of a physiological concentration of oxygen. When the hyperoxic stimulus is interrupted, the more significant scavenger presence than ROS could drive a hypoxia-like cellular response as lower reactive oxygen species molecules are available. Therefore, less HIF undergoes proteasomal degradation, promoting the transcription of EPO, vascular endothelial growth factor (VEGF), and all the other genes linked to the HIF cascade.

(3) Cyclical hyperoxic exposure causes a decrease in the ROS/scavenger ratio until this gradually becomes similar to the balance present under hypoxic conditions. From a molecular point of view, a reduction of hyperoxia generates a hypoxia-mimicking state by decreasing the percentage of ROS/scavenging capacity.

However, several remarks may be raised against this mechanism.

First, several studies evaluated the possible effects of ROS on the complex regulation of HIF and identified conflicting roles. Some results support the possible HIF stabilization through the inhibition of the proteins which are supposed to degrade it; others indicate that ROS induce the degradation of HIF through the proteasome pathway [50–52]. Moreover, the cellular response to hyperoxia-normoxia is mastered by the interplay between the activation of two transcription factors, HIF and NRF2. These, some inflammatory reactions, and other factors, such as NF-κB, are of course of major interest in the mechanism responding to hyperoxia. Their dynamic balance could lead and potentiate the whole mechanism [16,17].

Surely, the biological mechanism which lies beneath this phenomenon and all of the delicate regulations of the cellular response to oxygen and oxidative stress is complicated and has not been completely clarified yet. The significance of ROS in mediating this response remains unclear. Many other actors have a role in the redox balance of the cell and may also play a role in the explanation of the normobaric oxygen paradox.

The upper third of Figure 2 describes what happens during normoxia (redrawing of Figure 1). After a hyperoxic exposure (middle third), the increased presence of reactive oxygen species (ROS) determines an increase in the scavenging activity, which keeps the oxidative conditions of the cells under control, thus preventing the potential harm caused by reactive species to DNA and other pivotal molecules. After returning to normoxia from a hyperoxic state (lower third), extra scavengers induced by hyperoxia neutralize all the reactive oxygen species (ROS). The more significant scavenger presence than ROS could drive a hypoxia-like cellular response: less HIF-1α is hydroxylated, and thus it can now dimerize and translate for several genes. The duration of the hyperoxic stimulus, its frequency and the exact timing, which optimally elicits this mechanism, are still unknown (represented by the clock and the question mark).

4. Methods

A narrative approach was chosen for this review. A literature search was initially performed in PubMed, Scopus, and Google Scholar to identify studies, conducted in the last 20 years, that explored the normobaric oxygen paradox. The following search string was used: ("Hyperoxic" AND "Hypoxic") OR ("Normobaric" AND ("oxygen" OR "hyperoxic")) AND "paradox". The review was focused on humans both experimental and in-hospital settings with a preference for a clinical approach. We considered studies testing hyperbaric or normobaric hyperoxic–normoxic stimulus in adult healthy subjects and studies which evaluated potential oxygen effects on adult patients scheduled for general or cardiac surgery. Although it was of interest to our group, only a few studies involving critically ill patients have been found. The search was restricted to articles published in English in peer-reviewed journals. No restriction on study design was imposed. Abstract presentations, conference proceedings, and reviews were excluded.

Studies were manually selected based on title and abstract. Selected studies were read thoroughly to identify those suitable for inclusion in this narrative review. We extracted the demographic and experimental data from the selected studies. For each study, the following relevant information was extracted and summarized: characteristics of the investigated population; oxygen administration protocols (hyperbaric vs. normobaric; hyperoxia to normoxia or mild hypoxia); the experimental and/or clinical settings of application; and the main results of the studies in terms of body response to hypoxia and enhancing effect on HIF-1α pathway.

A schematic flow of the study selection is represented in Figure 3.

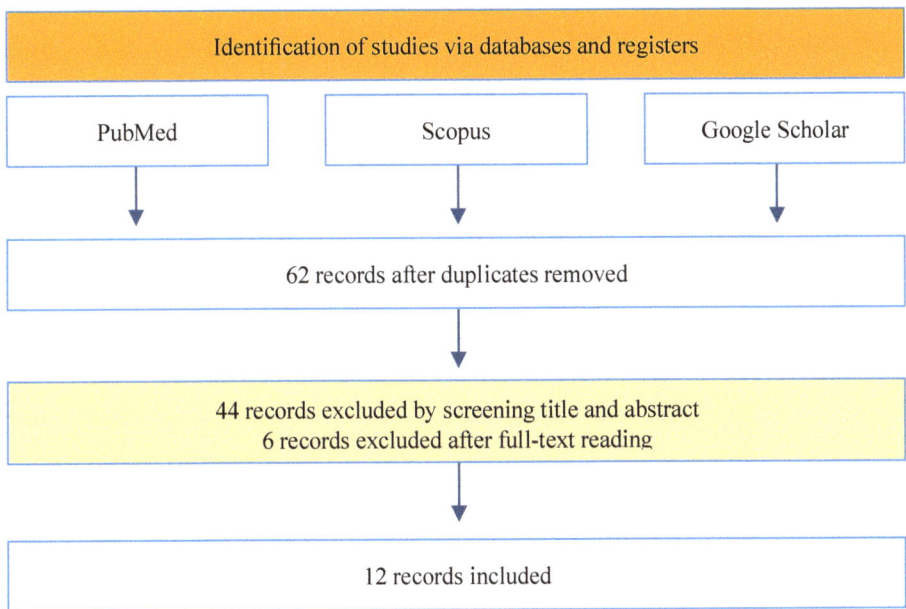

Figure 3. Flow diagram of the review.

5. Human Studies

Available studies dealing with NOP administration to humans are shown in Table 1.

Table 1. A summary of the main human studies on the normobaric oxygen paradox.

Author (Year)	Type of Study	No. of Patients	Intervention	Main Results
Balestra (2006) [15]	Human experimental study	16 healthy adults	Exposure to normobaric oxygen at FiO_2 1.0 for 2 h vs. exposure to hyperbaric oxygen 2.5 ATA FiO_2 1.0 for 1.5 h	Increase in EPO after normobaric oxygen exposure and decrease in EPO after hyperbaric oxygen exposure
Keramidas (2011) [53]	Single-blinded experimental study	10 healthy males	Exposure to normobaric oxygen at FiO_2 1 for 2 h × 7 d	Decrease in EPO levels after hyperoxic exposure compared with control group
Ciccarella (2011) [54]	Double-blind prospective pilot study	20 post cardiac surgery patients who had intraoperative CPB and MV	Exposure to normobaric oxygen at FiO_2 1.0 for 2 h vs. FiO_2 0.5 for 2 h	Increase in EPO in both groups but slope of the increase in the EPO plasma level significantly higher in those exposed to hyperoxia and relative hypoxia
Debevec (2011) [55]	Human experimental study	18 healthy male adults	Single exposure to 1 h normobaric oxygen FiO_2 1.0 followed by 1 h normobaric FiO_2 0.15	Exposure to hyperoxia followed by mild hypoxia led to temporary decrease in EPO levels. No difference in late time points for EPO levels Compared to control group

Table 1. Cont.

Author (Year)	Type of Study	No. of Patients	Intervention	Main Results
Lafere (2013) [56]	Double-blind multicenter clinical study	85 ASA 1 and 2 patients undergoing surgery for traumatic hip fracture	Exposure to 30 min of FiO$_2$ 1.0 normobaric oxygen vs. Air from POD 1 until discharge	Increase in reticulocytes count and reduction in hospital LOS and RBC transfusion in the experimental group.
Revelli (2013) [57]	Human experimental study	6 scuba divers	14-days of diving (8–10 m) with air at 1.8–2 ATA	Significant rise in serum EPO observed at 24 h post emersion
Donati (2017) [19]	Prospective observational pilot study	40 mechanical ventilated patients	Exposure to normobaric oxygen at FiO$_2$ 1.0 for 2 h	ROS increase after 1 h and glutathione level after 2 h from hyperoxia exposure. Reduction of microvascular density and perfusion during oxygen exposure rapidly normalized after returning to ambient air. EPO level rise after 48 h.
Kiboub (2018) [58]	Human experimental study	13 scuba divers	Decompression to surface pressure after long (from 25 to 27 days) professional saturation dive at 80–90 m depth	EPO markedly increased within 24 h after decompression
Perović (2020) [59]	Human experimental study	14 scuba divers	One dive per week over 5 weeks at a depth of 20–30 m for 30 min	A significant EPO increase before and after the third and the fifth dive compared to the level before and after the first dive.
Fratantonio (2021) [17]	Human experimental study	12 healthy adults	1 h exposure to normobaric oxygen FiO$_2$ 0.3 vs. normobaric oxygen FiO$_2$ 1.0 vs. hyperbaric oxygen 1.4 bar FiO$_2$ 1.4	Exposure to lower level of FiO$_2$ associated with a stronger response in HIF1-α synthesis and a lower level of inflammation and oxidative stress which was also less persistent than exposure to hyperbaric 1.4 FiO$_2$ oxygen
Khalife (2021) [18]	Prospective randomized clinical study	26 female patients undergoing breast surgery	1 h per day of normobaric oxygen FiO$_2$ 1.0 from POD 1 for 8 consecutive days	No difference in EPO or hemoglobin levels between the groups
Balestra (2022) [20]	Human experimental study	48 healthy adults	Single 1 h exposure to FiO$_2$ 0.10, 0.15, 0.3 or 1.0 normobaric oxygen and 1.4, 2.5 ATA hyperbaric oxygen	Significant elevation in microparticles from different cells was observed after exposure to every different oxygen concentration except after hyperbaric 1.4 ATA oxygen exposure.

In 2006, 16 healthy volunteers were studied by Balestra et al. before and after a 2 h period of breathing 100% normobaric oxygen and a 90-min period of breathing 100% hyperbaric oxygen at 2.5 ATA [15]. Serum EPO concentrations were measured at various time points during the subsequent 24–36 h. The authors observed a 60% increase in serum EPO 36 h after normobaric oxygen. By contrast, a 53% decrease in serum EPO concentration was observed 24 h after hyperbaric oxygen, suggesting that normobaric oxygen evokes a higher response in EPO production than hyperbaric oxygen. These results were unexpected since one could imagine that a higher stimulus should induce a higher response, paradoxically it was not the case. For this reason, they introduced the term *"normobaric oxygen paradox"*.

In 2011, Keramidas et al. published conflicting results [53]. In this single-blinded crossover trial, 10 healthy male volunteers breathed for 2 h ambient air (NOR group) first and then 100% normobaric O_2 (HYPER group). Blood samples were collected pre, mid, and post-exposure, and at 3, 5, 8, 24, 32, 48, 72, 96 h, 1 and 2 weeks after the exposure to determine serum EPO concentration. The authors observed an increase in serum EPO concentration at 8 and 32 h after ambient air (by 58% and 52%, respectively, $p < 0.05$), but in the discussion, this increase was attributed to natural EPO diurnal variation. Conversely, in the HYPER group, there was a 36% decrease in EPO 3 h after the exposure ($p < 0.05$). Moreover, EPO concentration was significantly lower in the HYPER than in the NOR group at 3, 5 and 8 h after the breathing intervention. Despite these significant results, it must be noted that the authors did not adjust their results to individual diurnal variations in EPO as carried out by others [15].

Several studies have been performed in the clinical setting. Lafère and colleagues [56] found that the normobaric oxygen paradox effectively increased the reticulocyte count after traumatic hip surgery. Patients were randomly assigned to a control group ($n = 40$) receiving 30 min of air or an O_2 group ($n = 40$) where patients were exposed to 100% normobaric oxygen 15 L/min for 30 min every day from the first postoperative day until discharge. On day 7, the O_2 group showed a significant increase in reticulocyte count and percent variation (184.9% ± 41.4%) compared to the air group (104.7% ± 32.6%). Even though no differences were found in hemoglobin or hematocrit levels, red blood cell (RBC) transfusions were significantly lower in the O_2 group than in the air group. However, this latter finding was not attributed to the increase in reticulocytes, since blood was administered before that variation, but probably to a better anemia/hypoxia tolerance or better coagulation related to oxygen stimuli.

Ciccarella et al. [54] presented, in a letter to the editor, results from a prospective, randomized, double-blind pilot trial, in which they evaluated 20 cardiac surgery patients divided into two groups. In the first group ($n = 10$), patients received FiO_2 1.0 of normobaric O_2 for 2 h, followed by exposure to FiO_2 0.5 normobaric O_2 post-cardiac surgery. The second group ($n = 10$) received FiO_2 0.5 of normobaric O_2 for 2 h. The slope of the increase in the plasmatic EPO level was significantly higher in the FiO_2 1.0 group than in the FiO_2 0.5 group, confirming that this stimulus may be helpful to enhance the endogenous production of EPO (eliciting cardioprotection and neuroprotection) in postoperative conditions.

In 2017, Donati et al. evaluated 20 hemodynamically stable, mechanically ventilated patients with inspired oxygen concentration (FiO_2) ≤ 0.5 and $PaO_2/FiO_2 \geq 200$ mmHg; the patients had a 2-h exposure to hyperoxia (FiO_2 1.0) [19]. A group of 20 patients with similar characteristics was chosen as a control. Blood samples were collected from both groups at 24 and 48 h to measure serum EPO concentration, and at baseline (t0), after 2 h of hyperoxia (t1) and 2 h after return to the initial FiO_2 concentration (t2) to measure serum glutathione and ROS levels. In addition, the microvascular sublingual response to hyperoxia was assessed. Serum ROS increased transiently at t1, and glutathione increased at t2. Interestingly, EPO levels increased in the hyperoxia group ($p < 0.05$) and were significantly higher at 48 h compared to baseline; no changes were seen in the control group. By contrast, there was no increase in the reticulocyte count, which decreased after 48 h, apparently in conflict with the results of Lafère et al. [56]. However, as discussed by the authors themselves, the 48-h observational period is too short to detect an increase in reticulocyte count and Hb, after one single hyperoxia exposure.

In 2021, Fratantonio et al. [17] randomized 12 healthy adult individuals to three groups of different oxygen FiO_2 exposure: the first group received one hour of FiO_2 0.3 (mild hyperoxia, MH), the second received one hour of FiO_2 1.0 for normobaric hyperoxia (high hyperoxia, HH), and the third received one hour of FiO_2 1.4 (FiO_2 1 inspired at 1.4 ATA in a hyperbaric chamber) for high hyperbaric hyperoxia (very high hyperoxia, VHH). The authors observed, in the nucleus of the peripheral blood mononuclear cells (PBMC), that the return to normoxia after MH was sensed as a hypoxic trigger characterized by HIF-1α activation. By contrast, in the HH and VHH groups, there was a shift toward an oxidative stress response, characterized by nuclear factor E2-related factor 2 (NRF2) and nuclear factor-kappa B (NF-κB) activation in the first 24 h post-exposure.

Interestingly, in another study evaluating the effects of hypoxemia on the human body, a similar increased activity of the transcriptional factor NRF2 (but not of NF-κB) was found after 24 h and 72 h of hypobaric hypoxia [21], highlighting again similar cellular responses of hyperoxia and hypoxia.

The same year, Khalife et al. [18] proposed a study similar to that by Fratantonio et al. [17] with apparently contrasting results. A group of 22 adult post-abdominal surgery patients was randomized to receive FiO_2 1.0 for one hour per day for eight consecutive days or no change in oxygen. Serum EPO, hemoglobin, and reticulocyte count were measured on admission to the ICU and on postoperative days seven and nine. EPO concentration at day nine was significantly higher in both groups compared to the baseline measurement on postoperative day 1. However, there were no differences between the groups in serum EPO concentration, hemoglobin, or reticulocyte count. As a possible confounder to these results, standard anesthesiology protocols were applied to both groups including the administration of $FiO_2 > 0.21$ in the perioperative period, potentially influencing the results as seen in other works [16,17].

Debevec et al. investigated the effect of consecutive 1 h hyperoxic (FiO_2 1.0) and hypoxic (FiO_2 0.15) breathing interventions in 18 healthy adult individuals [55]. The authors found a reduction in EPO concentrations within the initial 8 h after the hyperoxic/hypoxic exposure compared to controls, suggesting that their results contradicted the normobaric oxygen paradox. However, the results should be interpreted in light of the findings of Fratantonio et al. [17], i.e., an excessive oxygen stimulus (such as FiO_2 1.0) does not elicit a paradoxical hyperoxic-hypoxic response during the same time-lapse.

EPO elevation was found in scuba divers, performing a dive at a depth of 20–30 m (FiO_2 about 0.6–0.8) for 30 min once a week for 5 consecutive weeks [59]. These results are coherent with the ones obtained by studying six scuba divers after a 14-day dive (8–10 m) breathing air at 1.8–2 ATA (roughly FiO_2 0.4) [57], and with the ones studying professional saturation divers, after decompression to the surface pressure, after long (from 25 to 27 days) saturation procedure at 80–90 m depth (Breathing Helium-Oxygen mixture (Heliox) FiO_2 about 0.44) [58]. The recurrent exposure to normobaric oxygen breathing after hyperoxic conditions during diving could be the trigger for EPO production, even if other reasons may increase EPO production in this type of population which can even explain the lack in the increase of hemoglobin concentration (for example, the plasma volume changes during diving), as adequately pointed by the authors.

In one of their most recent studies, Balestra et al. investigated the metabolic response to a single 1 h exposure to different FiO_2 values (0.1, 0.15, 0.3, 1.0) at normobaric and hyperbaric conditions (1.4 ATA, 2.5 ATA), in 48 healthy subjects [20]. Blood samples were collected from each participant before and 120 min after oxygen exposure. The expression of microparticles (MPs) specific to platelets (CD41), neutrophils (CD66b), endothelial cells (CD146), and microglia (TMEM) was measured. There was a significant increase in MPs after all O_2 exposures, except after mild hyperbaric (1.4 ATA) conditions, for which there was a significant decrease in MPs. Surprisingly, during the normobaric oxygen exposure, FiO_2 0.3 elicited similar responses to FiO_2 1.0.

6. Discussion

A hyperoxic stimulus followed by a return to a normoxic state seems to produce an organic response similar to that of a hypoxic steady state, prompting the expression of a variety of proteins, initiated by the activation of HIF-1a. The expression of HIF-1a represents an upstream response to the production of EPO, which is just one of the results of a real or mimic hypoxic state. Interestingly, this effect is faster than that needed to trigger EPO release during exposure to altitude and low atmospheric pressure (36–48 h vs. days, respectively) [60].

EPO has complex activities other than RBC production, including neuroprotection via its action as a neurotrophic factor in the central nervous system [61], cardioprotective properties [61], cardioprotective properties [62], and vasoactive effects through the increased production of endothelin [63], highlighting the potential beneficial effects of the hyperoxic-normoxic stimulus. Nevertheless, if it is true that a hyperoxic stimulus recreates the benefits of a hypoxic-like response without inducing a detrimental hypoxic status, it needs to be demonstrated that the benefit of this stimulus (short hyperoxic sessions) would overwhelm the known harmful effects of prolonged hyperoxia.

The studies presented in this review have yielded contrasting results regarding the use of this approach. First, EPO baseline is not easy to assess, and individual circadian rhythm may impact the results [53], so unique patient matching should be used in clinical trials. This approach was not followed in several studies, and the mean serum EPO values may mask real differences before and after a hyperoxic stimulus in the same subject. Second, the increase in EPO concentrations may be absent in some individuals due to the depletion of intracellular glutathione reserves; N-acetyl-l-cysteine (NAC) supplementation has been demonstrated to increase EPO with and without oxygen [64,65]. The explanation could lie in the fact that N-acetyl-l-cysteine (NAC) is a major precursor of glutathione [66], thus it is effective in promoting a redox balance within the cells [67]. In addition, it contributes to stabilizing HIF-1α subunit in the cytosol and thus favoring its translocation [68,69]. Overall, in case of depletion of the intracellular glutathione reserve NAC, recreating an adequate redox environment and stabilizing HIF results in EPO increasing [65]. Third, the optimum concentration and time of the oxygen stimulus needed to obtain the maximal response in EPO synthesis as well as the time needed between intermittent exposures to optimize the outcome are unknown. On the contrary, exposure to excessively high oxygen concentrations acts against the production of EPO [53] at least after similar post-exposure time lapses. Of course, if the outcome aims for a reduction of HIF stimulation, higher concentration, and probably closer repetitions, may be needed. Finally, in some clinical studies, EPO serum concentration had similar changes in both the oxygen group and the control group (not exposed to high levels of extra oxygen). It does not necessarily go against the normobaric oxygen paradox since even minor O_2 variations (e.g., routine post-operative oxygen supply) may trigger the mechanism

An intermittent normobaric hyperoxic stimulus elicits a hypoxic-like response as it has been proven in the study of Cimino et al. [14]. The increase in the activity of HIF represents an upstream response to the production of EPO and Hemoglobin, which is just one of the results of a hypoxic real or mimic state. Anyway, if it is true that a hyperoxic stimulus re-creates the benefits of a hypoxic-like response without inducing a detrimental hypoxic status, it still has yet to be proven that the benefit of this stimulus overwhelms the known harmful effects of hyperoxia although such a short time of exposure is not likely to enter toxic levels, especially in pathologic situations.

Future Perspectives

Although the strength of this stimulus must still be measured, this paradox could have several clinical implications, from the treatment of anemia, thus limiting blood transfusions [70], to adjuvant therapy for septic patients [71], to precondition agent for sports training [72,73], to therapy in critical care settings in which a HIF response without an actual hypoxic state could be effective in cardio and neuroprotection [74,75].

Another potential future field of application concerns the therapeutic role of oxygen in tumor growth and spread. New evidence about oncologic progression has shown that cancer cells may evolve into a hypermetabolic state, which can be sustained even in the presence of a limited oxygen supply [76,77]. Genetical changes and uncontrolled cancer growth, which generate intra-tumor hypoxic areas (used by the innovative hypoxia-responsive drug delivery nanoplatforms [78]), cause HIF-1α overexpression enhancing neo-angiogenesis through VEGF synthesis and therefore favoring cancer progression and metastasis [79]. Only recently has the possible role of hyperoxia in tumor necrosis or development started to be investigated [80,81]. For example, leukemia cell lines exposed to a hyperoxic stimulus have been shown to increase the expression of caspase 3, and committing themselves to programmed death and apoptosis preceded morphological modifications of T and B cells [82].

In an animal model of breast cancer, Raa et al. [83] observed that normobaric and hyperbaric oxygen treatments showed more efficacy than conventional chemotherapy alone in reducing tumor growth, limiting neo-angiogenesis, decreasing cancer vascularization and inducing apoptosis.

The different response to the increased oxygen concentration in cancer cells, compared to healthy cells, may be linked to several mechanisms:

- A maladaptive response to hyperoxia, as well as to modification in adenosine pathways able to trigger anticancer effects of T cells and NK cells [84,85];
- Incapacity to deal with the overproduction of ROS during hyperoxia, ultimately leading to necrosis and apoptosis [83];
- A disequilibrium between antioxidants and reactive oxygen species [86].

7. Conclusions

Oxygen is a drug that is used in patients around the world on a daily basis. It is inexpensive and generally safe and may have more beneficial effects than just increasing the blood oxygen content. In the future, oxygen therapy could be implemented as a coadjutant in new frontiers of therapeutic schemes to treat several diseases. Evidence shows that a dynamic change in oxygen caused by a normobaric hyperoxia stimulus has a different effect to that of a steady state. The optimal timing and intensity of the O_2 stimulus still have to be determined. Efforts should be directed to further confirm this phenomenon, as a promising, cheap, and easy-access contribution in several clinical situations.

Author Contributions: Conceptualization, M.S., C.B.; methodology, M.S., G.C., G.S., F.S.T., C.B.; writing—original draft preparation, M.S., G.C., C.B.; writing—review and editing, M.S., G.C., G.S., F.S.T., S.M.-S., M.R., M.K., C.B.; visualization, M.S., G.C., F.S.T., C.B.; supervision, C.B. All authors have read and agreed to the published version of the manuscript.

Funding: This research received no external funding.

Institutional Review Board Statement: Not applicable.

Informed Consent Statement: Not applicable.

Conflicts of Interest: The authors declare no conflict of interest.

Abbreviations

ASA	American Society of Anesthesiologists physical status classification system
ARE	Antioxidant Response Elements
ATA	Atmosphere Absolute
EPO	Erythropoietin
FIH	Factor Inhibiting HIF
FiO_2	Inspired Fraction of Oxygen
GSH	Glutathione Reduced
GSSG	Glutathione Oxidized
HIF	Hypoxia Inducible Factor
HRE	Hypoxia Responsive Element
LOS	Length of Stay
NF-κB	Nuclear Factor-kappa B

NOP	Normobaric Oxygen Paradox
NRF2	Nuclear Factor Erythroid 2 Related—Factor 2
PaO$_2$	Oxygen Arterial Partial Pressure
PHD	Prolyl Hydroxylase domain
POD	Post-Operative Day
RBC	Red Blood Cells
ROS	Reactive Oxygen Species
SOD	Superoxide Dismutase
VHL	Von Hippen Lindau protein

References

1. Bhutta, B.S.; Alghoula, F.; Berim, I. *Hypoxia*; StatPearls: Tampa, FL, USA, 2022.
2. Mallat, J.; Rahman, N.; Hamed, F.; Hernandez, G.; Fischer, M.O. Pathophysiology, Mechanisms, and Managements of Tissue Hypoxia. *Anaesth. Crit. Care Pain Med.* **2022**, *41*, 101087. [CrossRef] [PubMed]
3. Semenza, G.L. Hypoxia-Inducible Factors in Physiology and Medicine. *Cell* **2012**, *148*, 399–408. [CrossRef] [PubMed]
4. Angus, D.C. Oxygen Therapy for the Critically Ill. *N. Engl. J. Med.* **2020**, *382*, 1054–1056. [CrossRef] [PubMed]
5. Helmerhorst, H.J.F.; Roos-Blom, M.J.; van Westerloo, D.J.; de Jonge, E. Association Between Arterial Hyperoxia and Outcome in Subsets of Critical Illness: A Systematic Review, Meta-Analysis, and Meta-Regression of Cohort Studies. *Crit. Care Med.* **2015**, *43*, 1508–1519. [CrossRef] [PubMed]
6. Damiani, E.; Donati, A.; Girardis, M. Oxygen in the Critically Ill: Friend or Foe? *Curr. Opin. Anaesthesiol.* **2018**, *31*, 129–135. [CrossRef]
7. Ariyaratnam, P.; Loubani, M.; Bennett, R.; Griffin, S.; Chaudhry, M.A.; Cowen, M.E.; Guvendik, L.; Cale, A.R.J.; Morice, A.H. Hyperoxic Vasoconstriction of Human Pulmonary Arteries: A Novel Insight into Acute Ventricular Septal Defects. *ISRN Cardiol.* **2013**, *2013*, 685735. [CrossRef]
8. Brueckl, C.; Kaestle, S.; Kerem, A.; Habazettl, H.; Krombach, F.; Kuppe, H.; Kuebler, W.M. Hyperoxia-Induced Reactive Oxygen Species Formation in Pulmonary Capillary Endothelial Cells in Situ. *Am. J. Respir. Cell Mol. Biol.* **2006**, *34*, 453–463. [CrossRef]
9. Johnson, N.J.; Dodampahala, K.; Rosselot, B.; Perman, S.M.; Mikkelsen, M.E.; Goyal, M.; Gaieski, D.F.; Grossestreuer, A.V. The Association Between Arterial Oxygen Tension and Neurological Outcome After Cardiac Arrest. *Ther. Hypothermia Temp. Manag.* **2017**, *7*, 36–41. [CrossRef]
10. Shah, J. Hyperbaric Oxygen Therapy. *J. Am. Coll. Certif. Wound Spec.* **2010**, *2*, 9–13. [CrossRef]
11. Pelaia, C.; Bruni, A.; Garofalo, E.; Rovida, S.; Arrighi, E.; Cammarota, G.; Navalesi, P.; Pelaia, G.; Longhini, F. Oxygenation Strategies during Flexible Bronchoscopy: A Review of the Literature. *Respir. Res.* **2021**, *22*, 253. [CrossRef]
12. Balestra, C.; Kot, J. Oxygen: A Stimulus, Not "Only" a Drug. *Medicina* **2021**, *57*, 1161. [CrossRef]
13. Fu, Q.; Duan, R.; Sun, Y.; Li, Q. Hyperbaric Oxygen Therapy for Healthy Aging: From Mechanisms to Therapeutics. *Redox Biol.* **2022**, *53*, 102352. [CrossRef]
14. Cimino, F.; Balestra, C.; Germonpré, P.; de Bels, D.; Tillmans, F.; Saija, A.; Speciale, A.; Virgili, F. Pulsed High Oxygen Induces a Hypoxic-like Response in Human Umbilical Endothelial Cells and in Humans. *J. Appl. Physiol.* **2012**, *113*, 1684–1689. [CrossRef]
15. Balestra, C.; Germonpré, P.; Poortmans, J.R.; Marroni, A. Serum Erythropoietin Levels in Healthy Humans after a Short Period of Normobaric and Hyperbaric Oxygen Breathing: The "Normobaric Oxygen Paradox". *J. Appl. Physiol.* **2006**, *100*, 512–518. [CrossRef]
16. Balestra, C.; Lambrechts, K.; Mrakic-Sposta, S.; Vezzoli, A.; Levenez, M.; Germonpré, P.; Virgili, F.; Bosco, G.; Lafère, P. Hypoxic and Hyperoxic Breathing as a Complement to Low-Intensity Physical Exercise Programs: A Proof-of-Principle Study. *Int. J. Mol. Sci.* **2021**, *22*, 9600. [CrossRef]
17. Fratantonio, D.; Virgili, F.; Zucchi, A.; Lambrechts, K.; Latronico, T.; Lafère, P.; Germonpré, P.; Balestra, C. Increasing Oxygen Partial Pressures Induce a Distinct Transcriptional Response in Human PBMC: A Pilot Study on the "Normobaric Oxygen Paradox". *Int. J. Mol. Sci.* **2021**, *22*, 458. [CrossRef]
18. Khalife, M.; ben Aziz, M.; Balestra, C.; Valsamis, J.; Sosnowski, M. Physiological and Clinical Impact of Repeated Inhaled Oxygen Variation on Erythropoietin Levels in Patients After Surgery. *Front. Physiol.* **2021**, *12*, 744074. [CrossRef]
19. Donati, A.; Damiani, E.; Zuccari, S.; Domizi, R.; Scorcella, C.; Girardis, M.; Giulietti, A.; Vignini, A.; Adrario, E.; Romano, R.; et al. Effects of Short-Term Hyperoxia on Erythropoietin Levels and Microcirculation in Critically Ill Patients: A Prospective Observational Pilot Study. *BMC Anesthesiol.* **2017**, *17*, 49. [CrossRef]
20. Balestra, C.; Arya, A.K.; Leveque, C.; Virgili, F.; Germonpré, P.; Lambrechts, K.; Lafère, P.; Thom, S.R. Varying Oxygen Partial Pressure Elicits Blood-Borne Microparticles Expressing Different Cell-Specific Proteins—Toward a Targeted Use of Oxygen? *Int. J. Mol. Sci.* **2022**, *23*, 7888. [CrossRef]
21. Malacrida, S.; Giannella, A.; Ceolotto, G.; Reggiani, C.; Vezzoli, A.; Mrakic-Sposta, S.; Moretti, S.; Turner, R.; Falla, M.; Brugger, H.; et al. Transcription Factors Regulation in Human Peripheral White Blood Cells during Hypobaric Hypoxia Exposure: An in-Vivo Experimental Study. *Sci. Rep.* **2019**, *9*, 9901. [CrossRef] [PubMed]
22. Majmundar, A.J.; Wong, W.J.; Simon, M.C. Hypoxia-Inducible Factors and the Response to Hypoxic Stress. *Mol. Cell* **2010**, *40*, 294–309. [CrossRef] [PubMed]

23. The Nobel Prize in Physiology or Medicine 2019—Advanced Information—NobelPrize.Org. Available online: https://www.nobelprize.org/prizes/medicine/2019/advanced-information/ (accessed on 7 November 2022).
24. Wang, G.L.; Semenza, G.L. Purification and Characterization of Hypoxia-Inducible Factor 1. *J. Biol. Chem.* **1995**, *270*, 1230–1237. [CrossRef] [PubMed]
25. Wang, G.L.; Jiang, B.H.; Rue, E.A.; Semenza, G.L. Hypoxia-Inducible Factor 1 Is a Basic-Helix-Loop-Helix-PAS Heterodimer Regulated by Cellular O2 Tension. *Proc. Natl. Acad. Sci. USA* **1995**, *92*, 5510. [CrossRef] [PubMed]
26. Zhe, N.; Chen, S.; Zhou, Z.; Liu, P.; Lin, X.; Yu, M.; Cheng, B.; Zhang, Y.; Wang, J. HIF-1α Inhibition by 2-Methoxyestradiol Induces Cell Death via Activation of the Mitochondrial Apoptotic Pathway in Acute Myeloid Leukemia. *Cancer Biol. Ther.* **2016**, *17*, 625. [CrossRef] [PubMed]
27. Wiesener, M.S.; Jürgensen, J.S.; Rosenberger, C.; Scholze, C.; Hörstrup, J.H.; Warnecke, C.; Mandriota, S.; Bechmann, I.; Frei, U.A.; Pugh, C.W.; et al. Widespread, Hypoxia-Inducible Expression of HIF-2α in Distinct Cell Populations of Different Organs. *FASEB J.* **2003**, *17*, 271–273. [CrossRef]
28. Shomento, S.H.; Wan, C.; Cao, X.; Faugere, M.C.; Bouxsein, M.L.; Clemens, T.L.; Riddle, R.C. Hypoxia-Inducible Factors 1α and 2α Exert Both Distinct and Overlapping Functions in Long Bone Development. *J. Cell. Biochem.* **2010**, *109*, 196–204. [CrossRef]
29. Choudhry, H.; Harris, A.L. Advances in Hypoxia-Inducible Factor Biology. *Cell Metab.* **2018**, *27*, 281–298. [CrossRef]
30. Simon, M.C. The Hypoxia Response Pathways—Hats Off! *N. Eng. J. Med.* **2016**, *375*, 1687–1689. [CrossRef]
31. Briggs, K.J.J.; Koivunen, P.; Cao, S.; Backus, K.M.M.; Olenchock, B.A.A.; Patel, H.; Zhang, Q.; Signoretti, S.; Gerfen, G.J.J.; Richardson, A.L.L.; et al. Paracrine Induction of HIF by Glutamate in Breast Cancer: EglN1 Senses Cysteine. *Cell* **2016**, *166*, 126–139. [CrossRef]
32. Fujita, N.; Markova, D.; Greg Anderson, D.; Chiba, K.; Toyama, Y.; Shapiro, I.M.; Risbud, M.V. Expression of Prolyl Hydroxylases (PHDs) Is Selectively Controlled by HIF-1 and HIF-2 Proteins in Nucleus Pulposus Cells of the Intervertebral Disc. *J. Biol. Chem.* **2012**, *287*, 16975–16986. [CrossRef]
33. Hadanny, A.; Efrati, S. The Hyperoxic-Hypoxic Paradox. *Biomolecules* **2020**, *10*, 958. [CrossRef]
34. Mahon, P.C.; Hirota, K.; Semenza, G.L. FIH-1: A Novel Protein That Interacts with HIF-1alpha and VHL to Mediate Repression of HIF-1 Transcriptional Activity. *Genes Dev.* **2001**, *15*, 2675–2686. [CrossRef]
35. Wenger, R.H.; Stiehl, D.P.; Camenisch, G. Integration of Oxygen Signaling at the Consensus HRE. *Sci. STKE* **2005**, *2005*, re12. [CrossRef]
36. Xia, O.; Lemieux, M.E.; Li, W.; Carroll, J.S.; Brown, M.; Shirley Liu, X.; Kung, A.L. Integrative Analysis of HIF Binding and Transactivation Reveals Its Role in Maintaining Histone Methylation Homeostasis. *Proc. Natl. Acad. Sci. USA* **2009**, *106*, 4260–4265. [CrossRef]
37. Fratantonio, D.; Cimino, F.; Speciale, A.; Virgili, F. Need (More than) Two to Tango: Multiple Tools to Adapt to Changes in Oxygen Availability. *BioFactors* **2018**, *44*, 207–218. [CrossRef]
38. Tonelli, C.; Chio, I.I.C.; Tuveson, D.A. Transcriptional Regulation by Nrf2. *Antioxid. Redox Signal.* **2018**, *29*, 1727–1745. [CrossRef]
39. Green, D.E.; Tzagoloff, A. The Mitochondrial Electron Transfer Chain. *Arch. Biochem. Biophys.* **1966**, *116*, 293–304. [CrossRef]
40. Auten, R.L.; Davis, J.M. Oxygen Toxicity and Reactive Oxygen Species: The Devil Is in the Details. *Pediatr. Res.* **2009**, *66*, 121–127. [CrossRef]
41. Das, K.; Roychoudhury, A. Reactive Oxygen Species (ROS) and Response of Antioxidants as ROS-Scavengers during Environmental Stress in Plants. *Front. Environ. Sci.* **2014**, *2*, 53. [CrossRef]
42. Wu, G.; Fang, Y.Z.; Yang, S.; Lupton, J.R.; Turner, N.D. Glutathione Metabolism and Its Implications for Health. *J. Nutr.* **2004**, *134*, 489–492. [CrossRef]
43. Reed, M.; Thomas, R.L.; Pavisic, J.; James, S.J.; Ulrich, C.M.; Nijhout, H.F. A Mathematical Model of Glutathione Metabolism. *Theor. Biol. Med. Model.* **2008**, *5*, 8. [CrossRef] [PubMed]
44. Buettner, G.R. Superoxide Dismutase in Redox Biology: The Roles of Superoxide and Hydrogen Peroxide. *Anticancer Agents Med. Chem.* **2011**, *11*, 341. [CrossRef] [PubMed]
45. Fuhrmann, D.C.; Brüne, B. Mitochondrial Composition and Function under the Control of Hypoxia. *Redox Biol.* **2017**, *12*, 208–215. [CrossRef]
46. Jones, D.P.; Sies, H. The Redox Code. *Antioxid. Redox Signal.* **2015**, *23*, 734–746. [CrossRef] [PubMed]
47. Cyran, A.M.; Zhitkovich, A. HIF1, HSF1, and NRF2: Oxidant-Responsive Trio Raising Cellular Defenses and Engaging Immune System. *Chem. Res. Toxicol.* **2022**, *35*, 1690–1700. [CrossRef]
48. Lee, P.; Chandel, N.S.; Simon, M.C. Cellular Adaptation to Hypoxia through Hypoxia Inducible Factors and Beyond. *Nat. Rev. Mol. Cell Biol.* **2020**, *21*, 268–283. [CrossRef]
49. Rocco, M.; D'Itri, L.; de Bels, D.; Corazza, F.; Balestra, C. The "Normobaric Oxygen Paradox": A New Tool for the Anesthetist. *Minerva Anestesiol.* **2014**, *80*, 366–372.
50. Corrado, C.; Fontana, S. Hypoxia and HIF Signaling: One Axis with Divergent Effects. *Int. J. Mol. Sci.* **2020**, *21*, 5611. [CrossRef]
51. Greer, S.N.; Metcalf, J.L.; Wang, Y.; Ohh, M. The Updated Biology of Hypoxia-Inducible Factor. *EMBO J.* **2012**, *31*, 2448–2460. [CrossRef]
52. Shvetsova, A.N.; Mennerich, D.; Kerätär, J.M.; Hiltunen, J.K.; Kietzmann, T. Non-Electron Transfer Chain Mitochondrial Defects Differently Regulate HIF-1α Degradation and Transcription. *Redox Biol.* **2017**, *12*, 1052. [CrossRef]

53. Keramidas, M.E.; Kounalakis, S.N.; Debevec, T.; Norman, B.; Gustafsson, T.; Eiken, O.; Mekjavic, I.B. Acute Normobaric Hyperoxia Transiently Attenuates Plasma Erythropoietin Concentration in Healthy Males: Evidence against the "normobaric Oxygen Paradox" Theory. *Acta Physiol.* **2011**, *202*, 91–98. [CrossRef]
54. Ciccarella, Y.; Balestra, C.; Valsamis, J.; van der Linden, P. Increase in Endogenous Erythropoietin Synthesis through the Normobaric Oxygen Paradox in Cardiac Surgery Patients. *Br. J. Anaesth.* **2011**, *106*, 752–753. [CrossRef]
55. Debevec, T.; Keramidas, M.E.; Norman, B.; Gustafsson, T.; Eiken, O.; Mekjavic, I.B.; Ferretti, G. Acute Short-Term Hyperoxia Followed by Mild Hypoxia Does Not Increase EPO Production: Resolving the "Normobaric Oxygen Paradox". *Eur. J. Appl. Physiol.* **2012**, *112*, 1059–1065. [CrossRef]
56. Lafère, P.; Schubert, T.; de Bels, D.; Germonpré, P.; Balestra, C. Can the Normobaric Oxygen Paradox (NOP) Increase Reticulocyte Count after Traumatic Hip Surgery? *J. Clin. Anesth.* **2013**, *25*, 129–134. [CrossRef]
57. Revelli, L.; Vagnoni, S.; D'Amore, A.; di Stasio, E.; Lombardi, C.P.; Storti, G.; Proietti, R.; Balestra, C.; Ricerca, B.M. EPO Modulation in a 14-Days Undersea Scuba Dive. *Int. J. Sports Med.* **2013**, *34*, 856–860. [CrossRef]
58. Kiboub, F.Z.; Balestra, C.; Loennechen, Ø.; Eftedal, I. Hemoglobin and Erythropoietin After Commercial Saturation Diving. *Front. Physiol.* **2018**, *9*, 1176. [CrossRef]
59. Perović, A.; Žarak, M.; Bratičević, M.N.; Dumić, J. Effects of Recreational Scuba Diving on Erythropoiesis-"normobaric Oxygen Paradox" or "Plasma Volume Regulation" as a Trigger for Erythropoietin? *Eur. J. Appl. Physiol.* **2020**, *120*, 1689–1697. [CrossRef]
60. Christoulas, K.; Karamouzis, M.; Mandroukas, K. "Living High—Training Low" vs. "Living High—Training High": Erythropoietic Responses and Performance of Adolescent Cross-Country Skiers. *J. Sports Med. Phys. Fitness* **2011**, *51*, 74–81.
61. Rey, F.; Balsari, A.; Giallongo, T.; Ottolenghi, S.; di Giulio, A.M.; Samaja, M.; Carelli, S. Erythropoietin as a Neuroprotective Molecule: An Overview of Its Therapeutic Potential in Neurodegenerative Diseases. *ASN Neuro* **2019**, *11*, 1759091419871420. [CrossRef]
62. Teng, R.; Calvert, J.W.; Sibmooh, N.; Piknova, B.; Suzuki, N.; Sun, J.; Martinez, K.; Yamamoto, M.; Schechter, A.N.; Lefer, D.J.; et al. Acute Erythropoietin Cardioprotection Is Mediated by Endothelial Response. *Basic Res. Cardiol* **2011**, *106*, 343–354. [CrossRef]
63. Vogel, V.; Kramer, H.J.; Bäcker, A.; Meyer-Lehnert, H.; Jelkmann, W.; Fandrey, J. Effects of Erythropoietin on Endothelin-1 Synthesis and the Cellular Calcium Messenger System in Vascular Endothelial Cells. *Am. J. Hypertens.* **1997**, *10*, 289–296. [CrossRef] [PubMed]
64. Momeni, M.; de Kock, M.; Devuyst, O.; Liistro, G. Effect of N-Acetyl-Cysteine and Hyperoxia on Erythropoietin Production. *Eur. J. Appl. Physiol.* **2011**, *111*, 2681–2686. [CrossRef] [PubMed]
65. Zembron-Lacny, A.; Slowinska-Lisowska, M.; Szygula, Z.; Witkowski, K.; Szyszka, K. The Comparison of Antioxidant and Hematological Properties of N-Acetylcysteine and Alpha-Lipoic Acid in Physically Active Males. *Physiol. Res.* **2009**, *58*, 855–861. [CrossRef] [PubMed]
66. Mokhtari, V.; Afsharian, P.; Shahhoseini, M.; Kalantar, S.M.; Moini, A. A Review on Various Uses of N-Acetyl Cysteine. *Cell J. (Yakhteh)* **2017**, *19*, 11. [CrossRef]
67. Medved, I.; Brown, M.J.; Bjorksten, A.R.; Leppik, J.A.; Sostaric, S.; McKenna, M.J. N-Acetylcysteine Infusion Alters Blood Redox Status but Not Time to Fatigue during Intense Exercise in Humans. *J. Appl. Physiol.* **2003**, *94*, 1572–1582. [CrossRef]
68. Haddad, J.J.E.; Olver, R.E.; Land, S.C. Antioxidant/pro-Oxidant Equilibrium Regulates HIF-1alpha and NF-Kappa B Redox Sensitivity. Evidence for Inhibition by Glutathione Oxidation in Alveolar Epithelial Cells. *J. Biol. Chem.* **2000**, *275*, 21130–21139. [CrossRef]
69. Zhang, Z.; Yan, J.; Taheri, S.; Liu, K.J.; Shi, H. Hypoxia-Inducible Factor 1 Contributes to N-Acetylcysteine's Protection in Stroke. *Free Radic. Biol. Med.* **2014**, *68*, 8–21. [CrossRef]
70. Viikinkoski, E.; Jalkanen, J.; Gunn, J.; Vasankari, T.; Lehto, J.; Valtonen, M.; Biancari, F.; Jalkanen, S.; Airaksinen, K.E.J.; Hollmén, M.; et al. Red Blood Cell Transfusion Induces Abnormal HIF-1α Response to Cytokine Storm after Adult Cardiac Surgery. *Sci. Rep.* **2021**, *11*, 22230. [CrossRef]
71. Calzia, E.; Asfar, P.; Hauser, B.; Matejovic, M.; Ballestra, C.; Radermacher, P.; Georgieff, M. Hyperoxia May Be Beneficial. *Crit. Care Med.* **2010**, *38*, S559–S568. [CrossRef]
72. Smeyne, M.; Sladen, P.; Jiao, Y.; Dragatsis, I.; Smeyne, R.J. HIF1α Is Necessary for Exercise-Induced Neuroprotection While HIF2α Is Needed for Dopaminergic Neuron Survival in the Substantia Nigra Pars Compacta. *Neuroscience* **2015**, *295*, 23–38. [CrossRef]
73. Brugniaux, J.V.; Coombs, G.B.; Barak, O.F.; Dujic, Z.; Sekhon, M.S.; Ainslie, P.N. Highs and Lows of Hyperoxia: Physiological, Performance, and Clinical Aspects. *Am. J. Physiol. Regul. Integr. Comp. Physiol.* **2018**, *315*, R1–R27. [CrossRef]
74. Zhu, T.; Zhan, L.; Liang, D.; Hu, J.; Lu, Z.; Zhu, X.; Sun, W.; Liu, L.; Xu, E. Hypoxia-Inducible Factor 1α Mediates Neuroprotection of Hypoxic Postconditioning against Global Cerebral Ischemia. *J. Neuropathol. Exp. Neurol.* **2014**, *73*, 975–986. [CrossRef]
75. Tekin, D.; Dursun, A.D.; Xi, L. Hypoxia Inducible Factor 1 (HIF-1) and Cardioprotection. *Acta Pharmacol. Sin.* **2010**, *31*, 1085–1094. [CrossRef]
76. D'Anselmi, F.; Valerio, M.; Cucina, A.; Galli, L.; Proietti, S.; Dinicola, S.; Pasqualato, A.; Manetti, C.; Ricci, G.; Giuliani, A.; et al. Metabolism and Cell Shape in Cancer: A Fractal Analysis. *Int. J. Biochem. Cell Biol.* **2011**, *43*, 1052–1058. [CrossRef]
77. Davies, J.M.S.; Cillard, J.; Friguet, B.; Cadenas, E.; Cadet, J.; Cayce, R.; Fishmann, A.; Liao, D.; Bulteau, A.L.; Derbré, F.; et al. The Oxygen Paradox, the French Paradox, and Age-Related Diseases. *Geroscience* **2017**, *39*, 499–550. [CrossRef]

78. Yang, K.; Yu, G.; Tian, R.; Zhou, Z.; Deng, H.; Li, L.; Yang, Z.; Zhang, G.; Liu, D.; Wei, J.; et al. Oxygen-Evolving Manganese Ferrite Nanovesicles for Hypoxia-Responsive Drug Delivery and Enhanced Cancer Chemoimmunotherapy. *Adv. Funct. Mater.* **2021**, *31*, 2008078. [CrossRef]
79. Höckel, M.; Vaupel, P. Tumor Hypoxia: Definitions and Current Clinical, Biologic, and Molecular Aspects. *J. Natl. Cancer Inst.* **2001**, *93*, 266–276. [CrossRef]
80. Herrera-Campos, A.B.; Zamudio-Martinez, E.; Delgado-Bellido, D.; Fernández-Cortés, M.; Montuenga, L.M.; Oliver, F.J.; Garcia-Diaz, A. Implications of Hyperoxia over the Tumor Microenvironment: An Overview Highlighting the Importance of the Immune System. *Cancers* **2022**, *14*, 2740. [CrossRef]
81. Terraneo, L.; Virgili, E.; Caretti, A.; Bianciardi, P.; Samaja, M. In Vivo Hyperoxia Induces Hypoxia-Inducible Factor-1α Overexpression in LNCaP Tumors without Affecting the Tumor Growth Rate. *Int. J. Biochem. Cell Biol.* **2014**, *51*, 65–74. [CrossRef] [PubMed]
82. de Bels, D.; Tillmans, F.; Corazza, F.; Bizzari, M.; Germonpre, P.; Radermacher, P.; Orman, K.G.; Balestra, C. Hyperoxia Alters Ultrastructure and Induces Apoptosis in Leukemia Cell Lines. *Biomolecules* **2020**, *10*, 282. [CrossRef] [PubMed]
83. Raa, A.; Stansberg, C.; Steen, V.M.; Bjerkvig, R.; Reed, R.K.; Stuhr, L.E.B. Hyperoxia Retards Growth and Induces Apoptosis and Loss of Glands and Blood Vessels in DMBA-Induced Rat Mammary Tumors. *BMC Cancer* **2007**, *7*, 23. [CrossRef] [PubMed]
84. Lee, H.Y.; Kim, I.K.; Lee, H.I.; Lee, H.Y.; Kang, H.S.; Yeo, C.D.; Kang, H.H.; Moon, H.S.; Lee, S.H. Combination of Carboplatin and Intermittent Normobaric Hyperoxia Synergistically Suppresses Benzo[a]Pyrene-Induced Lung Cancer. *Korean J. Intern. Med.* **2018**, *33*, 541–551. [CrossRef]
85. Hatfield, S.M.; Kjaergaard, J.; Lukashev, D.; Schreiber, T.H.; Belikoff, B.; Abbott, R.; Sethumadhavan, S.; Philbrook, P.; Ko, K.; Cannici, R.; et al. Immunological Mechanisms of the Antitumor Effects of Supplemental Oxygenation. *Sci. Transl. Med.* **2015**, *7*, 277ra30. [CrossRef]
86. de Bels, D.; Corazza, F.; Germonpré, P.; Balestra, C. The Normobaric Oxygen Paradox: A Novel Way to Administer Oxygen as an Adjuvant Treatment for Cancer? *Med. Hypotheses* **2011**, *76*, 467–470. [CrossRef]

Disclaimer/Publisher's Note: The statements, opinions and data contained in all publications are solely those of the individual author(s) and contributor(s) and not of MDPI and/or the editor(s). MDPI and/or the editor(s) disclaim responsibility for any injury to people or property resulting from any ideas, methods, instructions or products referred to in the content.

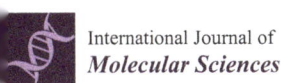

Review

Kidney Injuries and Evolution of Chronic Kidney Diseases Due to Neonatal Hyperoxia Exposure Based on Animal Studies

Liang-Ti Huang [1,2] and Chung-Ming Chen [2,3,*]

1. Department of Pediatrics, Wan Fang Hospital, Taipei Medical University, Taipei 110, Taiwan; a9309@tmu.edu.tw
2. Department of Pediatrics, School of Medicine, College of Medicine, Taipei Medical University, 250 Wu-Hsing Street, Taipei 110, Taiwan
3. Department of Pediatrics, Taipei Medical University Hospital, Taipei 110, Taiwan
* Correspondence: cmchen@tmu.edu.tw

Abstract: Preterm birth interrupts the development and maturation of the kidneys during the critical growth period. The kidneys can also exhibit structural defects and functional impairment due to hyperoxia, as demonstrated by various animal studies. Furthermore, hyperoxia during nephrogenesis impairs renal tubular development and induces glomerular and tubular injuries, which manifest as renal corpuscle enlargement, renal tubular necrosis, interstitial inflammation, and kidney fibrosis. Preterm birth along with hyperoxia exposure induces a pathological predisposition to chronic kidney disease. Hyperoxia-induced kidney injuries are influenced by several molecular factors, including hypoxia-inducible factor-1α and interleukin-6/Smad2/transforming growth factor-β, and Wnt/β-catenin signaling pathways; these are key to cell proliferation, tissue inflammation, and cell membrane repair. Hyperoxia-induced oxidative stress is characterized by the attenuation or the induction of multiple molecular factors associated with kidney damage. This review focuses on the molecular pathways involved in the pathogenesis of hyperoxia-induced kidney injuries to establish a framework for potential interventions.

Keywords: chronic kidney disease; hyperoxia; kidney injury; nephrogenesis; kidney fibrosis; prematurity

1. Introduction

The prevalence rate of preterm birth is approximately 15 million infants worldwide each year. A recent cohort study reported that the incidence rate of chronic kidney disease (CKD) by gestational age at birth is 9.24 per 1,000,000 for preterm infants (<28 weeks), indicating a threefold risk of CKD with respect to term infants; no difference was found between male and female infants [1]. Preterm births vary in terms of gestational age and causes, with inadequate gestational age being a common cause. Furthermore, an adverse intrauterine environment causes 38% of preterm births, and other conditions such as preeclampsia, multiple births, and chorioamnionitis may also be involved [2]. Exposure postnatally to factors such as high oxygen concentrations [3], medications [4], and inadequate nutrition [5] likely adversely influence postnatal growth and ongoing organ development. The renal consequences of preterm births have attracted increasing attention and include a high risk of (CKD) [1], a quick progression of renal pathology [6], and predisposition toward hypertension [7]. The third trimester of pregnancy is the most active period of fetal nephrogenesis, during which more than 60% of nephrons are formed [8,9]. Preterm birth (within <37 gestational weeks) interrupts the development and maturation of the kidneys during the critical growth period. Neonates born preterm have an immature antioxidant defense system [10] and present an imbalance between the oxidant and the antioxidant system leading to an increased level of free radicals (FR), with subsequent oxidative damage to organs [11]. Moreover, oxygen resuscitation [12] and intensive care maneuvers

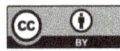

such as assisted ventilation, surfactant administration [13], total parenteral nutrition [14], and blood transfusions [15] enhance FR production, which further increments oxidative stress. Experimental hyperoxic exposure has been used in various previous studies to investigate the effects of oxidative stress on preterm neonates [16,17]. Hyperoxia during the neonatal period impairs renal tubular development. Human and animal studies have demonstrated that neonatal hyperoxia increases oxidative stress and induces glomerular and tubular injuries, which are manifested as renal corpuscle enlargement, renal tubular necrosis, interstitial inflammation, and kidney fibrosis during the perinatal period [18–22]. Through the suppression of antioxidants such as glutathione peroxidase, catalase, and superoxide dismutase activity [23,24], hyperoxia exposure augments free radical and reactive oxygen species (ROS) production, which leads to increased oxidative stress. Human kidney development is completed in utero in 36 gestational weeks [25], whereas nephrogenesis in rats begins on the 12th embryonic day and is completed within 10 to 15 days after birth [26]. Rats are born with immature kidneys; the first two postnatal weeks correspond to the second and third trimesters of human pregnancy during which fetal nephrogenesis occurs. Studies conducted using neonatal rat models have demonstrated the mechanism of fetal nephrogenesis in humans. Although previous studies have clearly demonstrated the presence of renal anomalies after hyperoxic exposure, the corresponding renal diseases and progression to CKD have yet to be investigated. Thus, this review focuses on CKD among prematurely born infants who were exposed to hyperoxia and discusses the theory, experimental evidence, and indicators reported in the literature. In general, vigilant surveillance and therapeutic interventions must be available to these infants.

2. Experimental Oxygen Studies and Kidney Injury

Hyperoxia causes structural defects and functional impairment [22,27–32], thereby predisposing newborns to hypertension and CKD [33–35]. Studies have demonstrated—using different animal models, including rat and mice models—that exposure to hyperoxia can cause renal corpuscle enlargement, tubular injuries, reduced glomerular filtration rate (GFR), and electrolyte derailment, as well as increased collagen content, kidney fibrosis, and apoptosis [21,22,36] (Table 1). In a mouse model based on hyperoxia gas exposure (85% O_2) in the early neonatal period (postnatal days 1 to 28), Mohr et al. showed that hyperoxia-induced neonatal renal injuries involve two phases: the acute and the regenerative phases. The acute renal injury phase is characterized by deregulated mitochondrial biogenesis, reduced renal cortical growth, reduced cell proliferation, and the activation of interleukin-6/Stat3 signaling coupled with active Smad2/transforming growth factor-β (TGF-β) signaling. The regenerative phase is characterized by renal cortical catch-up growth with reduced glomeruli relative to the renal cortical area, thereby causing glomerular and tubular dysfunction [37]. A previously developed rat model showed that hyperoxia exposure (80% O_2) in the early neonatal period (postnatal days 3–10) was associated with a 25% reduction in nephron number in adulthood [38]. Popeseu et al. also discovered a considerable decrease in both nephrogenic zone width and glomerular diameter and a considerable increase in apoptotic cell count using a similar rat model [36]. Compared with rats exposed to ambient air, rats exposed to neonatal hyperoxia (85% O_2 for 14 days) exhibited a notably lower glomerular number, a higher kidney injury score, and elevated expression of toll-like receptor 4 (TLR-4), myeloperoxidase (MPO), and 8-hydroxy-2-deoxyguanosine (8-OHdG) [39]. A similar study demonstrated that newborn rat exposure to hyperoxia caused tubular atrophy, dilatation of the tubular lumen, vacuolar degeneration of the tubular epithelium, and increased space between the renal tubules in conjunction with collagen deposition and macrophage infiltration [40]. In both short-term (1 week in Chen and in Chou et al.) [39,40] and long-term (3 weeks in Jiang et al.; 95% O_2 for 7 days and 60% O_2 for following 14 days) [22] studies, hyperoxic exposure resulted in increased collagen I and tissue connective tissue growth factor (CTGF) expression leading to renal tubular damage. In addition, the results of long-term studies on the effects of neonatal rats exposed to hyperoxia (85% O_2 for 14 days, then 21% O_2 till P 60 d) indicated impaired proximal tubular development [41,42], increased glomerular injury [43], decreased glomerular volume, and decreased nephron number [44]. Thus, neonatal hyperoxia exposure may cause transient apoptosis, renal fibrosis, and long-term glomerular and tubular damage and dysfunction in the kidneys. In contrast, however, in a mouse model, exposure to 65% O_2 from postnatal day 1 to 7, and to >98% O_2 from day 0 to 4 then to 21% for the following 4 days, did not lead to any significant alterations in renal development or nephron number [18,21]. The contribution of hyperoxia-induced neonatal kidney damage to vulnerability to adult CKD has yet to be clearly understood.

Table 1. Experimental models of hyperoxia exposure and kidney injury.

Model	Species	Primary Target Lesion	Molecules	Ref
85% O_2, P1 to P28, 21% O_2 till P70 (Mohr et al.)	mouse	Glomerular filtration rate Kidney cortex area Glomerular number Glomerular diameter Proximal tubular proliferation	IL-6 Collagen IV PAI-1 CTGF Smad2	[37]
80% O_2 P3 to P10 (Popeseu et al.)	rat	Nephrogenic zone Glomerular diameter Glomerular apoptotic cells	HIF-1α	[36]
95% O_2, P1 to P7, 60% O_2 till P21 (Jiang et al.)	rat	Tubular injury score Glomerular size	Total collagen 8-oHdG CTGF	[22]
80% O_2, P1 to P14 (Chen et al.)	rat	Kidney injury score Glomerular number Glomerular injury score	8-OHdG MPO activity TLR4 IL-1β M1 macrophage	[39]
85% O_2, P1 to P7 (Chou et al.)	rat	Tubular injury score	8-OHdG Collagen NF-κB MAPK/ERK	[40]
85% O_2, P0 to P14; 21% O_2 till P60 (Xu et al.)	rat	Nephrogenic zone Epithelial cells of mature proximal tubules Tubular cell apoptosis	HIF-1α Catalase IL-6 TNF-α Claudin-4 Occludin Zonula occluden-1 (ZO-1)	[41,42]
65% O_2, P1 to P7; 21% O_2 till P56 and P10m (Sutherland et al.)	mouse	Nephron number Renal corpuscles	-	[21]
80% O_2, P3 to P10; 21% O_2 till P11ms (Sutherland et al.)	rat	Glomerular injury Creatinine clearance	-	[43]
85% O_2, P3 to P15; 21% O_2 till P9ms (Kumar et al.)	mouse	Glomerular diameter Glomerular volume Nephron number	-	[44]
80% O_2, P3 to P10; 21% O_2 till P15wks (Yzydorczyk et al.)	rat	Blood pressure Microvascular rarefaction Nephron number	Superoxide dismutase analogue	[38]
>98% O_2 P0 to P4; 21% O_2 till P5, P8 (Torbati et al.)	rat	Tubular necrosis, dilation, and degeneration, Interstitial inflammation	-	[18]

Abbreviations: IL-6: interleukin-6; PAI-1: plasminogen activator inhibitor-1; CTGF: connective tissue growth factor; HIF-1α: hypoxia inducible factor-1α; 8-OHdG: 8-hydroxydeoxyguanosine; MPO: myeloperoxidase; TLR4: toll like receptor; IL-1β: interleukin-1β; MAPK/ERK: mitogen-activated protein kinase, extracellular signal-regulated kinase; TNF-α: tumor necrosis factor-α.

3. Predisposition to CKD Due to Hyperoxia-Induced Kidney Injuries

3.1. Proximal Tubular Injury and Interstitial Fibrosis

CKD affecting 13% of the global population is a growing epidemic resulting from renal insults caused by, e.g., hypertension, inflammatory glomerular diseases, diabetes mellitus, genetic disorders, and toxins [45]. Although CKD can be triggered by various factors, glomerulosclerosis, vascular sclerosis, and tubulointerstitial fibrosis are common in CKD, indicating that progressive injury occurs through a common final pathway [46]. CKD is the common endpoint of different etiologies including glomerular injuries, repeated acute kidney injury (AKI), and chronic tubulointerstitial injuries. The progression of CKD follows a common pathway whereby the normal renal parenchyma is replaced with matrix proteins such as collagen I, III, IV and fibronectin. The basic functional unit of the kidney is the nephron which filters the blood in the glomerulus. The resulting ultrafiltrate passes through the tubules, composed of a highly specialized epithelium, which reabsorb water and electrolytes [47]. With regard to histopathology, tubulointerstitial fibrosis (TIF) is characterized by extracellular matrix (ECM) accumulation, tubular atrophy, inflammatory cell infiltration, and peritubular microvascular loss, which are typically observed in CKD [48,49]. Matrix proteins accumulation in the glomerulus is termed glomerulosclerosis, whereas TIF describes the presence of matrix proteins replacing the tubules and/or surrounding the interstitium. The tubular epithelium, especially in the proximal tubules, is affected by acute and chronic injuries. The injured epithelium dedifferentiates and proliferates, thereby promoting healing after AKI [50]. Repetitive or persistent epithelial injuries may cause tubular apoptosis, which leads to progressive TIF. The dying epithelial cells may produce proinflammatory cytokines and other growth factors that promote inflammation and fibrosis. Renal fibrosis is typically preceded by the infiltration of inflammatory cells, including lymphocytes, monocytes/macrophages, dendritic cells, and mast cells. Fibrosis is primarily promoted by persistent inflammation [51]. Experimental models and human pathological studies of TIF have demonstrated that the activation of tubular epithelial cells and interstitial fibroblasts causes the excessive generation of ECM, which is constituted mostly by collagen, and the formation of scar tissue. Injured proximal tubular epithelial cells synthesize collagen, which promotes basement membrane thickening (collagen IV) and interstitial fibrosis (collagen I, III, IV) [52]. The dedifferentiated epithelial cells exhibit a partially mesenchymal phenotype, which is associated with an increased production of profibrotic cytokines. Renal injury alters the epithelial cell cycle, and these cell cycle changes may also impact TIF progression and the transition from AKI to CKD [47]. Most proximal tubule epithelial cells in uninjured kidney are quiescent (cell cycle stage G0). However, during injury, the cells may enter the cell cycle (G1, S, G2, M) to help replace cells lost to apoptosis/necrosis, and some cells become arrested in either G1 or G2. Cell arrest is adaptive to allow time for repair of any DNA damage and prevent the propagation of mutations that occur in injured cells. Chronically injured epithelial cells are arrested in G2/M; this cell cycle dysfunction is also associated with the excessive production of profibrotic growth factors [53]. G2/M cell cycle arrest results in increased activity of c-jun N-terminal kinase (JNK), which promotes the production of TGF-β and CTGF/CCN2 [53]. The augmented production of epithelial TGF-β may induce the interaction of other growth factors with fibroblasts, thereby promoting TIF progression.

3.2. Nephron Number Loss and Increase in Glomeruli Diameter

Studies have revealed that early exposure to hyperoxia causes a decrease in nephron number and an increase in glomeruli diameter as well as an increase in the incidence of glomerular injuries and in the number of apoptotic cells [37,38,43]. As nephron number decreases, the filtration capacity of nephrons increases. The number of functional nephrons decreases, creating more metabolic work for the remaining tubules. In agreement with Brenner's hypothesis about declining renal function and glomerular hyperfiltration [54], the remaining proximal tubules become hypertrophic to meet the increased demand of water and solutes reabsorption [55]. Although total energy expenditure in the CKD kidney decreases, the metabolism of the surviving nephrons increases to support the compensatory changes in reabsorption [56,57]. Protein intake correlates positively with proximal tubule hypertrophy and, in the rat subtotal nephrectomy model, led to more oxidative stress [58]. The increase in perfusion pressure above the normal physiological range may affect the structural filtration stability and cause glomerulosclerosis and nephron loss [59]. In a study on the effects of a low-protein diet during pregnancy and lactation, reduced nephron number, increased glomerulus volume, and enhanced TGF-β and collagen I expression and STAT3 phosphorylation were observed in children [60]. Srivastava et al. investigated the role of biomechanical forces in hyperfiltration-mediated glomerular injuries due to congenital anomalies in the kidney and urinary tract (CAKUT) by analyzing the effects of biomechanical forces on glomerular podocytes [61]. Moreover, children with CAKUT may progressively develop CKD because of early renal changes due to maladaptive hyperfiltration that leads to increased fluid flow shear stress [61]. Although the long-term consequences of preterm birth in the kidneys have yet to be discovered, evolutionary adaption may explain other responses in the CKD kidney that are initially adaptive but lead to dysfunction, such as senescence and inflammation. The decrease in nephron number and proliferation of tubular cells can induce functional changes in the kidneys later in life [37]. The available evidence indicates that preterm birth increases the risk of CKD [30,32], and neonatal hyperoxia exposure induces changes in renal structure and a decrease in GFR as well as glomerular and tubular damage, thereby increasing the chances of renal disorders in adulthood.

3.3. Glomerular and Podocyte Injury

The glomerulus contains four different cell types. Fenestrated endothelial cells cover the glomerular basement membrane (GBM) from the vascular side, and podocytes from the outside (urinary side), all together building the glomerular filtration barrier [62]. Mesangial cells produce extracellular matrix and scaffold the capillaries. The fourth cell type, parietal epithelial cells, lines the outer aspect of the glomerulus and thereby defines the Bowman's space from where primary urine flows into the tubule [63]. Mature podocytes do not proliferate in vivo due to their highly differentiated phenotype; thus, they respond to different types of injury through detachment from the glomerular basement membrane, dedifferentiation, autophagy, and apoptosis [64]. The mechanisms underlying podocyte injury are complex and include hemodynamic and metabolic pathways as well as the interplay of vasoactive molecules, growth factors, and cytokines [64,65]. Accumulating experimental and clinical evidence suggests that podocytes are quite vulnerable to oxidative damage, and amplification of oxidative stress seems to be a final and common pathway shared by different aggressors at the cellular level. Glomerular injury leads to podocyte loss and induces adhesion between the glomerular basement membrane and the parietal epithelium. A protein-rich ultrafiltrate usually passes from the capillaries to the Bowmans space and tubular lumen, but increased adhesion in the tuft and breaks in the parietal epithelium misdirect the protein ultrafiltrate to the interstitium [66]. Podocyte injury can induce their detachment from the GBM and thus their loss, which is the major determinant of progressive glomerular injury and glomerulosclerosis [67]. The loss of podocytes will also induce endothelial stress and injury, since podocyte-derived angiogenic factors such as VEGF are essential for normal endothelial homeostasis [63]. Paracrine signaling from injured podocytes induces the activation of parietal epithelial cells and mesangial cells, which directly facilitates the onset of glomerulosclerosis. Glomerular injury increases the filtered load of albumin, and this augmented proximal tubular protein reabsorption can have both direct toxic and paracrine effects that may promote TIF, which leads to CKD.

3.4. Similarities and Differences between Hyperoxia- and Other Factors-Induced Pathomechanisms in CKD

There are some similarities and differences in CKD induced by hyperoxia or by other factors, such as diabetes, hypertension, or obstructive uropapthy. CKD induced by hyperoxia and other factors CKD is characterized by nephron loss, nephron hypertrophy, proximal tubular injury, and interstitial fibrosis, which are originated from oxidative stress and inflammatory processes. CKD due to other factors presents dominant podocyte injury and detachment, focal segmental glomerulosclerosis, global glomerulosclerosis, and subsequent nephron atrophy, which are caused by direct toxicity, local or systemic infection, and genetic factors. Nephron loss involves a nonspecific wound-healing response that includes interstitial fibrosis. Infiltrating immune cells, albuminuria, and, in diabetes, glucosuria, activate proximal tubular epithelial cells, resulting in the secretion of proinflammatory and profibrotic mediators, and promote interstitial inflammation and fibrosis [68]. The increased tubular transport load of remnant nephrons also involves anerobic metabolism, intracelluar acidosis, and endoplasmic reticulum stress, which promote secondary tubular injury [69]. In other forms of CKD, angiotensin II plays an important role through the mechanistic targeting of rapamycin signaling, maintaining persistent podocyte hypertrophy and glomerular hyperfiltration and ultimately aggravating podocyte loss and proteinuria. Angiotensin II possibly also contributes to the dysregulated response of progenitor parietal epithelial cells along Bowman's capsule, generating FSGS lesions instead of replacing lost podocytes [70]. This structural remodelling of the glomerulus presents clinically as proteinuria, which is a marker of nephron damage and is predictive of CKD progression [71].

4. Cellular and Molecular Aspects

4.1. Influence of Hyperoxia-Inducible Factor-1a (HIF-1α) on Tubular Development

Several biomolecular factors including TGF-β, HIF-1α, and integrin-linked kinase have been found to influence in vivo epithelial–mesenchymal transformation [72–74]. The prevention of TGF-β-mediated signaling by bone morphogenetic protein-7 aids the reversal of TGF-β-mediated TIF [72] (Figure 1).

Hyperoxia-inducible factors (HIFs) are heterodimers comprising one of three O_2-sensitive alpha subunits (HIF-1α, HIF-2α, and HIF-3α) and a constitutively expressed beta-subunit HIF-1β [75]. HIF-1α and HIF-1β are the key regulators of oxygen homeostasis. HIF-1α promotes organogenesis [76,77] by regulating the expression of various factors involved in angiogenesis, cellular proliferation, and apoptosis [78,79]. Within the developing kidney, HIF-1α is expressed weakly in the outer cortex and strongly in some tubular and collecting duct epithelial cells. Mice genetically deficient in HIF-1α die at midgestation (embryonic day 9.5 [E9.5]) show vascular and neural tube defects [76,80]. Popeseu et al. investigated the influence of transient hyperoxia exposure on nephrogenesis in neonatal rats. Transient hyperoxia during nephrogenesis suppressed HIF-1α, reduced nephrogenic zone width and glomerular diameter, and increased apoptotic cell count, which were reversed by a HIF-1α stabilizer; however, no changes were observed in nephron number after nephrogenesis [36]. Xu et al. discovered that neonatal hyperoxia impaired proximal tubular development in conjunction with downregulated HIF-1α and altered mitogen-activated protein kinase (MAPK)/extracellular signal-regulated kinase (ERK) signaling and catalase [41]. MAPK/ERK signaling is crucial to the proliferation and differentiation of nephron progenitors. The catalase enzyme is key to protecting the cell from oxidative damage due to ROS [81]. Nephrectomized animals exhibited significant elevated levels of proinflammatory and profibrotic factors, activation of NF-κB, and increased activation of TGF-β/Smad3 and MAPK signaling pathways [82]. ROS activate a broad variety of hypertrophy signaling kinases and transcription factors, such as MAPK and NF-κB, as well as proliferation of activation of matrix metalloproteinases (MMPs) [83]. Thus, early exposure to hyperoxia can impair nephrogenesis and induce proximal tubular injuries through HIF-1α attenuation, predisposing infants to adult CKD.

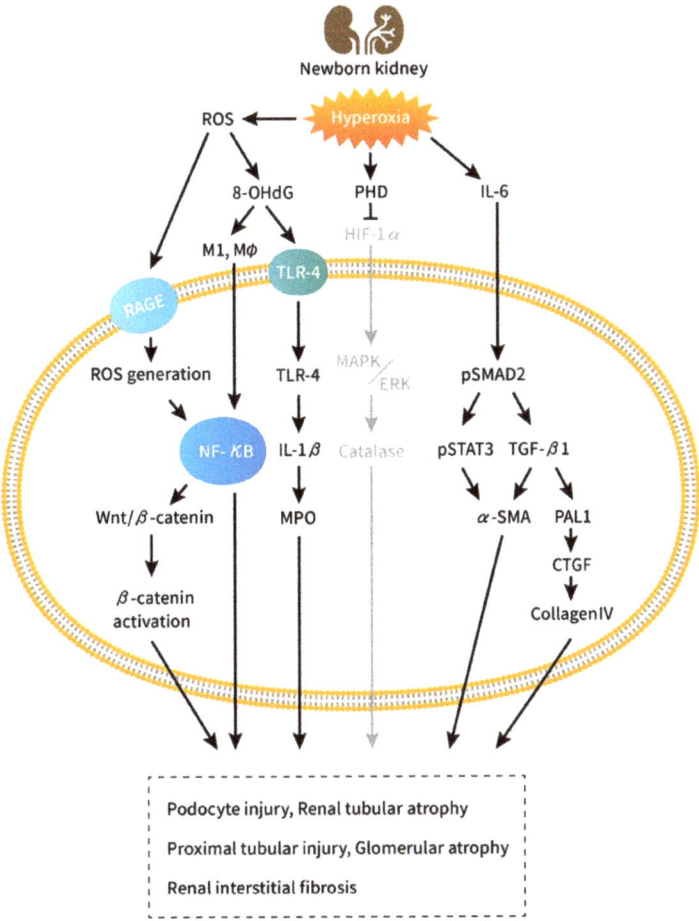

Figure 1. Schematic of the mechanism of hyperoxia-induced kidney injury and renal interstitial fibrosis. Hyperoxia induces reactive oxidative stress; prolyl hydroxylases domain enzymes, which downregulate HIF-1α, upregulate IL-6, and trigger the activation of 8-OHdG, bind to the plasma membrane receptor RAGE and TLR-4, thereby enhancing the generation of ROS. This regulates the inflammatory transcription factors NF-κB, IL-1β, and MPO, which induce Wnt ligands and subsequently activate β-catenin. The activation of β-catenin triggers podocyte injury through dedifferentiation and mesenchymal transition. The downregulation of HIF-1α suppresses MAPK and ERK, thereby reducing catalase levels. The reduction of catalase triggers proximal tubular injury and impairs glomerular development. The upregulation of IL-6 triggers the activation of phosphorylated Smad2. This in turn induces the phosphorylation of STAT3, the activation of TGF-β1, and the formation of alpha SMA, PAL1, CTGF, and collagen IV. The activation of α-SMA and collagen IV subsequently induces renal mesangial and interstitial fibrosis. Abbreviations: PHD: prolyl hydroxylases domain enzyme; IL-6: interleukin-6; PAI-1: plasminogen activator inhibitor-1; CTGF: connective tissue growth factor; HIF-1α: hypoxia inducible factor-1α; 8-OHdG: 8-hydroxydeoxyguanosine; MPO: myeloperoxidase; TLR4: toll like receptor; IL-1β: interleukin-1β; MAPK/ERK: mitogen-activated protein kinase, extracellular signal-regulated kinase; TNF-α: tumor necrosis factor-α; STAT3: signal transducer and activator of transcription3; TGF-β1: transforming growth factor-β1; alpha SMA: alpha smooth muscle actin.

4.2. Role of the Proinflammatory Cytokine Interleukin-6

Cytokines aid the inflammatory response but may induce organ dysfunction when released in excess [84,85]. IL-6 is a pleiotropic cytokine that not only regulates immune and inflammatory responses but also affects hematopoiesis, metabolism, and organ development [86]. The level of IL-6 is high in the renal tissue of patients with kidney diseases, diabetic nephropathy, glomerulonephritis, or obstructive nephropathy. Renal cells that express and secrete IL-6 include podocytes, endothelial cells, mesangial cells, and tubular epithelial cells. IL-6 signaling can enhance cell proliferation, affect differentiation, and promote TIF [86]. After prolonged exposure to oxygen, the levels of IL-6, TGF-β, and 8-OHdG increase in the tracheal aspirates of infants, leading to chronic lung disease [87–89]. Neonatal rat exposed to hyperoxia also augmented the production of 8-OHdG and TLR-4, MPO activity, and the levels of IL-1β, NF-κB, M1 and M2 macrophage and collagen in the kidneys, which indicated increased oxidative stress (8-OHdG), neutrophil accumulation (MPO activity), inflammatory response (TLR-4, IL-1b, NF-kB, and M1 and M2 macrophage), and fibrotic reaction (collagen) [39,40]. Furthermore, neonatal hyperoxia exposure considerably increased IL-6 levels in the lungs [90,91], indicating that hyperoxia enhanced ROS production, and the subsequent oxidative stress induced an inflammatory cellular response [92]. Mohr et al. discovered that elevated levels of IL-6 induced transient changes in renal fibrosis and a considerable decrease in GFR, glomerular number, and cell proliferation in neonatal mice after prolonged exposure to oxygen. These changes did not occur in IL-$6^{-/-}$ animals [37]. Increased renal expression of IL-6 and a marked activation of IL-6/Stat3 signaling in the acute renal injury phase may thus remain unchanged after regeneration under normoxic conditions [37]. In addition to increasing IL-6 levels, hyperoxia induces a marked activation of Smad2 and subsequently increases the expression of plasminogen activator inhibitor-1 (PAI-1) and other downstream molecules, such as CTGF, collagen a-4 type IV (collagen IV), and elastin. Smad2, an indicator of the TGF-β pathway activation, enhances the synthesis of matrix proteins and the secretion of protease inhibitors, which results in matrix accumulation. TGF-β is a key profibrotic growth factor that is activated in AKI and is associated with cellular responses that lead to the development of CKD. TGF-β signaling may sustain proximal tubule injury by inducing cell dedifferentiation, cell cycle arrest, and increased susceptibility to apoptosis. Furthermore, TGF-β signaling promotes macrophage chemotaxis, endothelial injury, and myofibroblast differentiation after AKI [93]. Tubular overexpression of TGF-β led to tubular autophagy and degeneration as well as peritubular fibrosis [94]. PAI-1, CTGF, collagen IV, and smooth muscle alpha-actin are downstream profibrotic effectors of Smad2 and are associated with enhanced extracellular matrix remodeling and fibrosis; they are also associated with damage in several organs in humans [95–99]. The activation of both IL-6 and TGF-β signaling due to hyperoxia during a critical period of nephrogenesis could adversely affect energy metabolism, tubular growth, and nephron functioning, thereby predisposing infants to adult CKD.

4.3. Influence of Hyperoxia on Nephrogenesis and Renal Fibrosis through Wnt/β-Catenin Signaling

Wnts are a family of secretory proteins that, upon binding with their cellular membrane receptors, induce a series of downstream signaling events resulting in the phosphorylation of beta-catenin [100]. The Wnt/β-catenin signaling pathway is crucial for organ development, tissue homeostasis, and postinjury organ repair [101–103]. Transient Wnt/β-catenin signaling stimulates repair and regeneration after AKI, and the continuous activation of the pathway promotes CKD-related fibrogenesis [104]. The Wnt/β-catenin signaling pathway is inactive in normal kidneys but is activated after kidney injury in various CKD situations, such as in the presence of ischemia–reperfusion injury, 5/6 nephrectomy, unilateral ureteral obstruction, and doxorubicin nephropathy [105–107]. The upregulation of multiple Wnt ligands and the activation of β-catenin are observed in renal biopsies of individuals with diabetic nephropathy, IgA nephropathy, and lupus nephritis and make them prone to podocyte damage and oxidative stress [108–110]. Previous evidence suggests that the action of Wnt/β-catenin is dependent on the activation of receptor of advanced glycation end product (RAGE) by advanced oxidation protein products (AOPPs). This triggers a cascade of reactions, including induction of NADPH oxidase, generation of ROS, and NF-κB activation, which leads to the induction of Wnt ligands and the activation of β-catenin [111]. Zhou et al. discovered that Wnt/β-catenin is activated in CKD patients and mediates oxidative stress-triggered podocyte dysfunction and proteinuria through a series of signaling events involving the induction of ROS/p65 NF-κB and Wnt [100]. Lin et al. experimentally demonstrated that the suppressed antioxidant element Se may induce renal fibrosis by enhancing the Wnt/β-catenin signaling pathway [112]. Thus, oxidative stress may lead to CKD and kidney fibrosis through the activation of the Wnt/β-catenin signaling pathway.

5. Therapeutic Approach According to Molecular Markers

In addition to basic science studies elucidating the importance of kidney injury in hyperoxia-exposed animals, other studies have described a new class of therapeutic interventions or medications that target molecular factors and protect against hyperoxia-induced kidney injury in neonatal animals. Experimentally systemic administration of the HIF-1α stabilizer dimethyloxalylglycine (DMOG) resulted in enhanced expression of HIF-1α and improved nephrogenesis: kidneys from hyperoxia-exposed pups treated with DMOG exhibited a nephrogenic zone width and a glomerular diameter similar to those of controls [36]. Investigations also showed that cathelicidin treatment attenuated kidney injury, as evidenced by lower kidney injury scores, less 8-OHdG-positive cells, reduced collagen deposition, and reversion of hyperoxia-induced M1/M2 macrophage polarization, accompanied by decreased NF-kB levels [40]. IL-6 deficiency ameliorated experimental hyperoxia-induced glomerular and tubular dysfunction through the inhibition of inflammatory signaling. These observations may indicate new avenues to protect premature infants from CKD [37]. In a rat model of hyperoxia-induced lung injury, resveratrol alleviated hyperoxia-induced histological injury in the lungs, regulated the redox balance, decreased proinflammatory cytokine release, and downregulated the expression of fibrosis-associated proteins through Wnt/β-catenin signaling suppression [23]. These novel therapeutic approaches provided some targeting goals to reduce the risk of CKD in premature babies. Nevertheless, there are currently no effective approaches for neonates exposed to hyperoxia. Large studies in specifically selected patient cohorts with current endpoints will require a multicenter approach, with long recruitment time and duration, which will substantially increase the time and costs.

6. Future Studies on Hyperoxia-Induced Kidney Injuries

Glomerular and tubular injury and renal fibrosis are not a single process but indicate various pathologic and fibrotic processes in specific renal compartments with a particular cellular and molecular composition. They involve virtually all renal cells and a large number of molecules, albeit only few molecules are directly involved in fibrogenesis itself. Hyperoxia during the neonatal period in animals causes pathological changes including glomerular injuries and proximal tubular dysfunction. Kidney injuries due to hyperoxia exposure vary, depending on the injury phase (acute or regenerative) after recovery in ambient air. The results of long-term studies indicate that early exposure to hyperoxia results in glomerular reduction and proximal tubular dysfunction [28], whereas short-term studies have not demonstrated the occurrence of deleterious effects [10]. In addition, several groups have shown that β-catenin activation in fibroblasts or pericytes promote TIF progression [113,114]. In contrast, investigations also demonstrated that β-catenin activity in the proximal tubule protect against TIF [115]. Although an increment in HIF-1α expression improved nephrogenesis and hyperoxia-induced kidney injury [38], increased HIF expression was found in animal models of CKD and in renal biopsy material from patients with diabetic nephropathy and other forms of renal disease [116,117]. Another study identified epithelial HIF-1 as a promoter of renal fibrosis in experimental unilateral ureteral obstruction [73]. Thus, the implications of these results are unclear because of a lack of long-term cohort studies specifying the target markers. Although pathological changes in glomeruli and tubules and the enhancement of biomolecular pathways may be the major causes of CKD, further studies must investigate the correlation between damaged nephrons and renal interstitial fibrosis. Furthermore, advanced therapeutic strategies must be developed to prevent CKD in prematurely born infants.

In conclusion, preterm birth and low birth weight contribute to the increased risk of CKD in later life. Oxygen therapy to treat neonatal respiratory diseases can also lead to kidney injury during nephrogenesis. The injured kidney structure and dysfunction may lead to CKD through ROS- and inflammation-induced nephron loss, proximal tubular and glomerular injuries, and interstitial fibrosis. These mechanisms are similar to those activated by other factors that may cause CKD. Several molecular signaling pathways are involved in the pathogenesis of hyperoxia-induced CKD. Targeting pathomolecular regulators might provide the means to simultaneously regulate the activity of multiple pathways that coordinately regulate different aspects of CKD progression.

Author Contributions: L.-T.H. wrote the review. C.-M.C. edited and made contribution to this review. All authors have read and agreed to the published version of the manuscript.

Funding: This study was funded by a grant from Taipei Medical University, Taiwan (110TMU-WFH-18).

Data Availability Statement: Data sharing is not applicable to this article.

Conflicts of Interest: The authors declare no conflict of interest regarding to this review article.

References

1. Crump, C.; Sundquist, J.; Winkleby, M.A.; Sundquist, K. Preterm birth and risk of chronic kidney disease from childhood into midadulthood: National cohort study. *BMJ* **2019**, *365*, l1346. [CrossRef] [PubMed]
2. Frey, H.A.; Klebanoff, M.A. The epidemiology, etiology, and costs of preterm birth. *Semin. Fetal Neonatal Med.* **2016**, *21*, 68–73. [CrossRef] [PubMed]
3. Saugstad, O.D. Update on oxygen radical disease in neonatology. *Curr. Opin. Obstet. Gynecol.* **2001**, *2*, 147–153. [CrossRef] [PubMed]
4. Schreuder, M.F.; Bueters, R.R.; Huigen, M.C.; Russel, F.G.; Masereeuw, R.; van den Heuvel, L.P. Effect of drugs on renal development. *Clin. J. Am. Soc. Nephrol.* **2011**, *1*, 212–217. [CrossRef]
5. Martin, C.R.; Brown, Y.F.; Ehrenkranz, R.A.; O'Shea, T.M.; Allred, E.N.; Belfort, M.B.; McCormick, M.C.; Leviton, A. Extremely Low Gestational Age Newborns Study Investigators. Nutritional practices and growth velocity in the first month of life in extremely premature infants. *Pediatrics* **2009**, *2*, 649–657. [CrossRef]
6. Luyckx, V.A.; Brenner, B.M. The clinical importance of nephron mass. *J. Am. Soc. Nephrol.* **2010**, *21*, 898–910. [CrossRef] [PubMed]
7. Paquette, K.; Fernandes, R.O.; Xie, L.F.; Cloutier, A.; Fallaha, C.; Girard-Bock, C.; Mian, M.O.R.; Lukaszewski, M.A.; Mâsse, B.; El-Jalbout, R.; et al. Kidney size, renal function, ang (angiotensin) peptides, and blood pressure in young adults born preterm. *Hypertension* **2018**, *72*, 918–928. [CrossRef]
8. Faa, G.; Gerosa, C.; Fanni, D.; Monga, G.; Zaffanello, M.; Van Eyken, P.; Fanos, V. Morphogenesis and molecular mechanisms involved in human kidney development. *J. Cell. Physiol.* **2012**, *227*, 1257–1268. [CrossRef] [PubMed]
9. Hinchliffe, S.A.; Sargent, P.H.; Howard, C.V.; Chan, Y.F.; van Velzen, D. Human intrauterine renal growth expressed in absolute number of glomeruli assessed by the disector method and Cavalieri principle. *Lab. Investig.* **1991**, *64*, 777–784. [PubMed]
10. Georgeson, G.D.; Szony, B.J.; Streitman, K.; Varga, I.S.; Kovács, A.; Kovács, L.; László, A. Antioxidant enzyme activities are decreased in preterm infants and in neonates born via caesarean section. *Eur. J. Obstet. Gynecol. Reprod. Biol.* **2002**, *103*, 136–139. [CrossRef]
11. Saugstad, O. Mechanisms of tissue injury by oxygen radicals: Implications for neonatal disease. *Acta Paediatr.* **1996**, *85*, 1–4. [CrossRef] [PubMed]
12. Vento, M.; Moro, M.; Escrig, R.; Arruza, L.; Villar, G.; Izquierdo, I.; Roberts, L.J.; Arduini, A.; Escobar, J.; Sastre, J.; et al. Preterm Resuscitation with Low Oxygen Causes Less Oxidative Stress, Inflammation, and Chronic Lung Disease. *Pediatrics* **2009**, *124*, e439–e449. [CrossRef] [PubMed]
13. Buonocore, G.; Perrone, S.; Longini, M.; Vezzosi, P.; Marzocchi, B.; Paffetti, P.; Bracci, R. Oxidative Stress in Preterm Neonates at Birth and on the Seventh Day of Life. *Pediatr. Res.* **2002**, *52*, 46–49. [CrossRef] [PubMed]
14. Perrone, S.; Salvi, G.; Bellieni, C.V.; Buonocore, G. Oxidative Stress and Nutrition in the Preterm Newborn. *J. Pediatr. Gastroenterol. Nutr.* **2007**, *45*, S178–S182. [CrossRef]
15. Hirano, K.; Morinobu, T.; Kim, H.; Hiroi, M.; Ban, R.; Ogawa, S.; Ogihara, H.; Tamai, H.; Ogihara, T. Blood transfusion increases radical promoting non-transferrin bound iron in preterm infants. *Arch. Dis. Child.-Fetal Neonatal Ed.* **2001**, *84*, F188–F193. [CrossRef]

16. Andresen, J.H.; Saugstad, O.D. Oxygen metabolism and oxygenation of the newborn. *Semin. Fetal Neonatal Med.* **2020**, *2*, 101078. [CrossRef]
17. Ma, D.; Gao, W.; Liu, J.; Kong, D.; Zhang, Y.; Qian, M. Mechanism of oxidative stress and Keap-1/Nrf2 signaling pathway in bronchopulmonary dysplasia. *Medicine* **2020**, *26*, e20433. [CrossRef] [PubMed]
18. Torbati, D.; Tan, G.H.; Smith, S.; Frazier, K.S.; Gelvez, J.; Fakioglu, H.; Totapally, B.R. Multiple-organ effect of normobaric hyperoxia in neonatal rats. *J. Crit. Care* **2006**, *21*, 85–94. [CrossRef]
19. Vento, M.; Sastre, J.; Asensi, M.A.; Viña, J. Room-air resuscitation causes less damage to heart and kidney than 100% oxygen. *Am. J. Respir. Crit. Care Med.* **2005**, *172*, 1393–1398. [CrossRef]
20. Perrone, S.; Mussap, M.; Longini, M.; Fanos, V.; Bellieni, C.V.; Proietti, F.; Cataldi, L.; Buonocore, G. Oxidative kidney damage in preterm newborns during perinatal period. *Clin. Biochem.* **2007**, *40*, 656–660. [CrossRef]
21. Sutherland, M.R.; O'Reilly, M.; Kenna, K.; Ong, K.; Harding, R.; Sozo, F.; Black, M.J. Neonatal hyperoxia: Effects on nephrogenesis and long term glomerular structure. *Am. J. Physiol. Ren. Physiol.* **2013**, *304*, F1308–F1316. [CrossRef] [PubMed]
22. Jiang, J.S.; Chou, H.C.; Yeh, T.F.; Chen, C.M. Neonatal hy.yperoxia exposure induces kidney fibrosis in rats. *Pediatr. Neonatol.* **2015**, *56*, 235–241. [CrossRef] [PubMed]
23. Xu, W.; Zhao, Y.; Zhang, B.; Xu, B.; Yang, Y.; Wang, Y.; Liu, C. Resveratrol attenuates hyperoxia-induced oxidative stress, inflammation and fibrosis and suppresses Wnt/β-catenin signalling in lungs of neonatal rats. *Clin. Exp. Pharmacol. Physiol.* **2015**, *10*, 1075–1083. [CrossRef] [PubMed]
24. Lembo, C.; Buonocore, G.; Perrone, S. Oxidative Stress in Preterm Newborns. *Antioxidants* **2021**, *11*, 1672. [CrossRef] [PubMed]
25. Zoetis, T.; Hurtt, M.E. Species comparison of anatomical and functional renal development. *Birth Defects Res. B Dev. Reprod. Toxicol.* **2003**, *68*, 111–120. [CrossRef] [PubMed]
26. Seely, J.C. A brief review of kidney development, maturation, developmental abnormalities, and drug toxicity: Juvenile animal relevancy. *J. Toxicol. Pathol.* **2017**, *30*, 125–133. [CrossRef] [PubMed]
27. Goldstein, R.S.; Tarloff, J.B.; Hook, J.B. Age-related nephropathy in laboratory rats. *FASEB J.* **1988**, *2*, 2241–2251. [CrossRef] [PubMed]
28. Reckelhoff, J.F. Age-related changes in renal hemodynamics in female rats: Role of multiple pregnancy and NO. *Am. J. Physiol.* **1997**, *272*, R1985–R1989. [CrossRef] [PubMed]
29. Black, M.J.; Lim, K.; Zimanyi, M.A.; Sampson, A.K.; Bubb, K.J.; Flower, R.L.; Parkington, H.C.; Tare, M.; Denton, K.M. Accelerated age-related decline in renal and vascular function in female rats following early-life growth restriction. *Am. J. Physiol. Regul. Integr. Comp. Physiol.* **2015**, *309*, R1153–R1161. [CrossRef]
30. Bacchetta, J.; Harambat, J.; Dubourg, L.; Guy, B.; Liutkus, A.; Canterino, I.; Kassaï, B.; Putet, G.; Cochat, P. Both extrauterine and intrauterine growth restriction impair renal function in children born very preterm. *Kidney Int.* **2009**, *76*, 445–452. [CrossRef] [PubMed]
31. Sen, N.; Satija, Y.K.; Das, S. PGC-1α, a key modulator of p53 promotes cell survival upon metabolic stress. *Mol. Cell* **2011**, *44*, 621–634. [CrossRef] [PubMed]
32. Keijzer-Veen, M.G.; Schrevel, M.; Finken, M.J.J.; Dekker, F.W.; Nauta, J.; Hille, E.T.M.; Frölich, M.; van der Heijden, B.J.; Dutch POPS-19 Collaborative Study Group. Microalbuminuria and lower glomerular filtration rate at young adult age in subjects born very premature and after intrauterine growth retardation. *J. Am. Soc. Nephrol.* **2005**, *16*, 2762–2768. [CrossRef] [PubMed]
33. Dalziel, S.R.; Parag, V.; Rodgers, A.; Harding, J.E. Cardiovascular risk factors at age 30 following pre-term birth. *Int. J. Epidemiol.* **2007**, *36*, 907–915. [CrossRef] [PubMed]
34. Cooper, R.; Atherton, K.; Power, C. Gestational age and risk factors for cardiovascular disease: Evidence from the 1958 British birth cohort followed to mid-life. *Int. J. Epidemiol.* **2009**, *38*, 235–244. [CrossRef] [PubMed]
35. De Jong, F.; Monuteaux, M.C.; van Elburg, R.M.; Gillman, M.W.; Belfort, M.B. Systematic review and meta-analysis of preterm birth and later systolic blood pressure. *Hypertension* **2012**, *59*, 226–234. [CrossRef]
36. Popescu, C.R.; Sutherland, M.R.; Cloutier, A.; Benoît, G.; Bertagnolli, M.; Yzydorczyk, C.; Germain, N.; Phan, V.; Lelièvre-Pegorier, M.; Sartelet, H.; et al. Hyperoxia exposure impairs nephrogenesis in the neonatal rat: Role of HIF-1α. *PLoS ONE* **2013**, *8*, e82421. [CrossRef]
37. Mohr, J.; Voggel, J.; Vohlen, C.; Dinger, K.; Dafinger, C.; Fink, G.; Göbel, H.; Liebau, M.C.; Dötsch, J.; Alejandre Alcazar, M.A. IL-6/Smad2 signaling mediates acute kidney injury and regeneration in a murine model of neonatal hyperoxia. *FASEB J.* **2019**, *33*, 5887–5902. [CrossRef]
38. Yzydorczyk, C.; Comte, B.; Cambonie, G.; Lavoie, J.C.; Germain, N.; Ting Shun, Y.; Wolff, J.; Deschepper, C.; Touyz, R.M.; Lelièvre-Pegorier, M.; et al. Neonatal oxygen exposure in rats leads to cardiovascular and renal alterations in adulthood. *Hypertension* **2008**, *5*, 889–895. [CrossRef]
39. Chen, C.M.; Chou, H.C. Maternal inflammation exacerbates neonatal hyperoxia-induced kidney injury in rat offspring. *Pediatr. Res.* **2019**, *86*, 174–180. [CrossRef]
40. Chou, H.C.; Chen, C.M. Cathelicidin attenuates hyperoxia-induced kidney injury in newborn rats. *Ren. Fail.* **2019**, *41*, 733–741. [CrossRef]
41. Xu, X.; You, K.; Bu, R. Proximal Tubular Development Is Impaired with Downregulation of MAPK/ERK Signaling, HIF-1α, and Catalase by Hyperoxia Exposure in Neonatal Rats. *Oxidative Med. Cell Longev.* **2019**, *2019*, 9219847. [CrossRef] [PubMed]

42. Xu, X.; Zhang, X.; Gao, L.; Liu, C.; You, K. Neonatal Hyperoxia Downregulates Claudin-4, Occludin, and ZO-1 Expression in Rat Kidney Accompanied by Impaired Proximal Tubular Development. *Oxidative Med. Cell Longev.* **2020**, *2020*, 2641461. [CrossRef] [PubMed]
43. Sutherland, M.R.; Béland, C.; Lukaszewski, M.A.; Cloutier, A.; Bertagnolli, M.; Nuyt, A.M. Age- and sex-related changes in rat renal function and pathology following neonatal hyperoxia exposure. *Physiol. Rep.* **2016**, *15*, e12887. [CrossRef] [PubMed]
44. Kumar, V.H.S.; Wang, H.; Kishkurno, S.; Paturi, B.S.; Nielsen, L.; Ryan, R.M. Long-Term Effects of Neonatal Hyperoxia in Adult Mice. *Anat. Rec.* **2018**, *301*, 717–726. [CrossRef] [PubMed]
45. Hill, N.R.; Fatoba, S.T.; Oke, J.L.; Hirst, J.A.; O'Callaghan, C.A.; Lasserson, D.S.; Hobbs, F.D. Global Prevalence of Chronic Kidney Disease–A Systematic Review and Meta-Analysis. *PLoS ONE* **2016**, *7*, e0158765. [CrossRef]
46. Fogo, A.B. Mechanisms of progression of chronic kidney disease. *Pediatr. Nephrol.* **2007**, *22*, 2011–2022. [CrossRef] [PubMed]
47. Gewin, L.S. Renal fibrosis: Primacy of the proximal tubule. *Matrix Biol.* **2018**, *68–69*, 248–262. [CrossRef]
48. Gewin, L.; Zent, R.; Pozzi, A. Progression of chronic kidney disease: Too much cellular talk causes damage. *Kidney Int.* **2017**, *3*, 552–560. [CrossRef]
49. Oliveira, E.A.; Mak, R.H. Progression of chronic kidney disease in children-role of glomerular hemodynamics and interstitial fibrosis. *Curr. Opin. Pediatr.* **2018**, *2*, 220–227. [CrossRef] [PubMed]
50. Ishibe, S.; Cantley, L.G. Epithelial-mesenchymal-epithelial cycling in kidney repair. *Curr. Opin. Nephrol. Hypertens* **2008**, *17*, 379–385. [CrossRef] [PubMed]
51. Liu, Y. Cellular and molecular mechanisms of renal fibrosis. *Nat. Rev. Nephrol.* **2011**, *7*, 684–696. [CrossRef] [PubMed]
52. Hewitson, T.D.; Holt, S.G.; Smith, E.R. Progression of tubulointerstitial fibrosis and the chronic kidney disease phenotype-role of risk factors and epigenetics. *Front. Pharmacol.* **2017**, *8*, 520. [CrossRef] [PubMed]
53. Yang, L.; Besschetnova, T.Y.; Brooks, C.R.; Shah, J.V.; Bonventre, J.V. Epithelial cell cycle arrest in G2/M mediates kidney fibrosis after injury. *Nat. Med.* **2010**, *16*, 535–543. [CrossRef] [PubMed]
54. Hostetter, T.H.; Olson, J.L.; Rennke, H.G.; Venkatachalam, M.A.; Brenner, B.M. Hyperfiltration in remnant nephrons: A potentially adverse response to renal ablation. *Am. J. Physiol.* **1981**, *1*, F85–F93. [CrossRef] [PubMed]
55. Johnston, J.R.; Brenner, B.M.; Hebert, S.C. Uninephrectomy and dietary protein affect fluid absorption in rabbit proximal straight tubules. *Am. J. Physiol.* **1987**, *2 Pt 2*, F222–F233. [CrossRef] [PubMed]
56. Harris, D.C.; Chan, L.; Schrier, R.W. Remnant kidney hypermetabolism and progression of chronic renal failure. *Am. J. Phys.* **1988**, *2 Pt 2*, F267–F276. [CrossRef]
57. Chevalier, R.L. The proximal tubule is the primary target of injury and progression of kidney disease: Role of the glomerulotubular junction. *Am. J. Physiol. Ren. Physiol.* **2016**, *1*, F145–F161. [CrossRef]
58. Nath, K.A.; Croatt, A.J.; Hostetter, T.H. Oxygen consumption and oxidant stress in surviving nephrons. *Am. J. Physiol.* **1990**, *5 Pt 2*, F1354–F1362. [CrossRef]
59. Kriz, W.; Lemley, K.V. Mechanical challenges to the glomerular filtration barrier: Adaptations and pathway to sclerosis. *Pediatr. Nephrol.* **2017**, *32*, 405–417. [CrossRef]
60. Lamana, G.L.; Ferrari, A.L.L.; Gontijo, J.A.R.; Boer, P.A. Gestational and Breastfeeding Low-Protein Intake on Blood Pressure, Kidney Structure, and Renal Function in Male Rat Offspring in Adulthood. *Front. Physiol.* **2021**, *12*, 658431. [CrossRef]
61. Srivastava, T.; Thiagarajan, G.; Alon, U.S.; Sharma, R.; El-Meanawy, A.; McCarthy, E.T.; Savin, V.J.; Sharma, M. Role of biomechanical forces in hyperfiltration-mediated glomerular injury in congenital anomalies of the kidney and urinary tract. *Nephrol. Dial. Transplant.* **2017**, *32*, 759–765. [CrossRef]
62. Henderson, N.C.; Mackinnon, A.C.; Farnworth, S.L.; Kipari, T.; Haslett, C.; Iredale, J.P.; Liu, F.T.; Hughes, J.; Sethi, T. Galectin-3 expression and secretion links macrophages to the promotion of renal fibrosis. *Am. J. Pathol.* **2008**, *172*, 288–298. [CrossRef] [PubMed]
63. Bartlett, C.S.; Jeansson, M.; Quaggin, S.E. Vascular growth factors and glomerular disease. *Annu. Rev. Physiol.* **2016**, *78*, 437–461. [CrossRef]
64. Nagata, M. Podocyte injury and its consequences. *Kidney Int.* **2016**, *89*, 1221–1230. [CrossRef] [PubMed]
65. Miner, J.H. Podocyte biology in 2015: New insights into the mechanisms of podocyte health. *Nat. Rev. Nephrol.* **2016**, *12*, 63–64. [CrossRef]
66. Kriz, W.; LeHir, M. Pathways to nephron loss starting from glomerular diseases-insights from animal models. *Kidney Int.* **2005**, *2*, 404–419. [CrossRef] [PubMed]
67. Grahammer, F.; Wanner, N.; Huber, T.B. Podocyte regeneration: Who can become a podocyte? *Am. J. Pathol.* **2013**, *183*, 333–335. [CrossRef] [PubMed]
68. Schnaper, H.W. The Tubulointerstitial Pathophysiology of Progressive Kidney Disease. *Adv. Chronic. Kidney Dis.* **2017**, *2*, 107–116. [CrossRef]
69. Peired, A.; Angelotti, M.L.; Ronconi, E.; la Marca, G.; Mazzinghi, B.; Sisti, A.; Lombardi, D.; Giocaliere, E.; Della Bona, M.; Villanelli, F.; et al. Proteinuria impairs podocyte regeneration by sequestering retinoic acid. *J. Am. Soc. Nephrol.* **2013**, *11*, 1756–1768. [CrossRef]
70. Rizzo, P.; Perico, N.; Gagliardini, E.; Novelli, R.; Alison, M.R.; Remuzzi, G.; Benigni, A. Nature and mediators of parietal epithelial cell activation in glomerulonephritides of human and rat. *Am. J. Pathol.* **2013**, *6*, 1769–1778. [CrossRef]

71. Clark, W.F.; Macnab, J.J.; Sontrop, J.M.; Jain, A.K.; Moist, L.; Salvadori, M.; Suri, R.; Garg, A.X. Dipstick proteinuria as a screening strategy to identify rapid renal decline. *J. Am. Soc. Nephrol.* **2011**, *9*, 1729–1736. [CrossRef] [PubMed]
72. Zeisberg, M.; Hanai, J.; Sugimoto, H.; Mammoto, T.; Charytan, D.; Strutz, F.; Kalluri, R. BMP-7 counteracts TGF-beta1-induced epithelial-to-mesenchymal transition and reverses chronic renal injury. *Nat. Med.* **2003**, *9*, 964–968. [CrossRef] [PubMed]
73. Higgins, D.F.; Kimura, K.; Bernhardt, W.M.; Shrimanker, N.; Akai, Y.; Hohenstein, B.; Saito, Y.; Johnson, R.S.; Kretzler, M.; Cohen, C.D.; et al. Hypoxia promotes fibrogenesis in vivo via HIF-1 stimulation of epithelial-to-mesenchymal transition. *J. Clin. Investig.* **2007**, *117*, 3810–3820. [CrossRef]
74. Li, Y.; Yang, J.; Dai, C.; Wu, C.; Liu, Y. Role for integrin-linked kinase in mediating tubular epithelial to mesenchymal transition and renal interstitial fibrogenesis. *J. Clin. Investig.* **2003**, *112*, 503–516. [CrossRef] [PubMed]
75. Semenza, G.L. Hypoxia-inducible factors in physiology and medicine. *Cell* **2012**, *148*, 399.e408. [CrossRef]
76. Iyer, N.V.; Kotch, L.E.; Agani, F.; Leung, S.W.; Laughner, E.; Wenger, R.H.; Gassmann, M.; Gearhart, J.D.; Lawler, A.M.; Yu, A.Y.; et al. Cellular and developmental control of O_2 homeostasis by hypoxia-inducible factor 1 alpha. *Genes Dev.* **1998**, *12*, 149–162. [CrossRef] [PubMed]
77. Compernolle, V.; Brusselman, K.; Franco, D.; Moorman, A.; Dewerchin, M.; Collen, D.; Carmeliet, P. Cardia bifida, defective heart development and abnormal neural crest migration in embryos lacking hypoxia-inducible factor-1alpha. *Cardiovasc. Res.* **2003**, *60*, 569–579. [CrossRef] [PubMed]
78. Pugh, C.W.; Ratcliffe, P.J. Regulation of angiogenesis by hypoxia: Role of the HIF system. *Nat. Med.* **2003**, *9*, 677–684. [CrossRef]
79. Carmeliet, P.; Dor, Y.; Herbert, J.M.; Fukumura, D.; Brusselmans, K.; Dewerchin, M.; Neeman, M.; Bono, F.; Abramovitch, R.; Maxwell, P.; et al. Role of HIF-1alpha in hypoxia-mediated apoptosis, cell proliferation and tumour angiogenesis. *Nature* **1998**, *394*, 485–490. [CrossRef]
80. Ryan, H.E.; Lo, J.; Johnson, R.S. HIF-1 alpha is required for solid tumor formation and embryonic vascularization. *EMBO J.* **1998**, *17*, 3005–3015. [CrossRef]
81. Nazıroğlu, M. Molecular role of catalase on oxidative stress-induced Ca (2+) signaling and TRP cation channel activation in nervous system. *J. Recept. Signal Transduct. Res.* **2012**, *3*, 134–141. [CrossRef]
82. Ding, W.; Wang, B.; Zhang, M.; Gu, Y. Tempol, a Superoxide Dismutase-Mimetic Drug, Ameliorates Progression of Renal Disease in CKD Mice. *Cell Physiol. Biochem.* **2015**, *6*, 2170–2182. [CrossRef] [PubMed]
83. Hafstad, A.D.; Nabeebaccus, A.A.; Shah, A.M. Novel aspects of ROS signalling in heart failure. *Basic Res. Cardiol.* **2013**, *108*, 359. [CrossRef] [PubMed]
84. Marshall, J.C. Inflammation, coagulopathy, and the pathogenesis of multiple organ dysfunction syndrome. *Crit. Care Med.* **2001**, *29*, S99–S106. [CrossRef] [PubMed]
85. Cohen, J. The immunopathogenesis of sepsis. *Nature* **2002**, *420*, 885–891. [CrossRef] [PubMed]
86. Su, H.; Lei, C.T.; Zhang, C. Interleukin-6 Signaling Pathway and Its Role in Kidney Disease: An Update. *Front. Immunol.* **2017**, *8*, 405. [CrossRef] [PubMed]
87. Choi, C.W.; Kim, B.I.; Kim, H.-S.; Park, J.D.; Choi, J.-H.; Son, D.W. Increase of interleukin-6 in tracheal aspirate at birth: A predictor of subsequent bronchopulmonary dysplasia in preterm infants. *Acta Paediatr.* **2006**, *95*, 38–43. [CrossRef]
88. Lecart, C.; Cayabyab, R.; Buckley, S.; Morrison, J.; Kwong, K.Y.; Warburton, D.; Ramanathan, R.; Jones, C.A.; Minoo, P. Bioactive transforming growth factor-beta in the lungs of extremely low birthweight neonates predicts the need for home oxygen supplementation. *Biol. Neonate* **2000**, *77*, 217–223. [CrossRef]
89. Hsiao, C.C.; Chang, J.C.; Tsao, L.Y.; Yang, R.C.; Chen, H.N.; Lee, C.H.; Lin, C.Y.; Tsai, Y.G. Correlates of Elevated Interleukin-6 and 8-Hydroxy-2′-Deoxyguanosine Levels in Tracheal Aspirates from Very Low Birth Weight Infants Who Develop Bronchopulmonary Dysplasia. *Pediatr. Neonatol.* **2017**, *1*, 63–69. [CrossRef]
90. Johnston, C.J.; Wright, T.W.; Reed, C.K.; Finkelstein, J.N. Comparison of adult and newborn pulmonary cytokine mRNA expression after hyperoxia. *Exp. Lung Res.* **1997**, *23*, 537–552. [CrossRef]
91. Jiang, J.S.; Chou, H.C.; Chen, C.M. Cathelicidin attenuates hyperoxia-induced lung injury by inhibiting oxidative stress in newborn rats. *Free Radic. Biol. Med.* **2020**, *150*, 23–29. [CrossRef] [PubMed]
92. Bowie, A.; O'Neill, L.A. Oxidative stress and nuclear factor-kappa B activation: A reassessment of the evidence in the light of recent discoveries. *Biochem. Pharmacol.* **2000**, *59*, 13–23. [CrossRef]
93. Gewin, L. The many talents of transforming growth factor-β in the kidney. *Curr. Opin. Nephrol. Hypertens* **2019**, *3*, 203–210. [CrossRef] [PubMed]
94. Koesters, R.; Kaissling, B.; Lehir, M.; Picard, N.; Theilig, F.; Gebhardt, R.; Glick, A.B.; Hähnel, B.; Hosser, H.; Gröne, H.J.; et al. Tubular overexpression of transforming growth factorbeta1 induces autophagy and fibrosis but not mesenchymal transition of renal epithelial cells. *Am. J. Pathol.* **2010**, *2*, 632–643. [CrossRef]
95. Samarakoon, R.; Higgins, P.J. The Cytoskeletal Network Regulates Expression of the Profibrotic Genes PAI-1 and CTGF in Vascular Smooth Muscle Cells. *Adv. Pharmacol.* **2018**, *81*, 79–94.
96. Chen, J.T.; Wang, C.Y.; Chen, M.H. Curcumin inhibits TGF-β1-induced connective tissue growth factor expression through the interruption of Smad2 signaling in human gingival fibroblasts. *J. Formos. Med. Assoc.* **2018**, *12*, 1115–1123. [CrossRef]
97. Sand, J.M.; Leeming, D.J.; Byrjalsen, I.; Bihlet, A.R.; Lange, P.; Tal-Singer, R.; Miller, B.E.; Karsdal, M.A.; Vestbo, J. High levels of biomarkers of collagen remodeling are associated with increased mortality in COPD-results from the ECLIPSE study. *Respir. Res.* **2016**, *1*, 125. [CrossRef] [PubMed]

98. Will, J.P.; Hirani, D.; Thielen, F.; Klein, F.; Vohlen, C.; Dinger, K.; Dötsch, J.; Alejandre Alcázar, M.A. Strain-dependent effects on lung structure, matrix remodeling, and Stat3/Smad2 signaling in C57BL/6N and C57BL/6J mice after neonatal hyperoxia. *Am. J. Physiol. Regul. Integr. Comp. Physiol.* **2019**, *1*, R169–R181. [CrossRef] [PubMed]
99. Dasgupta, C.; Sakurai, R.; Wang, Y.; Guo, P.; Ambalavanan, N.; Torday, J.S.; Rehan, V.K. Hyperoxia-induced neonatal rat lung injury involves activation of TGF-{beta} and Wnt signaling and is protected by rosiglitazone. *Am. J. Physiol. Lung Cell Mol. Physiol.* **2009**, *6*, L1031–L1041. [CrossRef] [PubMed]
100. Zhou, L.; Chen, X.; Lu, M.; Wu, Q.; Yuan, Q.; Hu, C.; Miao, J.; Zhang, Y.; Li, H.; Hou, F.F.; et al. Wnt/β-catenin links oxidative stress to podocyte injury and proteinuria. *Kidney Int.* **2019**, *4*, 830–845. [CrossRef]
101. Angers, S.; Moon, R.T. Proximal events in Wnt signal transduction. *Nat. Rev. Mol. Cell. Biol.* **2009**, *10*, 468–477. [CrossRef] [PubMed]
102. Clevers, H.; Nusse, R. Wnt/beta-catenin signaling and disease. *Cell* **2012**, *149*, 1192–1205. [CrossRef]
103. Zhou, D.; Tan, R.J.; Fu, H.; Liu, Y. Wnt/beta-catenin signaling in kidney injury and repair: A double-edged sword. *Lab. Investig.* **2016**, *96*, 156–167. [CrossRef]
104. Schunk, S.J.; Floege, J.; Fliser, D.; Speer, T. WNT-β-catenin signalling-A versatile player in kidney injury and repair. *Nat. Rev. Nephrol.* **2021**, *17*, 172–184. [CrossRef]
105. Zhou, L.; Li, Y.; Hao, S.; Zhou, D.; Tan, R.J.; Nie, J.; Hou, F.F.; Kahn, M.; Liu, Y. Multiple genes of the renin-angiotensin system are novel targets of Wnt/beta-catenin signaling. *J. Am. Soc. Nephrol.* **2015**, *26*, 107–120. [CrossRef] [PubMed]
106. Xiao, L.; Zhou, D.; Tan, R.J.; Fu, H.; Zhou, L.; Hou, F.F.; Liu, Y. Sustained activation of Wnt/beta-catenin signaling drives AKI to CKD progression. *J. Am. Soc. Nephrol.* **2016**, *27*, 1727–1740. [CrossRef] [PubMed]
107. Zhou, L.; Mo, H.; Miao, J.; Zhou, D.; Tan, R.J.; Hou, F.F.; Liu, Y. Klotho ameliorates kidney injury and fibrosis and normalizes blood pressure by targeting the renin-angiotensin system. *Am. J. Pathol.* **2015**, *185*, 3211–3223. [CrossRef]
108. Dai, C.; Stolz, D.B.; Kiss, L.P.; Monga, S.P.; Holzman, L.B.; Liu, Y. Wnt/beta-catenin signaling promotes podocyte dysfunction and albuminuria. *J. Am. Soc. Nephrol.* **2009**, *20*, 1997–2008. [CrossRef]
109. Cox, S.N.; Sallustio, F.; Serino, G.; Pontrelli, P.; Verrienti, R.; Pesce, F.; Torres, D.D.; Ancona, N.; Stifanelli, P.; Zaza, G.; et al. Altered modulation of WNT-beta catenin and PI3K/Akt pathways in IgA nephropathy. *Kidney Int.* **2010**, *78*, 396–407. [CrossRef]
110. Wang, X.D.; Huang, X.F.; Yan, Q.R.; Bao, C.D. Aberrant activation of the WNT/beta catenin signaling pathway in lupus nephritis. *PLoS ONE* **2014**, *9*, e84852.
111. Li, C.; Siragy, H.M. High glucose induces podocyte injury via enhanced (pro) renin receptor-Wnt-catenin-snail signaling pathway. *PLoS ONE* **2014**, *9*, e89233. [CrossRef] [PubMed]
112. Lin, T.; Tao, J.; Chen, Y.; Zhang, Y.; Li, F.; Zhang, Y.; Han, X.; Zhao, Z.; Liu, G.; Li, H. Selenium Deficiency Leads to Changes in Renal Fibrosis Marker Proteins and Wnt/β-Catenin Signaling Pathway Components. *Biol. Trace Elem. Res.* **2022**, *3*, 1127–1139. [CrossRef] [PubMed]
113. DiRocco, D.P.; Kobayashi, A.; Taketo, M.M.; McMahon, A.P.; Humphreys, B.D. Wnt4/β-catenin signaling in medullary kidney myofibroblasts. *J. Am. Soc. Nephrol.* **2013**, *9*, 1399–1412. [CrossRef] [PubMed]
114. Zhou, D.; Fu, H.; Zhang, L.; Zhang, K.; Min, Y.; Xiao, L.; Lin, L.; Bastacky, S.I.; Liu, Y. Tubule-derived Wnts are required for fibroblast activation and kidney fibrosis. *J. Am. Soc. Nephrol.* **2017**, *8*, 2322–2336. [CrossRef] [PubMed]
115. Nlandu-Khodo, S.; Neelisetty, S.; Phillips, M.; Manolopoulou, M.; Bhave, G.; May, L.; Clark, P.E.; Yang, H.; Fogo, A.B.; Harris, R.C.; et al. Blocking TGF-beta and beta-catenin epithelial crosstalk exacerbates CKD. *J. Am. Soc. Nephrol.* **2017**, *12*, 3490–3503. [CrossRef]
116. Fine, L.G.; Norman, J.T. Chronic hypoxia as a mechanism of progression of chronic kidney diseases: From hypothesis to novel therapeutics. *Kidney Int.* **2008**, *74*, 867–872. [CrossRef]
117. Neusser, M.A.; Lindenmeyer, M.T.; Moll, A.G.; Segerer, S.; Edenhofer, I.; Sen, K.; Stiehl, D.P.; Kretzler, M.; Grone, H.J.; Schlondorff, D.; et al. Human nephrosclerosis triggers a hypoxia-related glomerulopathy. *Am. J. Pathol.* **2010**, *176*, 594–607. [CrossRef]

Article

Oxidative Stress Response's Kinetics after 60 Minutes at Different (30% or 100%) Normobaric Hyperoxia Exposures

Clément Leveque [1,2], Simona Mrakic-Sposta [3], Pierre Lafère [1,2,4], Alessandra Vezzoli [3], Peter Germonpré [1,4,5], Alexandre Beer [1], Stéphane Mievis [1], Fabio Virgili [6], Kate Lambrechts [1], Sigrid Theunissen [1], François Guerrero [2] and Costantino Balestra [1,4,7,8,*]

1. Environmental, Occupational, Aging (Integrative) Physiology Laboratory, Haute Ecole Bruxelles-Brabant (HE2B), 1160 Brussels, Belgium
2. Laboratoire ORPHY, EA 4324, Université de Bretagne Occidentale, 29238 Brest, France
3. Institute of Clinical Physiology, National Research Council (CNR), 20162 Milan, Italy
4. DAN Europe Research Division (Roseto-Brussels), 1020 Brussels, Belgium
5. Hyperbaric Centre, Queen Astrid Military Hospital, 1120 Brussels, Belgium
6. Council for Agricultural Research and Economics-Food and Nutrition Research Centre (C.R.E.A.-AN), 00187 Rome, Italy
7. Anatomical Research and Clinical Studies, Vrije Universiteit Brussels (VUB), 1090 Brussels, Belgium
8. Motor Sciences Department, Physical Activity Teaching Unit, Université Libre de Bruxelles (ULB), 1050 Brussels, Belgium
* Correspondence: costantinobalestra@gmail.com

Abstract: Oxygen is a powerful trigger for cellular reactions and is used in many pathologies, including oxidative stress. However, the effects of oxygen over time and at different partial pressures remain poorly understood. In this study, the metabolic responses of normobaric oxygen intake for 1 h to mild (30%) and high (100%) inspired fractions were investigated. Fourteen healthy non-smoking subjects (7 males and 7 females; age: 29.9 ± 11.1 years; height: 168.2 ± 9.37 cm; weight: 64.4 ± 12.3 kg; BMI: 22.7 ± 4.1) were randomly assigned in the two groups. Blood samples were taken before the intake at 30 min, 2 h, 8 h, 24 h, and 48 h after the single oxygen exposure. The level of oxidation was evaluated by the rate of reactive oxygen species (ROS) and the levels of isoprostane. Antioxidant reactions were observed by total antioxidant capacity (TAC), superoxide dismutase (SOD), and catalase (CAT). The inflammatory response was measured using interleukin-6 (IL-6), neopterin, creatinine, and urates. Oxidation markers increased from 30 min on to reach a peak at 8 h. From 8 h post intake, the markers of inflammation took over, and more significantly with 100% than with 30%. This study suggests a biphasic response over time characterized by an initial "permissive oxidation" followed by increased inflammation. The antioxidant protection system seems not to be the leading actor in the first place. The kinetics of enzymatic reactions need to be better studied to establish therapeutic, training, or rehabilitation protocols aiming at a more targeted use of oxygen.

Keywords: normobaric oxygen paradox; hyperoxic–hypoxic paradox; hyperoxia; oxygen biology; cellular reactions; human; oxygen therapy; human performance; decompression; diving

1. Introduction

Oxygen, the third most abundant element in the biosphere, is mostly known for its role in the development and ability to sustain aerobic organisms [1], and it is administered as a therapeutic agent [2]. Indeed, oxygen is considered as a cornerstone of modern medical care within well-defined limits to mitigate adverse effects [3]. Nowadays, oxygen use is not only limited to counteract hypoxia or restore patient saturation. New research paths have coined the use of several inhaled oxygen fractions (FiO$_2$) in the physiology of aging [4,5], such as cartilage degeneration [6], prediabetes [7], or neuroprotection [8]. It must be acknowledged that variable FiO$_2$, hypoxic or hyperoxic, is already relatively common, for instance, for preconditioning in cardiovascular disease [9,10], sports training [11], and before exposure to challenging environments such as scuba diving [12], high altitude military parachute freefall [13,14], and space flight activities [15].

Under physiological conditions, unstable molecules derived from oxygen called reactive oxygen species (ROS; i.e., superoxide anions ($O_2\bullet-$), hydroxyl radicals ($\bullet OH$), peroxyl radicals ($ROO\bullet$), and alkoxy radicals ($RO\bullet$)), are primary signals to modulate several pathways involved in homeostasis and cell proliferation/differentiation/survival [16,17].

ROS increase due to environmental and/or chemical stimuli. When ROS increase and the endogenous antioxidant system (enzymatic and/or non-enzymatic) is perturbed, oxidative stress is triggered. This results in damage to lipids, proteins, and DNA [18–20].

Furthermore, it is known that oxidative stress, inflammation, the immune system, and metabolism are intricately intertwined [21,22]. Specific inflammatory cytokines utilize ROS as part of their signaling cascades, and these can contribute to the development and/or progression of acute or chronic inflammatory responses [23].

Our previous works highlighted the non-linearity of the dose–response curve, which makes the definition of an optimal oxygen dose difficult.

Based on the current literature, several factors such as FiO_2 [11,15,24,25], duration and frequency [26–28], or pressure of exposure—either normobaric, hypobaric, or hyperbaric [15,26,29]—may influence the ability to reach a specific clinical or molecular effect.

Although some mechanisms were identified, there is a lack of data regarding the kinetics of the cellular response to those different oxygen partial pressures.

Therefore, the objective of this study is to describe the kinetics of cell expression in response to a single exposure at different FiO_2 percentages (30% and 100%) in normobaric conditions only.

2. Results

2.1. Reactive Oxygen Species (ROS) Rate and Isoprostane Levels after One Hour of Oxygen Exposure at a FiO_2 of 30% or 100%

Both oxygen exposures, 30% and 100%, elicited a significant increase of plasmatic ROS production rate (Figure 1A). Both responses were similar in amplitude and shape, characterized by a significant increase with a peak at 8 h after exposure (30%: 0.24 ± 0.01 µmol.min^{-1}; 100%: 0.25 ± 0.04 µmol.min^{-1}) followed by a decrease after 30%, reaching a plateau after 100%. At 48 h, there was a significant difference between oxygen concentrations (30%: 0.21 ± 0.01 µmol.min^{-1}; 100%: 0.23 ± 0.01 µmol.min^{-1}; $p = 0.012$, unpaired t test). Isoprostane (8-iso-PGF 2α), a biomarker of lipid peroxidation (Figure 1B), followed the same trend for both oxygen exposures with a peak at 2 h after 30% exposure (498.7 $\pm$ 99.55 pg.mg^{-1}; 100%: 499.1 $\pm$ 164.0 pg.mg^{-1}; $p = 0.0078$). At 48 h the baseline was reached for both exposures (30%: 266.4 $\pm$ 95.67 pg.mg^{-1}; 100%: 281.2 $\pm$ 135.3 pg.mg^{-1}; $p = 0.63$ and 0.99, respectively).

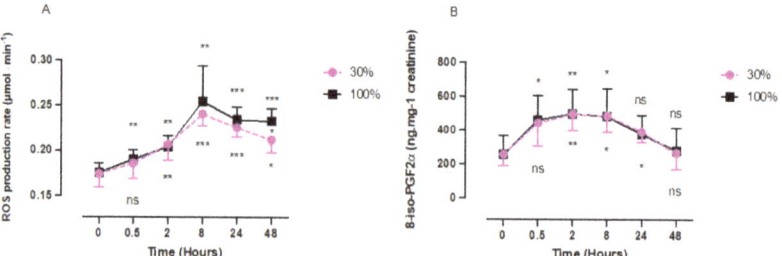

Figure 1. Evolution of ROS (**A**) production rate and isoprostane level (**B**) after 60 min of mild (30%, n = 6) or high (100%, n = 8) hyperoxia. Results are expressed as mean $\pm$ SD. T0 represents pre-exposure baseline (ns: not significant; *: $p < 0.05$, **: $p < 0.01$, ***: $p < 0.001$; intragroup: one-way ANOVA; intergroup: unpaired t test).

2.2. Antioxidant Response (TAC, SOD, CAT) after One Hour of Oxygen Exposure at a FiO$_2$ of 30% or 100%

Figure 2 illustrates the antioxidant response as a function of blood total antioxidant capacity (TAC), superoxide dismutase (SOD), and catalase (CAT) concentration. SOD and CAT activities were not modified by oxygen exposure (30%: 3.9 ± 0.9 U/mL and 25.9 ± 7.5 U/mL, respectively; 100%: 4.1 ± 0.9 U/mL and 24.7 ± 6.3 U/mL, respectively). Nonetheless, compared to 100%, after being exposed at 30%, the TAC was significantly increased 24 h after the end of exposure (3.8 ± 0.5 M vs. 2.9 ± 0.3 mM; $p = 0.004$, unpaired t test). However, compared to baseline, this difference was not significant ($p = 0.32$, one-way ANOVA).

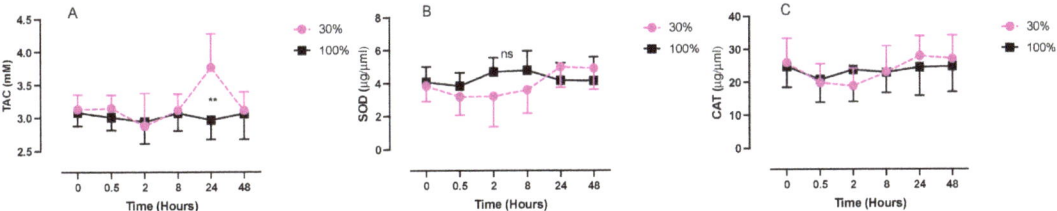

Figure 2. Evolution of the antioxidant response after 60 min of mild (30%, n = 6) or high hyperoxia (100%, n = 8). (**A**) Total antioxidant capacity (TAC). (**B**) Superoxide dismutase activity (SOD). (**C**) Catalase activity (CAT). Results are expressed as mean ± SD. T0 represents pre-exposure (ns: not significant, **: $p < 0.01$; intragroup one-way ANOVA; intergroup unpaired t test).

2.3. Inflammatory Response (IL-6, Neopterin, Creatinine, and Urates) after One Hour of Oxygen Exposure at a FiO$_2$ of 30% or 100%

Interleukin 6 (IL-6) was measured in plasma samples, while neopterin, creatinine, and urates were obtained from urine samples (Figure 3).

IL-6 followed a similar pattern in both conditions, although with a late higher amplitude after 100% exposure. It was characterized by a significant decrease in concentration followed by a rebound without returning to the baseline. The nadir was reach after 2 h (30%: 2.0 ± 1.0 pg/mL; 100%: 3.9 ± 2.7 pg/mL; $p = 0.017$ and $p = 0.015$, respectively, one-way ANOVA), while the acme was reached after 24 h (30%: 8.8 ± 4.6 pg/mL; 100%: 14.7 ± 2.7 pg/mL; $p > 0.99$ and $p = 0.001$, respectively, one-way ANOVA).

From 8 h post-exposure and beyond, the two curves significantly diverged (8 h: $p = 0.001$; 24 h: $p = 0.04$; 48 h: $p = 0.008$, unpaired t test).

Neopterin exhibited a similar pattern, although the magnitudes of the changes were reduced. These changes were not statistically significant.

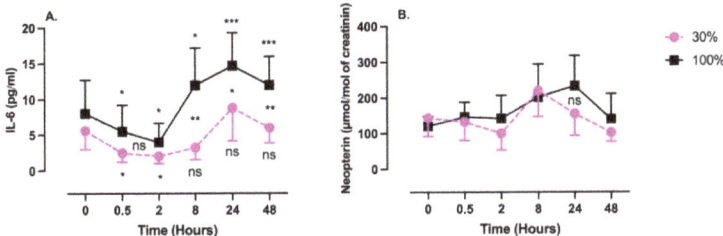

Figure 3. Evolution of the inflammatory response after 60 min of mild (30%, n = 6) or high hyperoxia (100%, n = 8). (**A**) Interleukin-6 (IL-6). (**B**) Neopterin. Results are expressed as mean ± SD. T0 represents pre-exposure (ns: not significant; *: $p < 0.05$, **: $p < 0.01$, ***: $p < 0.001$; intragroup: one-way ANOVA; intergroup: unpaired t test).

Creatinine and urates in urine exhibited opposite U-shaped responses, with a creatinine nadir between 2- and 8-h post-exposure and an urate acme within the same time frame (Figure 4), although compared to the baseline, these variations were not statistically significant (one-way ANOVA). There was, however, a significant difference in the urate's kinetics. It was characterized by a stronger initial response after exposure at 100% (30 min: 25.2 ± 5.5 mg/dL vs. 15.5 ± 3.8 mg/dL, p = 0.03; and 2 h, 35.2 ± 7.5 mg/dL vs. 18.7 ± 8.5 mg/dL, p = 0.005; unpaired t test).

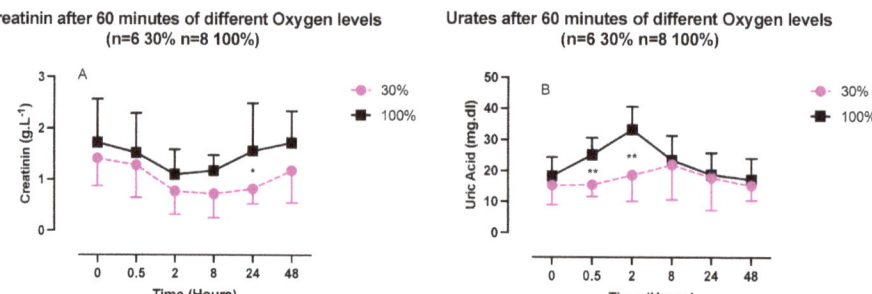

Figure 4. Evolution of urinary markers after 60 min of mild (30%, n = 6) or high hyperoxia (100%, n = 8). (A) Creatinine. (B) Uric Acid. Results are expressed as mean ± SD. T0 represents pre-exposure (ns: not significant; *: p < 0.05, **: p < 0.01; intragroup: one-way ANOVA; intergroup: unpaired t test).

2.4. Percent of Expressed Proteins and Reactive Oxygen Species (ROS) after One Hour of Oxygen Exposure at a FiO_2 of 30% or 100%

The magnitude and direction of changes among all results are illustrated in Figure 5.

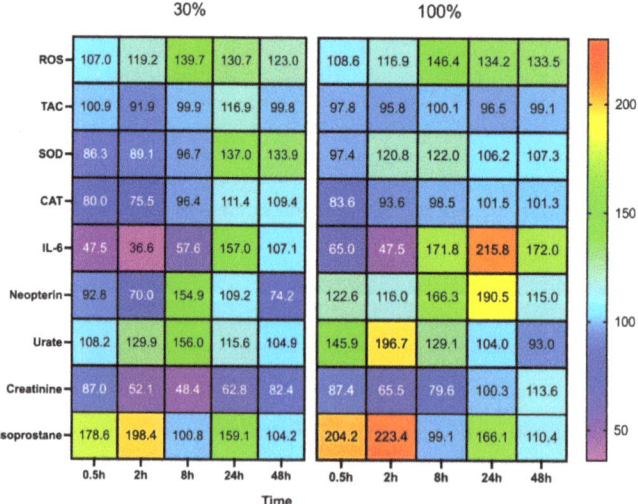

Figure 5. Heat map of percent changes compared to baseline, derived responses after 60 min of mild (30%, n = 6) or high hyperoxia (100%, n = 8). Each measurement is compared to baseline (T0), which was set at 100%. Results are given as mean change.

3. Discussion

Hormesis in mammals is defined as an adaptation capacity to different stresses, which encompasses dynamic processes of repair, recovery, and toxicity that occur over time [30]. At the most basic level, it is mediated through "dose–response" and "dose–time" combinations to oxidative stress, metabolic changes, and inflammation [31]. This is a well-known process in pathological situations [32] or ageing. Indeed, the age-related imbalance between pro- and anti-inflammatory factors is a recognized etiology for metabolic, cardiovascular, and neurodegenerative diseases [33].

Until a decade ago, ROS were thought to cause exclusively toxic effects and were associated with various pathologies [34]; with time, this view has changed, considering that the presence of ROS in cells indicates that ROS production was evolutionarily selected in order to achieve certain useful roles [35]. It is now accepted that biological specificity of ROS action is achieved through the amount, duration, and localization of their production, as we underline in this study.

More recent data have encouraged us to investigate a new paradigm, namely, to consider oxygen as a potent stimulus of molecular complex reactions rather than a simple drug [36].

Several studies exploring the effect of pulsed hyperoxia demonstrated that it is possible to stimulate the production of hypoxia inducible factor (HIF-1α), which was believed to be expressed only under hypoxic conditions—hence its name.

This phenomenon is called the "normobaric oxygen paradox" [25,26,37] or the "hyperoxic–hypoxic paradox" [24] (for a global view of the mechanisms, see Figure 6).

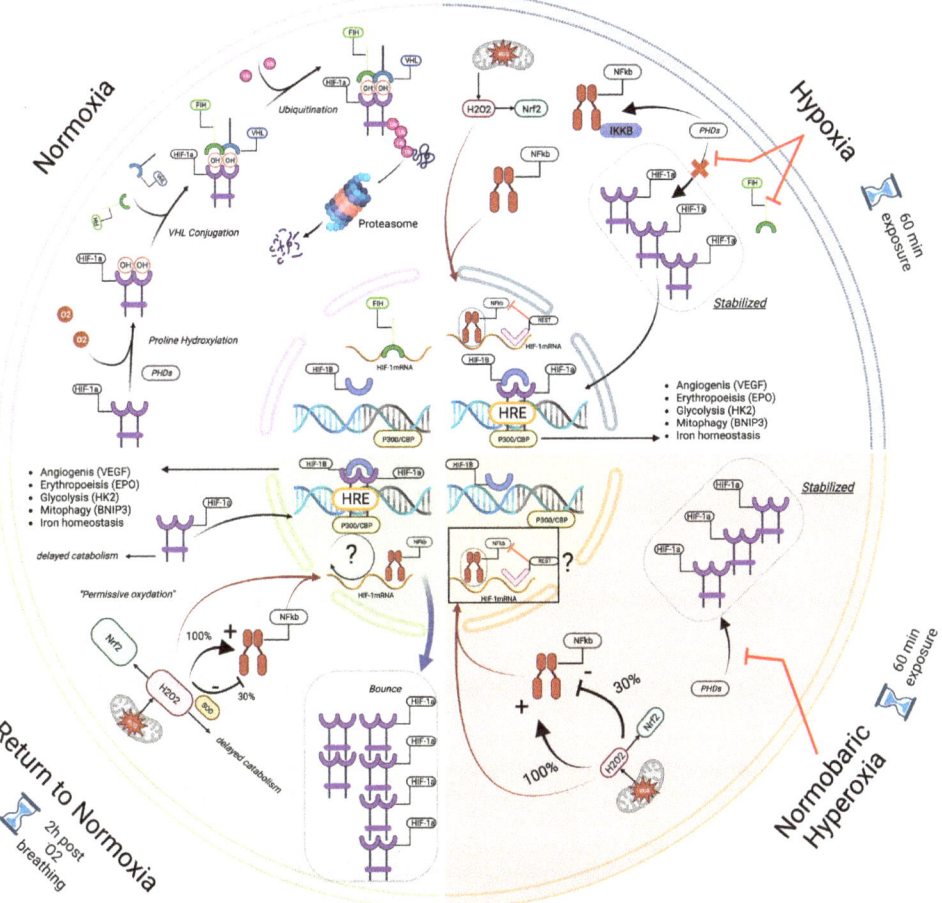

Figure 6. Illustration (created with Biorender.com) of the mechanisms involved during the normobaric oxygen paradox: First, in normoxia, HIF−1α is constantly produced and destroyed by the intervention

of PHDs and FIH. During hypoxia and intermittent hyperoxia, the stabilization in the cytosol of HIF−1α protein is improved by repressing the activity of isoforms 1 to 3 of prolyly hydroxylase (PHDs) and of FIH (only in hypoxia), whereas nuclear synthesis is blocked by inhibiting proteins such as REST. Therefore, during these altered oxygen states, immune activation seems to start earlier than antioxidant defenses, allowing subtle kinetics between inflammation and ROS, in their role similar to a "second messenger". Upon the return to normoxia, the destabilization of HIF−1α by the intervention of PHD and FIH is delayed by the late activation of antioxidant protection, leaving the cell in a state of "permissive oxidation". Following this, nuclear synthesis begins earlier, explaining the rebound phenomenon encountered in the production of HIF−1α. NRF2 and NF-κB are overexpressed after 100%, whereas under 30% only NRF2 is stimulated.

During these interventions, the return to normoxia after mild hyperoxia is sensed as a hypoxic stress without significant NF-κB activation [29]. On the contrary, high and very high hyperoxia induce a shift toward an oxidative stress response, characterized by NRF2 and NF-κB activation in the first 24 h post-exposure. These observations suggest a modulated cellular response to targeted oxygen exposure [29]. This is further confirmed by microparticle expression under different oxygen partial pressures. All tested exposures demonstrated significant elevations of CD41, CD66b, TMEM, and expression and phalloidin binding, except for 1.4 ATA, which elicited the total opposite response with significant decreases of all measured parameters [15].

As shown in previous studies, oxygen breathing induced a hormetic stimulus, eliciting increased ROS production starting from 30 min post-exposure.

Our results suggest that there is no difference in the initial response intensity between the two groups (100% and 30%). However, after the acme, which is reached 8 h post-exposure, the kinetics starts to diverge with a between-group statistical difference at 48 h. In addition, the increase of isoprostanes testifies that the production rate of ROS is already significant enough to produce lipid peroxidation. This must be considered together with the kinetics of the antioxidant response of SOD and CAT.

The absence of an intracellular antioxidant response (CAT and SOD), despite the production of ROS over time, suggests that the cell abides a state of "permissive oxidation" and might be explained by the fact that some diurnal variations are possible and also that some circadian rhythms are opposite in males and females for some antioxidants or enzymes [38]; we may consider that since our group was a mix of males and females, at a given point some concomitant situations may result in non-statistically significant changes.

The significantly higher total antioxidant capacity for a low level of hyperoxia such as 30% recorded at 24 h might be caused by food intake. Furthermore, TAC variations are probably not the most reliable measurement in our experimental setting, given the fact that we followed the participants for 48 h without diet restriction. Some other hyperoxia-induced oxidative stress or transient hypoxia resulting from sleep apnea may also increase myeloid cell recruitment and activation in the lungs. Activated myeloid cells produce myeloperoxidase (MPO), which oxidizes chloride ions to hypochlorous acid, causing oxidative damage and even cell dead [39]. This mechanism, even if important, has been analyzed upon prolonged exposures of several days and may not be preeminent in our experimental setting.

Our results could be explained by the cellular needs for second messengers, such as H_2O_2, as mediators likely to act through NRF2 activation, inducing the release of keap1 expression [40]. Although it is now accepted that HIF-1α is the leading agent in the regulation of homeostasis during hypoxia [41] and hyperoxia [26], other regulating factors must be considered, such as NRF2. For instance, repressor element 1-silencing transcription factor (REST) is a known nuclear inhibitor of HIF-1α synthesis [42]. During exposure to hypoxia, REST accumulates in the nucleus with a four-fold increase compared to normoxia. This can be quickly reversed by reoxygenation [43].

To the best of our knowledge, the evaluation of REST in hyperoxia has not yet been studied. However, keeping in mind that NOP has the capacity to mimic hypoxia [25,36,44] and is therefore a powerful tool to trigger a hormetic response, it may be used as a reasonable hypothesis to suggests that the lower the hyperoxia delta, the longer the permissive oxidative state, allowing the secondary cellular messengers [45] to potentiate their nuclear transcription role and trigger a strong and rapid response (within the first 3 h). Indeed, recent data demonstrate epigenic changes by methylation/demethylation upon gene expression are related to oxygen homeostasis [46]. The kinetics of these oxygen-induced activation/deactivation mechanisms are dependent upon enzymatic reactions where the role of 2-oxoglutarate dioxygenase seems to be decisive [47].

Alternatively, this could be also explained by a slower kinetics of intracellular defenses. Indeed, we have recently demonstrated that after 30% oxygen exposure, the synthesis of glutathione is effective only after 24 h, whereas after exposure at 100%, its synthesis and release occur earlier, approximately 3 h post-exposure [29].

This latter study also demonstrated that the inflammatory response was different between these two conditions (30% and 100%). Exposure at 30% of oxygen was associated with a significant increase in NRF2 without a significant increase in NF-κB, while an exposure at 100% elicited significant activation of inflammatory pathways mediated by NF-κB [29]. Interestingly, our results are consistent with this observation. First, Il-6 expression within the first two hours post-exposure can be explained by synthesis repression related to parallel NRF2 activation [48]. Second, the greater amplitude of IL-6 expression after the exposure at 100% suggests a shift in the cross-linked pathway of NRF2/NF-κB [49]. Although not significant, neopterin shares a similar pattern from inhibition to overexpression with a return to baseline within 24 h. Since this molecule is indicative of a pro-inflammatory with the recruitment of cellular immunity and the induction of apoptosis, its scheme might suggest the possibility that NOP is able to produce immunomodulation. However, to reach significant levels of modulation, more sessions will be needed, as has recently been shown for 30% and 100% FiO_2 after 5 weeks of regular sessions three times per week [11]. Isoprostane changes are parallel for both exposures, and lipid damage follows ROS production in both percentages (30% and 100%) of administered O_2.

Other recent data on platelet (CD41a)-, astrocyte (TMEM119)-, and neutrophil (CD66+)-related microparticle release after oxygen exposure (30% and 100%) [15] are consistent with this analysis.

The more potent initial inflammatory response triggered by exposure at 100% is also confirmed based on uric acid measurements. Circulating uric acid is a major aqueous antioxidant in humans, especially for peroxynitrites (ONOO–) in the hydrophilic environment. However, uric acid becomes a powerful pro-oxidant under hydrophobic conditions. Uric acid can induce intracellular and mitochondrial oxidative stress and stimulate expression of inflammatory cytokines [30].

Finally, although not significant, the creatinine pattern is consistent with other results of this study, especially ROS and uric acid. Indeed, creatine kinase is inhibited by ROS, especially H_2O_2 [31], while uric acid acts as an iron chelator in extracellular fluids, which is a co-factor to creatine kinase activity [30]. Evidently, urates may be related to ROS generation (particularly under oxidative stress conditions), for example, when interacting with peroxynitrite, resulting in the formation of active but less reactive products [50].

It can thus be assumed that the observed increase in the ROS level in plasma after moderate hyperoxia (FiO_2 of 30%) is associated not with the elevation of oxidative stress but with the protective mechanism harnessed by the body during the neutralization of highly reactive peroxynitrite with uric acid [51]. The results obtained by Gu et al. also suggest that hyperoxia-induced peroxynitrite formation causes endothelial cell apoptosis, disrupting key survival pathways, and that blocking peroxynitrite formation prevents apoptosis.

Limitations

Strengths:

— This study is to our knowledge one of the first to tackle the kinetics of responses to a single normobaric oxygen exposure at 30% and 100% of FiO_2.

- The measurements were conducted until 48 h post exposure and putatively open the door to new possible therapeutic outcomes for oxygen administration protocols.
- The sampling was a standard plasmatic withdrawal, and the analysis is possible in a usual clinical setting without very specialized machinery or procedures.

Weaknesses:

- The number of subjects is limited, but the sample can be considered to be homogenous since all were healthy young students and gender balanced.
- The analysis was not made in the nucleus of the cells but in the plasma; this could be considered a weakness for some, but analysis in the nucleus would need a thoroughly different experimental setting.

4. Materials and Methods

4.1. Experimental Protocol

Fourteen healthy subjects (7 females and 7 males) volunteered for this study, after approval from the Bio-Ethical Committee for Research and Higher Education, Brussels (No. B200-2020-088), and written informed consent was obtained. All experimental procedures were conducted in accordance with the Declaration of Helsinki [52].

After medical screening to exclude any comorbidity, participants were prospectively randomized into 2 groups to receive oxygen at different FiO_2 (Figure 7). As far as age (29.9 ± 11.1 years old (mean ± SD)), height (168.2 ± 9.37 cm) weight (64.4 ± 12.3 kg) BMI [22.7 ± 4.1 kg/m^2], gender ratio, and health status are concerned, groups were comparable.

Oxygen was administered for 1 h by means of an orofacial nonrebreather mask with a reservoir with care being taken to fit and tighten the mask on the subject's face. The mild hyperoxia group received 30% of oxygen (oxygen partial pressure (PO_2): 0.3 bar; 300 hPa, n = 6) from a pressurized gas tank with a gas flow set at 10 L/min, while the high hyperoxia group received 100% of oxygen (PO_2: 1.0 bar, 1000 hPa, n = 8) from an oxygen concentrator (NewLife Intensity, CAIRE Inc., Ball Ground, GA, USA).

Blood and urine samples were obtained before exposure (T0) and 30 min, 2 h, 8 h, 24 h, and 48 h after the end of oxygen administration.

Each blood sample consisted of approximately 15 mL of venous human blood collected in lithium heparin and EDTA tubes (Vacutainer, BD Diagnostic, Becton Dickinson, Italia S.p.a.). Plasma and red blood cells (RBCs) were separated by centrifugation (Eppendorf Centrifuge 5702R, Darmstadt Germany) at 1000× g at 4 °C for 10 min. The samples were then stored in multiple aliquots at −80 °C until assayed; analysis was performed within one month from collection.

Urine was collected by voluntary voiding in a sterile container and stored in multiple aliquots at −20 °C until assayed and thawed only before analysis.

4.2. Blood Sample Analysis

4.2.1. Determination of ROS and TAC by Electron Paramagnetic Resonance (EPR)

An electron paramagnetic resonance instrument (E-Scan—Bruker BioSpin, GmbH, Rheinstetten, Germany) X-band, with a controller temperature at 37 °C interfaced to the spectrometer, was adopted for ROS production rate and total antioxidant capacity (TAC) as already performed by some of the authors [53–56]. The EPR measurements are highly reproducible, as previously demonstrated [57].

Briefly, for ROS detection, 50 µL of plasma were treated with an equal volume of CMH (1-hydroxy-3-methoxycarbonyl-2,2,5,5-tetramethylpyrrolidine); then 50 µL of this solution was placed inside a glass EPR capillary tube in the spectrometer cavity for data acquisition. A stable radical CP (3-carboxy-2,2,5,5-tetramethyl-1-pyrrolidinyloxy) was used as an external reference to convert ROS determinations in absolute quantitative values (µmol/min). For TAC, we used the spin trap DPPH· (2,2-diphenyl-1-picrylhydrazyl), a free radical compound soluble and stable in ethanol. All operations were performed in the dark to avoid photochemical effects on DPPH·, and a calibration curve was computed from pure

Trolox-containing reactions. Finally, an equation was used to calculate the anti-oxidant capacity expressed in terms of Trolox equivalent antioxidant capacity (TAC, mM).

All EPR spectra were collected by adopting the same protocol and obtained by using software standardly supplied by Bruker (Billerica, MA, USA) (version 2.11, WinEPR System).

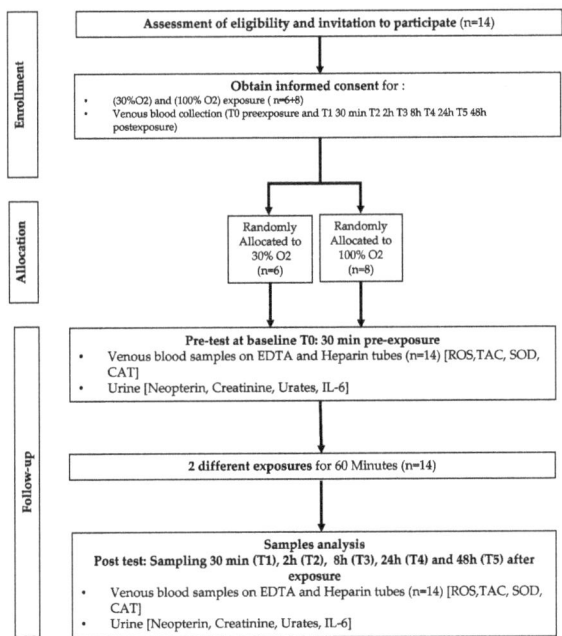

Figure 7. Experimental flowchart.

4.2.2. Super-Oxide Dismutase (SOD), Catalase (CAT)

SOD, CAT plasmatic levels were measured by enzyme-linked immunosorbent assay (ELISA kits) according to the manufacturer's instructions.

SOD activity was assessed by Cayman's SOD assay kit (706002) that utilizes a tetrazolium salt for detection of superoxide radicals generated by xanthine oxidase and hypoxathine.

One unit of SOD is defined as the amount of enzyme needed to exhibit 50% dismutation of the superoxide radical measured in change in absorbance (450 nm) per minute at 25° and pH 8.0.

CAT activity was assessed by Cayman's assay kit (707002) that utilizes the peroxidic function of CAT. The method is based on the reaction of enzyme with methanol in presence of an optimal concentration of H_2O_2.

The formaldehyde produced is measured colorimetrically with Purpald (540 nm) as chromogen. One unit of CAT is defined as the amount of enzyme that will cause the formation of 1 nmol of formaldehyde per minute at 25 °C.

All samples and standards were read by a microplate reader spectrophotometer (Infinite M200, Tecan Group Ltd., Männedorf, Switzerland).

The determinations were assessed in duplicate, and the inter-assay coefficient of variation was in the range indicated by the manufacturer.

4.3. Urine Sample Analysis

4.3.1. Lipid Peroxidation (8-iso-PGF2α)

Lipid peroxidation was assessed in urine by competitive immunoassay (Cayman Chemical, Ann Arbor, MI, USA) measuring 8-isoprostane (8-iso-PGF2α) concentration following the manufacturer's recommendations. Briefly, 50 µL of urine was placed in a well plate with mouse monoclonal antibody.

Therefore, 50 µL of 8-iso PGF2α-tracer and 8-iso PGF2α-antiserum were added and incubated for 18 h at 4 °C. After washing with buffer, 200 µL of Ellman's reagent containing the substrate of acetylcholinesterase was added.

The 8-iso-PGF2α concentrations were determined using a standard curve. Samples and standards were spectrophotometrically read at wavelengths between 405 and 420 nm.

4.3.2. Interleukin-6

IL-6 levels were determined using the ELISA assay kit (ThermoFisher Scientific, Waltham, MA, USA), based on the double-antibody "sandwich" technique in accordance with the manufacturer's instruction. All the above samples and standards were read by a microplate reader spectrophotometer (Infinite M200, Tecan Group Ltd., Männedorf, Switzerland). The determinations were assessed in duplicate, and the inter-assay coefficient of variation was in the range indicated by the manufacturer.

4.3.3. Creatinine, Neopterin, and Uric acid Concentrations

Urinary creatinine, neopterin, and uric acid concentrations were measured by the high-pressure liquid chromatography (HPLC) method, as previously described [58], by a Varian instrument (pump 240, autosampler ProStar 410) coupled to a UV–VIS detector (Shimadzu SPD 10-AV, λ = 240 nm for creatinine and uric acid; and JASCO FP-1520, λ_{ex} = 355 nm and at λ_{em} = 450 nm) for neopterin.

After urine centrifugation at 13,000 rpm at 4 °C for 5 min, analytic separations were performed at 50 °C on a 5 µm Discovery C18 analytical column (250 × 4.6 mm I.D., Supelco, Sigma-Aldrich) at a flow rate of 0.9 mL/min. The calibration curves were linear over the range of 0.125–1 µmol/L, 0.625–20 mmol/L, and 1.25–10 mmol/L for neopterin, uric acid, and creatinine levels, respectively. The inter-assay and intra-assay coefficients of variation were <5%.

4.4. Statistical Analysis

The normality of the data was verified by means of the Shapiro–Wilk test, which allowed us to assume a Gaussian distribution. Compared to baseline (T0—pre-exposure), data were analyzed with a one-way ANOVA for repeated measures with Dunnett's post hoc test for intragroup comparison. An unpaired t test was used for intergroup comparison. Taking the baseline measures as 100% (T0), percentage or fold changes were calculated for each oxygen protocol, allowing an appreciation of the magnitude of change rather than the absolute values. All data were presented as mean ± standard deviation (SD).

All statistical tests were performed using a standard computer statistical package, GraphPad Prism version 9.00 for Mac (GraphPad Software, San Diego, CA, USA). A threshold of $p < 0.05$ was considered statistically significant.

5. Conclusions

This study suggests a biphasic response over time characterized by an initial "permissive oxidation" followed by the overexpression of inflammation. The antioxidant protection system seems not to be the leading actor in the first place. It corroborates the concept that cellular hormesis is dependent on complex multimodal processes driven by an increase in ROS, inflammation, metabolism, and probably gene expression. This last point needs to be better studied, especially the kinetics of enzymatic reactions related to the expression or repression of intracellular molecular biogenesis, since it is for us important to have sufficient understanding of the exposure/repetition-related leading mechanisms in order to optimize the outcome. This would allow for the definition of proper training and therapeutic or rehabilitation protocols aiming at a more targeted use of oxygen.

Author Contributions: All authors listed have made a substantial, direct, and intellectual contribution to the work and approved it for publication. Conceptualization: C.B., P.L., P.G., C.L., S.T., K.L., F.V., S.M.-S., A.V. and A.B.; Investigation: P.L., C.L., S.T., C.B., K.L., P.G., S.M.-S., A.V. and A.B.; Writing: C.L.,P.L., C.B., P.G., F.V., S.M.-S., F.G. and S.M.; Funding: C.B., F.V., K.L. and S.T.; Data Analysis: C.L., S.M.-S., A.V., F.V., C.B., P.L., F.G., P.G. and S.M.-S. All authors have read and agreed to the published version of the manuscript.

Funding: This manuscript is part of the DELTO$_2$X Project and is funded by WBE (Wallonia-Brussels-Education) Belgium to the Environmental, Occupational, Aging (Integrative) Physiology Laboratory, Haute Ecole Bruxelles-Brabant (HE2B), Belgium. The sponsors had no role in the design and conduct of the study; the collection, management, analysis, and interpretation of the data; the preparation, review, or approval of the manuscript; and the decision to submit the manuscript for publication.

Institutional Review Board Statement: Ethics Committee approval from the Bio-Ethical Committee for Research and Higher Education, Brussels (No. B 200-2020-088).

Informed Consent Statement: Informed consent was obtained from all subjects involved in the study.

Data Availability Statement: Data are available upon request from the authors.

Acknowledgments: The authors are grateful to all volunteer participants, especially to students of the Haute Ecole Bruxelles-Brabant, Motor Sciences Department (Physiotherapy). Special acknowledgment is given to Maristella Gussoni for the accurate and in-depth expert contribution.

Conflicts of Interest: The authors declare no conflict of interest.

Abbreviations

FIH	Factor inhibiting HIF
PHD	Prolyl hydroxylase domain
REST	Repressor Element 1-Silencing Transcription factor
CAT	Catalase
FiO2	Inspired fraction of oxygen
HIF-1α	Hypoxia Inducible Factor-1α
IL-6	Interleukin-6
NOP	Normobaric oxygen paradox
NF-κB	Nuclear factor-kappa B
NRF2	Nuclear Factor Erythroid 2 Related–Factor 2
PO2	Oxygen partial pressure
ROS	Reactive oxygen species
SOD	Superoxide dismutase
TAC	Total antioxidant capacity
HRE	Hypoxia responsive element

References

1. Poulton, S.W.; Bekker, A.; Cumming, V.M.; Zerkle, A.L.; Canfield, D.E.; Johnston, D.T. A 200-million-year delay in permanent atmospheric oxygenation. *Nature* **2021**, *592*, 232–236. [CrossRef]
2. Bitterman, H. Bench-to-bedside review: Oxygen as a drug. *Crit. Care* **2009**, *13*, 205. [CrossRef]
3. Nakane, M. Biological effects of the oxygen molecule in critically ill patients. *J. Intensive Care* **2020**, *8*, 95. [CrossRef] [PubMed]
4. van Vliet, T.; Demaria, F.C.M. To breathe or not to breathe: Understanding how oxygen sensing contributes to age-related phenotypes. *Ageing Res. Rev.* **2021**, *67*, 101267. [CrossRef] [PubMed]
5. Fu, Q.; Duan, R.; Sun, Y.; Li, Q. Hyperbaric oxygen therapy for healthy aging: From mechanisms to therapeutics. *Redox Biol.* **2022**, *53*, 102352. [CrossRef] [PubMed]
6. Okada, K.; Mori, D.; Makii, Y.; Nakamoto, H.; Murahashi, Y.; Yano, F.; Chang, S.H.; Taniguchi, Y.; Kobayashi, H.; Semba, H.; et al. Hypoxia-inducible factor-1 alpha maintains mouse articular cartilage through suppression of NF-κB signaling. *Sci. Rep.* **2020**, *10*, 5425. [CrossRef] [PubMed]
7. Serebrovska, Z.O.; Serebrovska, T.V.; Kholin, V.A.; Tumanovska, L.V.; Shysh, A.M.; Pashevin, D.A.; Goncharov, S.V.; Stroy, D.; Grib, O.N.; Shatylo, V.B.; et al. Intermittent Hypoxia-Hyperoxia Training Improves Cognitive Function and Decreases Circulating Biomarkers of Alzheimer's Disease in Patients with Mild Cognitive Impairment: A Pilot Study. *Int. J. Mol. Sci.* **2019**, *20*, 5405. [CrossRef]
8. Burtscher, J.; Mallet, R.T.; Burtscher, M.; Millet, G.P. Hypoxia and brain aging: Neurodegeneration or neuroprotection? *Ageing Res. Rev.* **2021**, *68*, 101343. [CrossRef]

9. Bestavashvili, A.; Glazachev, O.; Bestavashvili, A.; Suvorov, A.; Zhang, Y.; Zhang, X.; Rozhkov, A.; Kuznetsova, N.; Pavlov, C.; Glushenkov, D.; et al. Intermittent Hypoxic-Hyperoxic Exposures Effects in Patients with Metabolic Syndrome: Correction of Cardiovascular and Metabolic Profile. *Biomedicines* **2022**, *10*, 566. [CrossRef]
10. Matta, A.; Nader, V.; Lebrin, M.; Gross, F.; Prats, A.C.; Cussac, D.; Galinier, M.; Roncalli, J. Pre-Conditioning Methods and Novel Approaches with Mesenchymal Stem Cells Therapy in Cardiovascular Disease. *Cells* **2022**, *11*, 1620. [CrossRef]
11. Balestra, C.; Lambrechts, K.; Mrakic-Sposta, S.; Vezzoli, A.; Levenez, M.; Germonpre, P.; Virgili, F.; Bosco, G.; Lafere, P. Hypoxic and Hyperoxic Breathing as a Complement to Low-Intensity Physical Exercise Programs: A Proof-of-Principle Study. *Int. J. Mol. Sci.* **2021**, *22*, 9600. [CrossRef] [PubMed]
12. Balestra, C.; Theunissen, S.; Papadopoulou, V.; Le Mener, C.; Germonpre, P.; Guerrero, F.; Lafere, P. Pre-dive Whole-Body Vibration Better Reduces Decompression-Induced Vascular Gas Emboli than Oxygenation or a Combination of Both. *Front. Physiol.* **2016**, *7*, 586. [CrossRef] [PubMed]
13. Webb, J.T.; Pilmanis, A.A. Fifty years of decompression sickness research at Brooks AFB, TX: 1960-2010. *Aviat. Space Env. Med.* **2011**, *82* (Suppl. S5), A1–A25. [CrossRef] [PubMed]
14. Sannigrahi, P.; Sushree, S.K.; Agarwal, A. Aeromedical Concerns and Lessons Learnt during Oxygen Jump at Dolma Sampa. *Indian J. Aerosp. Med.* **2018**, *62*, 16–20.
15. Balestra, C.; Arya, A.K.; Leveque, C.; Virgili, F.; Germonpre, P.; Lambrechts, K.; Lafere, P.; Thom, S.R. Varying Oxygen Partial Pressure Elicits Blood-Borne Microparticles Expressing Different Cell-Specific Proteins-Toward a Targeted Use of Oxygen? *Int. J. Mol. Sci.* **2022**, *23*, 7888. [CrossRef]
16. Halliwell, B.; Gutteridge, J.M.C. *Free Radicals in Biology and Medicine*; Oxford University Press: Oxford, UK, 2015.
17. Sies, H.; Belousov, V.V.; Chandel, N.S.; Davies, M.J.; Jones, D.P.; Mann, G.E.; Murphy, M.P.; Yamamoto, M.; Winterbourn, C. Defining roles of specific reactive oxygen species (ROS) in cell biology and physiology. *Nat. Rev. Mol. Cell Biol.* **2022**, *23*, 499–515. [CrossRef]
18. La Sala, L.; Tagliabue, E.; Mrakic-Sposta, S.; Uccellatore, A.C.; Senesi, P.; Terruzzi, I.; Trabucchi, E.; Rossi-Bernardi, L.; Luzi, L. Lower miR-21/ROS/HNE levels associate with lower glycemia after habit-intervention: DIAPASON study 1-year later. *Cardiovasc. Diabetol.* **2022**, *21*, 35. [CrossRef]
19. Cova, E.; Pandolfi, L.; Colombo, M.; Frangipane, V.; Inghilleri, S.; Morosini, M.; Mrakic-Sposta, S.; Moretti, S.; Monti, M.; Pignochino, Y.; et al. Pemetrexed-loaded nanoparticles targeted to malignant pleural mesothelioma cells: An in vitro study. *Int. J. Nanomed.* **2019**, *14*, 773–785. [CrossRef]
20. Mrakic-Sposta, S.; Vezzoli, A.; Maderna, L.; Gregorini, F.; Montorsi, M.; Moretti, S.; Greco, F.; Cova, E.; Gussoni, M. R(+)-Thioctic Acid Effects on Oxidative Stress and Peripheral Neuropathy in Type II Diabetic Patients: Preliminary Results by Electron Paramagnetic Resonance and Electroneurography. *Oxid. Med. Cell Longev.* **2018**, *2018*, 1767265. [CrossRef]
21. Calabrese, E.J.; Mattson, M.P. How does hormesis impact biology, toxicology, and medicine? *NPJ Aging Mech. Dis.* **2017**, *3*, 13. [CrossRef]
22. Lennicke, C.; Cochemé, H.M. Redox metabolism: ROS as specific molecular regulators of cell signaling and function. *Mol. Cell* **2021**, *81*, 3691–3707. [CrossRef] [PubMed]
23. Chelombitko, M.A. Role of Reactive Oxygen Species in Inflammation: A Minireview. *Mosc. Univ. Biol. Sci. Bull.* **2018**, *73*, 199–202. [CrossRef]
24. Hadanny, A.; Efrati, S. The Hyperoxic-Hypoxic Paradox. *Biomolecules* **2020**, *10*, 958. [CrossRef] [PubMed]
25. Balestra, C.; Germonpré, P.; Poortmans, J.R.; Marroni, A. Serum erythropoietin levels in healthy humans after a short period of normobaric and hyperbaric oxygen breathing: The "normobaric oxygen paradox". *J. Appl. Physiol.* **2006**, *100*, 512–518. [CrossRef] [PubMed]
26. Cimino, F.; Balestra, C.; Germonpre, P.; De Bels, D.; Tillmans, F.; Saija, A.; Speciale, A.; Virgili, F. Pulsed high oxygen induces a hypoxic-like response in human umbilical endothelial cells and in humans. *J. Appl. Physiol.* **2012**, *113*, 1684–1689. [CrossRef] [PubMed]
27. Khalife, M.; Ben Aziz, M.; Balestra, C.; Valsamis, J.; Sosnowski, M. Physiological and Clinical Impact of Repeated Inhaled Oxygen Variation on Erythropoietin Levels in Patients After Surgery. *Front. Physiol.* **2021**, *12*, 744074. [CrossRef] [PubMed]
28. Lafere, P.; Schubert, T.; De Bels, D.; Germonpre, P.; Balestra, C. Can the normobaric oxygen paradox (NOP) increase reticulocyte count after traumatic hip surgery? *J. Clin. Anesth.* **2013**, *25*, 129–134. [CrossRef]
29. Fratantonio, D.; Virgili, F.; Zucchi, A.; Lambrechts, K.; Latronico, T.; Lafere, P.; Germonpre, P.; Balestra, C. Increasing Oxygen Partial Pressures Induce a Distinct Transcriptional Response in Human PBMC: A Pilot Study on the "Normobaric Oxygen Paradox". *Int. J. Mol. Sci.* **2021**, *22*, 458. [CrossRef]
30. Calabrese, E. Hormesis: Path and Progression to Significance. *Int. J. Mol. Sci.* **2018**, *19*, 2871. [CrossRef]
31. Franceschi, C.; Bonafè, M.; Valensin, S.; Olivieri, F.; De Luca, M.; Ottaviani, E.; De Benedictis, G. Inflamm-aging. An evolutionary perspective on immunosenescence. *Ann. N. Y. Acad. Sci.* **2000**, *908*, 244–254. [CrossRef]
32. Franceschi, C.; Campisi, J. Chronic inflammation (inflammaging) and its potential contribution to age-associated diseases. *J. Gerontol. A Biol. Sci. Med. Sci.* **2014**, *69* (Suppl. S1), S4–S9. [CrossRef] [PubMed]
33. Furman, D.; Campisi, J.; Verdin, E.; Carrera-Bastos, P.; Targ, S.; Franceschi, C.; Ferrucci, L.; Gilroy, D.W.; Fasano, A.; Miller, G.W.; et al. Chronic inflammation in the etiology of disease across the life span. *Nat. Med.* **2019**, *25*, 1822–1832. [CrossRef] [PubMed]

34. Akhigbe, R.; Ajayi, A. The impact of reactive oxygen species in the development of cardiometabolic disorders: A review. *Lipids Health Dis.* **2021**, *20*, 23. [CrossRef] [PubMed]
35. Checa, J.; Aran, J.M. Reactive Oxygen Species: Drivers of Physiological and Pathological Processes. *J. Inflamm. Res.* **2020**, *13*, 1057–1073. [CrossRef]
36. Balestra, C.; Kot, J. Oxygen: A Stimulus, Not "Only" a Drug. *Medicina* **2021**, *57*, 1161. [CrossRef] [PubMed]
37. Rocco, M.; D'Itri, L.; De Bels, D.; Corazza, F.; Balestra, C. The "normobaric oxygen paradox": A new tool for the anesthetist? *Minerva Anestesiol.* **2014**, *80*, 366–372.
38. Bel'skaya, L.V.; Kosenok, V.K.; Sarf, E.A. Chronophysiological features of the normal mineral composition of human saliva. *Arch. Oral. Biol.* **2017**, *82*, 286–292. [CrossRef]
39. Teng, R.J.; Jing, X.; Martin, D.P.; Hogg, N.; Haefke, A.; Konduri, G.G.; Day, B.W.; Naylor, S.; Pritchard, K.A., Jr. N-acetyl-lysyltyrosylcysteine amide, a novel systems pharmacology agent, reduces bronchopulmonary dysplasia in hyperoxic neonatal rat pups. *Free Radic. Biol. Med.* **2021**, *166*, 73–89. [CrossRef]
40. Chen, C.; He, M.; Li, X.; Yu, L.; Liu, Y.; Yang, Y.; Li, L.; Jia, J.; Li, B. H2O2/DEM-Promoted Maft Promoter Demethylation Drives Nrf2/ARE Activation in Zebrafish. *Life* **2022**, *12*, 1436. [CrossRef]
41. Semenza, G.L. HIF-1: Mediator of physiological and pathological responses to hypoxia. *J. Appl. Physiol.* **2000**, *88*, 1474–1480. [CrossRef]
42. Cavadas, M.A.S.; Mesnieres, M.; Crifo, B.; Manresa, M.C.; Selfridge, A.C.; Scholz, C.C.; Cummins, E.P.; Cheong, A.; Taylor, C.T. REST mediates resolution of HIF-dependent gene expression in prolonged hypoxia. *Sci. Rep.* **2015**, *5*, 17851. [CrossRef] [PubMed]
43. Cavadas, M.A.S.; Mesnieres, M.; Crifo, B.; Manresa, M.C.; Selfridge, A.C.; Keogh, C.E.; Fabian, Z.; Scholz, C.C.; Nolan, K.A.; Rocha, L.M.A.; et al. REST is a hypoxia-responsive transcriptional repressor. *Sci. Rep.* **2016**, *6*, 31355. [CrossRef] [PubMed]
44. De Bels, D.; Corazza, F.; Germonpre, P.; Balestra, C. The normobaric oxygen paradox: A novel way to administer oxygen as an adjuvant treatment for cancer? *Med. Hypotheses* **2010**, *76*, 467–470. [CrossRef] [PubMed]
45. Sies, H. Role of Metabolic H2O2 Generation. *J. Biol. Chem.* **2014**, *289*, 8735–8741. [CrossRef] [PubMed]
46. Basang, Z.; Zhang, S.; Yang, L.; Quzong, D.; Li, Y.; Ma, Y.; Hao, M.; Pu, W.; Liu, X.; Xie, H.; et al. Correlation of DNA methylation patterns to the phenotypic features of Tibetan elite alpinists in extreme hypoxia. *J. Genet. Genom.* **2021**, *48*, 928–935. [CrossRef]
47. Wilson, J.W.; Shakir, D.; Batie, M.; Frost, M.; Rocha, S. Oxygen-sensing mechanisms in cells. *FEBS J.* **2020**, *287*, 3888–3906. [CrossRef]
48. Kobayashi, E.H.; Suzuki, T.; Funayama, R.; Nagashima, T.; Hayashi, M.; Sekine, H.; Tanaka, N.; Moriguchi, T.; Motohashi, H.; Nakayama, K.; et al. Nrf2 suppresses macrophage inflammatory response by blocking proinflammatory cytokine transcription. *Nat. Commun.* **2016**, *7*, 11624. [CrossRef]
49. Gao, W.; Guo, L.; Yang, Y.; Wang, Y.; Xia, S.; Gong, H.; Zhang, B.K.; Yan, M. Dissecting the Crosstalk Between Nrf2 and NF-κB Response Pathways in Drug-Induced Toxicity. *Front. Cell Dev. Biol.* **2021**, *9*, 809952. [CrossRef]
50. Kuzkaya, N.; Weissmann, N.; Harrison, D.G.; Dikalov, S. Interactions of peroxynitrite with uric acid in the presence of ascorbate and thiols: Implications for uncoupling endothelial nitric oxide synthase. *Biochem. Pharm.* **2005**, *70*, 343–354. [CrossRef]
51. Gu, X.; El-Remessy, A.B.; Brooks, S.E.; Al-Shabrawey, M.; Tsai, N.T.; Caldwell, R.B. Hyperoxia induces retinal vascular endothelial cell apoptosis through formation of peroxynitrite. *Am. J. Physiol. Cell Physiol.* **2003**, *285*, C546–C554. [CrossRef]
52. World Medical, A. World Medical Association Declaration of Helsinki: Ethical principles for medical research involving human subjects. *JAMA* **2013**, *310*, 2191–2194.
53. Mrakic-Sposta, S.; Vezzoli, A.; D'Alessandro, F.; Paganini, M.; Dellanoce, C.; Cialoni, D.; Bosco, G. Change in Oxidative Stress Biomarkers During 30 Days in Saturation Dive: A Pilot Study. *Int. J. Env. Res. Public Health* **2020**, *17*, 7118. [CrossRef] [PubMed]
54. Moretti, S.; Mrakic-Sposta, S.; Roncoroni, L.; Vezzoli, A.; Dellanoce, C.; Monguzzi, E.; Branchi, F.; Ferretti, F.; Lombardo, V.; Doneda, L.; et al. Oxidative stress as a biomarker for monitoring treated celiac disease. *Clin. Transl. Gastroenterol.* **2018**, *9*, 157. [CrossRef] [PubMed]
55. Mrakic-Sposta, S.; Vezzoli, A.; Rizzato, A.; Della Noce, C.; Malacrida, S.; Montorsi, M.; Paganini, M.; Cancellara, P.; Bosco, G. Oxidative stress assessment in breath-hold diving. *Eur. J. Appl. Physiol.* **2019**, *119*, 2449–2456. [CrossRef]
56. Bosco, G.; Rizzato, A.; Quartesan, S.; Camporesi, E.; Mrakic-Sposta, S.; Moretti, S.; Balestra, C.; Rubini, A. Spirometry and oxidative stress after rebreather diving in warm water. *Undersea Hyperb. Med.* **2018**, *45*, 191–198. [CrossRef]
57. Mrakic-Sposta, S.; Gussoni, M.; Montorsi, M.; Porcelli, S.; Vezzoli, A. A quantitative method to monitor reactive oxygen species production by electron paramagnetic resonance in physiological and pathological conditions. *Oxid. Med. Cell Longev.* **2014**, *2014*, 306179. [CrossRef] [PubMed]
58. Bosco, G.; Paganini, M.; Giacon, T.A.; Oppio, A.; Vezzoli, A.; Dellanoce, C.; Moro, T.; Paoli, A.; Zanotti, F.; Zavan, B.; et al. Oxidative Stress and Inflammation, MicroRNA, and Hemoglobin Variations after Administration of Oxygen at Different Pressures and Concentrations: A Randomized Trial. *Int. J. Env. Res. Public Health* **2021**, *18*, 9755. [CrossRef]

Disclaimer/Publisher's Note: The statements, opinions and data contained in all publications are solely those of the individual author(s) and contributor(s) and not of MDPI and/or the editor(s). MDPI and/or the editor(s) disclaim responsibility for any injury to people or property resulting from any ideas, methods, instructions or products referred to in the content.

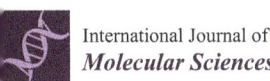

Article

The "ON-OFF" Switching Response of Reactive Oxygen Species in Acute Normobaric Hypoxia: Preliminary Outcome

Simona Mrakic-Sposta [1,*], Maristella Gussoni [2], Mauro Marzorati [3], Simone Porcelli [4], Gerardo Bosco [5], Costantino Balestra [6,7], Michela Montorsi [1,8], Claudio Lafortuna [1] and Alessandra Vezzoli [1]

1. Institute of Clinical Physiology, National Research Council (IFC-CNR), 20162 Milan, Italy
2. Institute of Chemical Sciences and Technologies "G. Natta", National Research Council (SCITEC-CNR), 20133 Milan, Italy
3. Institute of Biomedical Technologies, National Research Council (ITB-CNR), 20090 Milan, Italy
4. Department of Molecular Medicine, Università di Pavia, 27100 Pavia, Italy
5. Department of Biomedical Sciences, University of Padova, 35131 Padova, Italy
6. Environmental, Occupational, Aging (Integrative) Physiology Laboratory, Haute Ecole Bruxelles-Brabant (HE2B), 1090 Brussels, Belgium
7. Anatomical Research and Clinical Studies, Vrije Universiteit Brussels (VUB), 1090 Brussels, Belgium
8. Department of Human Sciences and Promotion of the Quality of Life, San Raffaele Roma Open University, 00166 Roma, Italy
* Correspondence: simona.mrakicsposta@cnr.it

Abstract: Exposure to acute normobaric hypoxia (NH) elicits reactive oxygen species (ROS) accumulation, whose production kinetics and oxidative damage were here investigated. Nine subjects were monitored while breathing an NH mixture (0.125 F_IO_2 in air, about 4100 m) and during recovery with room air. ROS production was assessed by Electron Paramagnetic Resonance in capillary blood. Total antioxidant capacity, lipid peroxidation (TBARS and 8-iso-PFG2α), protein oxidation (PC) and DNA oxidation (8-OH-dG) were measured in plasma and/or urine. The ROS production rate (μmol·min^{-1}) was monitored (5, 15, 30, 60, 120, 240 and 300 min). A production peak (+50%) was reached at 4 h. The on-transient kinetics, exponentially fitted ($t_{1/2} = 30$ min $r^2 = 0.995$), were ascribable to the low O_2 tension transition and the mirror-like related SpO_2 decrease: 15 min: −12%; 60 min: −18%. The exposure did not seem to affect the prooxidant/antioxidant balance. Significant increases in PC (+88%) and 8-OH-dG (+67%) at 4 h in TBARS (+33%) one hour after hypoxia offset were also observed. General malaise was described by most of the subjects. Under acute NH, ROS production and oxidative damage resulted in time and SpO_2-dependent reversible phenomena. The experimental model could be suitable for evaluating the acclimatation level, a key element in the context of mountain rescues in relation to technical/medical workers who have not had enough time for acclimatization—as, for example, during helicopter flights.

Keywords: oxidative stress; normobaric hypoxia; simulate altitude; ROS; electron paramagnetic resonance

Citation: Mrakic-Sposta, S.; Gussoni, M.; Marzorati, M.; Porcelli, S.; Bosco, G.; Balestra, C.; Montorsi, M.; Lafortuna, C.; Vezzoli, A. The "ON-OFF" Switching Response of Reactive Oxygen Species in Acute Normobaric Hypoxia: Preliminary Outcome. *Int. J. Mol. Sci.* **2023**, *24*, 4012. https://doi.org/10.3390/ijms24044012

Academic Editor: Thomas Kietzmann

Received: 21 January 2023
Revised: 10 February 2023
Accepted: 13 February 2023
Published: 16 February 2023

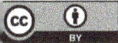

Copyright: © 2023 by the authors. Licensee MDPI, Basel, Switzerland. This article is an open access article distributed under the terms and conditions of the Creative Commons Attribution (CC BY) license (https://creativecommons.org/licenses/by/4.0/).

1. Introduction

Exposure to acute hypoxia elicits several functional changes in the human body to cope with the decreased oxygen availability [1]. Whereas some of these adjustments (increased pulmonary ventilation and heart rate) are well characterized, others are still poorly understood. Excesses in the accumulation of reactive oxygen species (ROS), generated within the mitochondria, drive mechanisms contributing to injury—including the induction of oxidative damage [2]. A growing body of evidence indicates that hypoxia decreases both the activity and effectiveness of the antioxidant system, as well as causing increased ROS production with a consequent increase in oxidative damage [3] to lipids [4–6], proteins and the DNA [5,7] of cellular compartments [8–10]. Most studies on the effects of hypoxia have been carried out at high altitude [9–16]. However, under such conditions, several factors other than hypoxia could induce oxidative damage; UV radiation, intense physical activity and cold may in fact produce an imbalance between ROS generation and antioxidant protection [17,18]. Indeed, a limited number of studies have been carried out in humans aimed at dissociating hypoxia from other potential environmental oxidative stressors and utilizing normobaric hypoxic gas mixtures in normobaric conditions [19–21]. Normobaric hypoxia (NH; 9 h simulating exposure at approximately 3800 m) was found to stimulate the production of cerebral ROS as well as associated biomarkers of oxidative stress [22]. However, to the best of our knowledge, the time course of changes in systemic ROS production, which represents the most valid tool for systemic oxidative stress evaluation during exposure to acute NH, has not still been assessed.

In recent years, our group has developed an Electron Paramagnetic Resonance (EPR) microinvasive method [23–30] capable of providing absolute ROS quantification using a drop of capillary blood taken from the fingertip. The small amount of blood requested for the analysis and the ease of the sample collection procedure makes this technique particularly suitable for performing repeated measures in a short time frame and thus for quantitatively monitoring the ROS response kinetics (on and off) to a particular stimulus. The aim of this study was to investigate the time-course changes in systemic ROS production in response to acute, severe and short-term normobaric hypoxia (NH) exposure. The temporal relationship between ROS and oxidative stress biomarkers production was assessed in parallel. The present study is a continuation of the research project started in 2012 [31] that was continued with a field study in the Alps [13,14].

2. Results

2.1. ROS Production and SpO$_2$ Kinetics

One subject dropped out during the experiment, after exactly 2 h of exposure to NH. The subject reported severe headache with dizziness and nausea. The other subjects completed the experimental session.

Exposure to acute NH induced EPR-detectable changes in the ROS production rate ($\mu mol \cdot min^{-1}$). ROS elicited by NH were measured at the different time points (5, 15, 30, 60, 120, 240 and 300 min) in subjects' capillary blood. The data calculated at the different time points in the protocol (before, during and after NH exposure) are shown in Figure 1A. A production peak (+50%) was reached at 4 h of hypoxia exposure, followed by a return to around the pre-hypoxia level during the recovery phase while breathing room air. The exponential fit of the percent data of the on-transient kinetics returned a $t_{1/2} = 30$ min ($r^2 = 0.995$; see insert at the right panel, bottom).

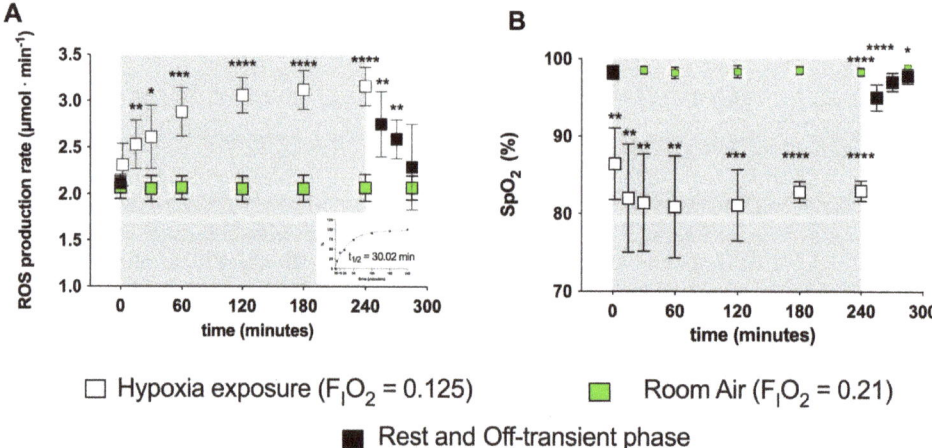

Figure 1. Cont.

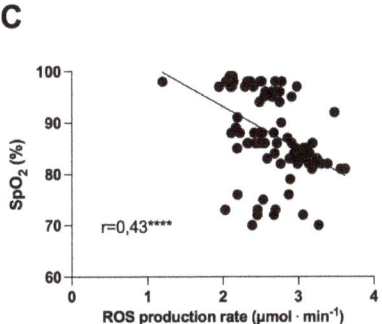

Figure 1. (**A**) Time course of the ROS production rate ($\mu mol \cdot min^{-1}$) assessed by EPR technique and (**B**) SpO_2 (%) during the transition from normoxia to acute normobaric hypoxia and back to normoxia during recovery. EXP group: full symbols are the data obtained before (0 min) and 15, 30, 45 min after hypoxia exposure (recovery); open symbols are the data during hypoxia status: at 5, 15, 30, 60, 120, 180, 240 min. Green symbols are the data obtained from the CTR (room air, normoxia state FiO_2 = 0.21) for ROS ($\mu mol \cdot min^{-1}$) and SpO_2 (%). In the inset at the right bottom of Figure A, the exponential fit of the on-transient kinetics data ($t_{1/2}$ = 30.02 min, r^2 = 0.995) is shown. Results are expressed as mean ± SD. (**C**) Data (full symbols) and linear correlation line (continuous line, r = 0.43) of the ROS production rate versus SpO_2. Changes over time were significantly different when compared to pre-exposure levels (* $p < 0.05$; ** $p < 0.01$; *** $p < 0.001$; **** $p < 0.0001$ symbols).

No significant differences in ROS production or SpO_2 were observed in the CTR group (Figure 1A, B) throughout the observational period. Compared to normoxia (0 min), acute NH induced a fast initial ROS production increase (15 min: +20%; 60 min: +36%) whose size appeared to be mirror-like in relation to the subjects' blood oxygen saturation decrease—15 min: −12%; 60 min: −18%; see Figure 1B). The SpO_2 (%) remained at a relatively constant level (85–90%) during the time course of the simulated hypoxia exposure. The relationship between the ROS production rate levels and the SpO_2 (%) resulted in a significant, mild, inverse linear correlation (r = 0.43, $p = 0.0001$), obtained by the Spearman product–moment correlation (see Figure 1C).

2.2. Oxidative Damage and Antioxidant Capacity Response

Average TAC values did not show any significant change (Figure 2A). Plasmatic PC concentration (nmol·mg^{-1} protein) significantly ($p < 0.05$) increased after four hours of hypoxia exposure (at 240 min: +88%), whereas TBARS (μM) significantly ($p < 0.05$) increased (+33%) one hour after hypoxia offset. Both variables returned back to pre-hypoxia values during recovery (Figure 2B, C). After four hours of hypoxia exposure, the urinary 8-OH-dG concentration, a biomarker of DNA damage, was significantly increased ($p < 0.05$; +67%; Figure 2D); otherwise, no changes in urinary 8-iso-PGF2α, a marker of lipid peroxidation, were observed (Figure 2E).

As shown in Figure 3, after 4 h of NH, subjects exposed to Hypoxia (F_IO_2 = 0.125) described a worsening of their feeling of overall wellness. With respect to the normoxia (black bars), a significant worsening in wellness and increase in tiredness and sleepiness—with no significant difference in the level of headache and nausea—were reported. In the CTR, only a little general malaise was reported—probably due to the 4 h spent sitting on the chair without the possibility of standing up. However, the items recorded in the VAS returned to the baseline within about a couple of hours.

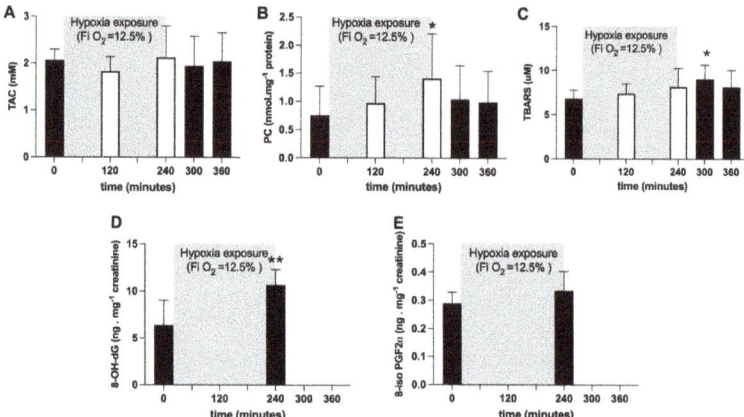

Figure 2. Histogram plots (mean ± SD) of (**A**) TAC (mM), (**B**) TBARS (μM) and (**C**) PC (nmol·mg^{-1} protein) concentration levels obtained from plasma samples collected at 0, 120 and 240 min of NH. Data at 60 and 120 min of the recovery time, when breathing normoxic room air, are also shown. (**D**) 8-OH-dG and (**E**) 8-iso-PGF2α (ng·mg^{-1} creatinine) data levels before and after NH. Changes over time were significantly different when compared to pre-exposure levels (* $p < 0.05$; ** $p < 0.01$ symbols).

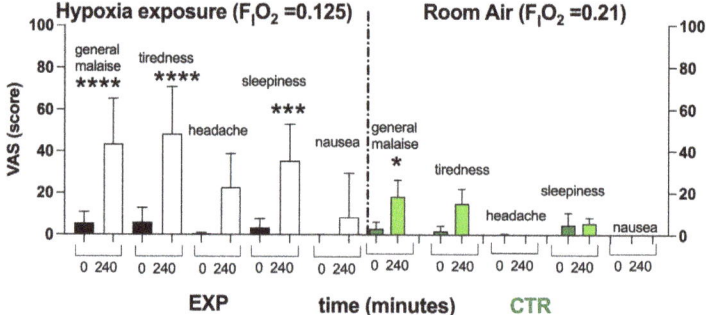

Figure 3. Histogram plot (mean ± SD) of the VAS score from the EXP and CTR. Data obtained Pre- (black and green bars respectively) and after 240 min of NH (white and light green bars, respectively) are shown. Changes over time were significantly different when compared to pre-exposure levels (* $p < 0.05$; *** $p < 0.001$; **** $p < 0.0001$ symbols).

3. Discussion

The present study was designed to analyze the kinetics of ROS production and oxidative damage in response to acute, severe and short-term normobaric hypoxia exposure. Nowadays, a number of reports have provided evidence for ROS production during acute hypoxia exposure, but a lack of information was found regarding its timing/on–off kinetics under a controlled environment, with the exclusion of the presence of external overlapping factors that can lead to confusion.

The main finding of the present study was the significant and fast increase (+17%) in ROS production that occurred when breathing the hypoxic mixture (0.125% O$_2$ in air). By the exponential fit of the transient on-kinetics, a $t_{1/2}$ of 30.02 min ($r^2 = 0.995$) was calculated. This was possibly ascribable to a transition to a low intracellular O$_2$ tension, as evidenced by the significant reduction in SpO$_2$. ROS production continued to increase, reaching a "plateau value" at 60 min that was maintained until the "turning off" of the hypoxia status. Thereafter, the ROS production returned to around normoxia levels (+9%

with respect to the basal level). Nevertheless, a short (4 h) NH exposure did not seem to affect the prooxidant/antioxidant balance; no significant differences were found in the total antioxidant capacity (Figure 2A). By contrast, the decrease in the TAC values previously reported in response to hypoxia [9,15,16] could be due both to a longer exposure (>24 h) and/or to hypobaric conditions.

As also highlighted by Millet et al. (2012) [32], normobaric hypoxia can induce responses different from hypobaric hypoxia (HH); in fact, the physiological/biological responses to HH suggest it is a more severe environmental condition, leading to different physiological adaptations [33].

The total antioxidant capacity data did not evidence substantial changes during the NH experimental session (see Figure 2A), suggesting good tissue and systemic responses to the hypoxic stimulus; this is in agreement with Ribon and colleagues' [33] data, who found that GPX and SOD activity was not significantly higher after NH. On the contrary, significant changes were observed after HH.

The findings presented here were consistent with the fast increase of ROS concentrations found in isolated systemic vessels exposed to hypoxia [34–36]. The increase in ROS production in response to hypoxia has important systemic implications [37]—particularly at the brain level, with damage to the vascular endothelium, neurons and glia and the downregulation of Na^+-K^+-ATPase, Ca^{2+}-ATPase and Na^+/Ca^{2+} exchanger activity [22,38]; these results have been recently confirmed by cellular microparticle production during acute hypoxia [39].

A possible explanation for the kinetics of this ROS production may be found in the autoxidation process of hemoglobin. As is well-known [40], hemoglobin continuously undergoes autoxidation by producing superoxide. In particular, a reduction in SpO_2 has been found to result in a dramatic increase in the rate of hemoglobin autoxidation [40–42]. Therefore, because of the hypoxic exposition, oxidative stress might result from an increase in the autoxidation rate of partially oxygenated hemoglobin—particularly to that formed at the microcirculation level, as shown by the post-occlusion hyperhaemia reaction during acute hypoxia exposure [43]. This hypothesis seems to be confirmed by the reported significant inverse relationship between SpO_2 and the ROS production rate presently detected.

Furthermore, no changes in ROS production and SaO_2 were observed in the CTR condition during the 4 h of the experiment, confirming that the data obtained from the EXP were not affected by variables (experiment duration, food restriction, tedium) other than the hypoxic status. Incidentally, these data also confirmed the high reproducibility of the EPR measurements and the stability of ROS production by biological samples in a full-rest context [23]. Indeed, the importance of an accurate and specific detection of reactive oxygen species in different biological samples is essential to the study of redox-regulated signaling in biological settings [44].

NH exposure induced an enhancement of oxidative damage, estimated by an increase in TBARS, PC and 8-OH-dG, that resulted in delays with respect to the ROS production increase. The late onset of oxidative stress damage might suggest to us that the oxidative damage phenomenon, evidenced by the production of some biomarkers, is a process growing in evidence over time. At the end of the NH exposure, in both markers of lipid peroxidation (TBARS in plasma and 8-iso-PGF2a in urine), no significant difference was found (see Figure 3C,E). One hour after the end of the experiment, the TBARS plasma concentration was found to be significantly (+33%) increased, returning to the pre-hypoxia control value in subsequent hours (Figure 2B). A similar behavior was also observed for PC plasma levels, which significantly increased during NH, attained their highest value (+88%) at 4 h, and then slowly decreased at hypoxia offset (Figure 2C). Finally, DNA underwent a 67% increase at 2 h of recovery from hypoxia (Figure 2D).

VAS has been demonstrated to be a suitable method in the field of medicine to measure pain [45], general wellness [37,46], nausea [47], feelings of fatigue [48] and sleep quality [49]. Nevertheless, VAS has been also used as an auxiliary diagnostic method for the Lake Louise score (LLS) for evaluating acute mountain sickness (AMS) [50–52]. In hypobaric chambers, VAS shows the changing severity of symptoms during the process of elevation increasing [50,52]. However, from the results of the present study, a general discomfort, tiredness, headache and sleepiness during the time of the experiments were reported during the EXP, while only a general discomfort was reported in the CTR. As already pointed out, this could probably be ascribable to the subjects being compelled to sit on a chair with their mask attached to the instrument, with the impossibility of moving. This discomfort could perhaps be avoided by other experimental setups—for example, setting the experiment up in an extreme environments simulator center (i.e., NOI Techpark in Bolzano, South Tyrol, Italy), where climate chambers differ in size and equipment and can accommodate people for prolonged periods.

Limitations

The present study had some experimental limitations, mainly concerning the number of participants, the duration of the experimental session (from four to six hours) and the investigated elevation, which was about 4100 m in altitude. The main purpose of the presently adopted protocol was to avoid any external and/or overlapping factors that can lead to confusion and in any way affect the results, such as those related to a prolonged permanence at high altitude. Indeed, the experimental design developed in the present study could be applied to a greater number of subjects, possibly of different age and/or levels of sport activity, and could increase both the amount and the duration of hypoxia.

Finally, colorimetric assays are common methods for evaluating plasma TAC and TBARS, but their principal limitation is the non-specificity of the test. Nevertheless, various kits based on these methods are commercially available, and results have also been published recently [53–55]; they represent a reasonable compromise in terms of costs and reliability.

4. Materials and Methods

4.1. Subjects

Nine healthy sedentary subjects (7 males and 2 females; age 26.8 ± 13.2 years; height 175.2 ± 7.26 cm; weight 76.9 ± 10.1 kg) participated in this study (EXP); only 6 of these subjects (6 males; age 25.3 ± 1.5 years; height 1.74 ± 0.08 m; weight 75.43 ± 6.0 kg) lent themselves to the control condition (CTR).

One week before the experimental session, all subjects underwent a clinical screening during which a physical examination and resting ECG were performed.

The exclusion criteria were regular smoking, hypertension, hypercholesterolemia, diabetes, cardiovascular or respiratory diseases, infections, supplementation of antioxidant or anti-inflammatory substances and habitual use of drugs.

All subjects resided below 500 m and, to minimize confounding effects, no subject had spent time above 1000 m of altitude in the four weeks preceding the study, nor was regularly engaged in a training program. Furthermore, participants were required to abstain from any strenuous physical activity and from alcohol and caffeine containing beverages, respectively, 2 weeks and 24 h prior to the study.

All subjects were informed about the aims, the experimental protocol and the potential risks of the investigation before giving written informed consent to take part in the study. This study was approved by the Local Ethical Committee (BESTA/IBFM, Report #27, 9 March 2016) and was carried out in accordance with the standard set by the Declaration of Helsinki [56].

4.2. Experimental Protocol

Participants arrived at the laboratory in Milan (122 m) early in the morning after a light breakfast and sat comfortably on a chair, breathing room air. The room temperature was kept constant at 21 °C. At time 0, the subjects in the EXP condition started breathing a normobaric hypoxic mixture (0.125 F_IO_2 in air, simulating about 4100 m altitude) obtained by removing oxygen from the air (MAG-10, Higher Peak LLC, Winchester, MA, USA). The gas mixture was delivered through a facemask at 30 L.min^{-1}. Excess airflow was diverted outside the mask to prevent inspired oxygen pressure from increasing above 90 Torr. Four hours later, subjects were switched to normoxic breathing conditions. During the entire session, pulse oxygen saturation (SpO$_2$, %) was monitored at the earlobe by an oximeter (Biox 3740 Pulse Oximeter, Ohmeda, Denver, CO, USA). Visual Analog Scale (VAS) scores were obtained both before the test session and at the end of the NH exposition to evaluate subjective general conditions.

The subjects that lent themselves to the CTR condition were tested for the same time duration in room air (0.21 F$_I$O$_2$).

4.3. Sample Collection

With concern to the hypoxic condition (EXP), capillary blood samples for ROS assessments were collected before the test session while the participants were breathing room air, during hypoxia exposure (at 5, 15, 30, 60, 120, 180 and 240 min) and during the subsequent recovery phase with room air (at 15, 30 and 45 min).

Venous blood samples for oxidative insult assessment (a cannula was placed into an antecubital vein) were withdrawn before the testing session while breathing room air, at different times during hypoxia (at 120 and 240 min) and during the recovery phase breathing room air (at 60 and 120 min). Blood samples (5 mL) were drawn and collected in heparinized tubes (Becton Dickinson Company, Swindon, UK) and centrifuged (Centrifuge 5702 R, Eppendorf, Hamburg, Germany) at 4000 rpm for 10 min at 4 °C. The separated plasma was stored in multiple aliquots at −80 °C.

Urine samples were collected before and after hypoxia exposure (4 h) by voluntary voiding into a sterile container and were stored at −20 °C until assayed. All samples were thawed only once before analysis. In the normoxic condition (CTR), for each subject, capillary blood was drawn from the fingertip before and during 4 h of breathing (room air and normoxia at 30, 60, 120, 180, 240 and 285 min) under the same conditions as the EXP. The time points for the blood and urine sampling are shown in Figure 4.

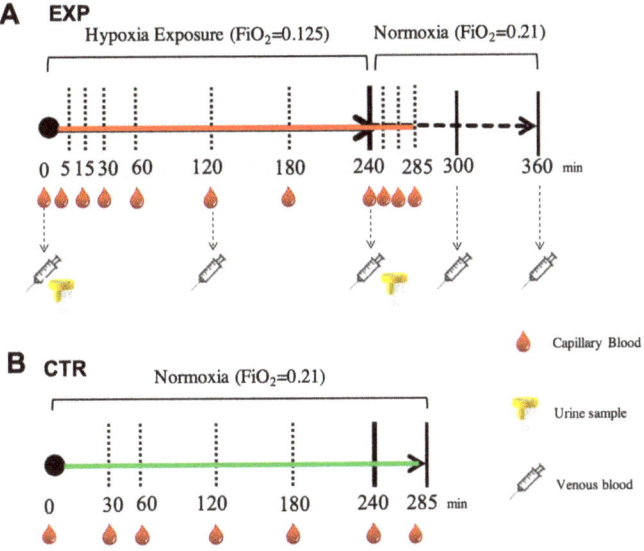

Figure 4. (**A**) EXP. Experimental timeline adopted for collecting each subject's blood sample (capillary (red drops), venous (syringes)) to measure ROS production by EPR, oxidative damage (PC and TBARS) by enzymatic assays and urine (glasses) to assess urinary 8-OH-dG and 8-iso-PGF2 alfa by ELISA. (**B**) CTR. Experimental timeline (continuous green line) adopted for collecting capillary blood samples (red drops) to measure ROS production by EPR.

4.4. Measurements

4.4.1. ROS Detection by Electron Paramagnetic Resonance

For both the experimental procedures, ROS assessments were carried out by a X-band EPR Spectrometer (e-scan, Bruker, Bremen, Germany) and a 1-hydroxy-3-methoxycarbonyl-2,2,5,5tetramethyl-pyrrolidine-hydrochloride (CMH, Noxygen Science Transfer & Diagnostics, Elzach, Germany) spin-probe at 1 mM was prepared in buffer solution—Krebs-Hepes buffer (KHB) containing 25 µM deferroxamine methane-sulfonate salt (DF) chelating agent and 5 µM sodium diethyldithio-carbamate trihydrate (DETC) at pH 7.4—which reacts with extra and intracellular one-electron oxidants, generating the EPR detectable radical CM•. Capillary blood was immediately treated with CMH (1:1) and put into an EPR capillary tube and then placed inside the cavity of the EPR spectrometer for acquisition at 37 °C by the temperature and Gas controller "Bio III" unit (Noxygen Science Transfer & Diagnostics GmbH, Germany), interfaced to the spectrometer.

All spectra were collected by adopting the same acquisition parameters: microwave frequency = 9.652 GHz; modulation frequency: 86 kHz; modulation amplitude: 2.28 G; center field: 3456.8 G; sweep width: 60 G; microwave power: 21.90 mW; number of scans: 10; receiver gain: 3.17×10. Data were converted in absolute concentration values ($\mu mol \cdot min^{-1}$) by using the CP• (3-carboxy-2,2,5,5-tetramethyl-1-pyrrolidinyloxy) stable radical as an external reference. Spectra acquired were recorded and analyzed using the Win EPR software (version 2.11) standardly supplied by Bruker.

Details on the procedures have been previously reported [9,10,23,24].

4.4.2. Total Antioxidant Capacity (TAC)

TAC was measured using a commercial enzymatic kit (Cayman Chemical, Ann Arbor, MI, USA). The assay relies on the ability of antioxidants present in plasma to inhibit the oxidation of ABTS (2,2′-Azino-di-[3-ethylbenzthiazoline sulphonate]). The TAC signal is proportional to the suppression of the oxidized ABTS absorbance signal at 750 nm and is evaluated by a Trolox standard curve [24,57].

4.4.3. Protein Carbonyls (PCs)

The accumulation of oxidized proteins was measured by their reactive carbonyl content. A protein carbonyl (PC) assay kit (Cayman Chemical, Ann Arbor, MI, USA) was used to colorimetrically evaluate the oxidized proteins at 370 nm. The obtained values were normalized to the total protein concentration (at 280 nm) to determine the protein loss during the washing steps, as suggested by the kit's user manual [9,10,23,24].

4.4.4. Thiobarbituric Acid-Reactive Substances (TBARS)

TBARS measurements were adopted to detect lipid peroxidation. An assay kit (Cayman Chemical, Ann Arbor, MI, USA) was used to allow a rapid photometric thiobarbituric acid malondialdehyde (TBAMDA) adduct detection at 532 nm. A linear calibration curve was computed from pure malondialdehyde-containing solutions [9,10,16,23,24,57,58].

4.4.5. 8-Isoprostane (8-iso-PGF2α)

Lipid peroxidation was assessed also using an immunoassay of 8-isoprostane concentration (Cayman Chemical, Ann Arbor, MI, USA) in urine, as previously described [9,10,14]. Samples and standard were read in duplicate at a wavelength of 512 nm. Results were normalized by urine creatinine values.

4.4.6. 8-OH-2-Deoxyguanosine (8-OH-dG)

Levels of 8-OH-dG were measured using an immunoassay EIA kit (Cayman Chemical, Ann Arbor, MI, USA) in urine. This is a biomarker for DNA damage assessment. Samples and standards were spectrophotometrically read at 412 nm. Results were normalized by urine creatinine values [10,29,59].

4.4.7. Visual Analog Scale (VAS)

Subjective mood, general wellness/malaise, rested/tired feelings, headaches, sleepiness and nausea were evaluated using a 0–100 mm visual analog scale (VAS). This scoring system has been previously suggested for assessing discomfort and/or general malaise [52]. Based on its usefulness in performing other clinical evaluations, VAS was deemed suitable for testing the subjective perception of normobaric hypoxia effects [20,37,60].

4.5. Statistical Analysis

All values are expressed as mean ± SD. Data were analyzed using parametric statistics following the mathematical confirmation of a normal distribution using the Shapiro–Wilks W test. To determine the statistical significance of the changes during hypoxia exposure, ANOVA for repeated measures was performed, followed by the Tukey's post-hoc test. Significant differences were set at $p < 0.05$. The relationships between the investigated variables were assessed using Spearman correlation coefficients. Change $\Delta\%$ estimation (([post value-pre value]/pre value) × 100)) was also reported in the text. Statistical analyses were performed using Prism 9.3.1 software for Mac (GraphPad, Software Inc., San Diego, CA, USA).

ROS production was considered as the primary outcome (no other parameters were taken into account) and prospective calculations of power to determine sample size were made using G power software (GPower 3.1) [61]. At 80% power, the sample size—calculated in preliminary studies [9,29]—was set at five subjects.

5. Conclusions

In conclusion, the results of the present study provide evidence that under short, acute, normobaric hypoxia, ROS production and oxidative damage are time as well as SpO_2-dependent and are reversible phenomena. At the same time, the increase in oxidative damage, measured by enzymatic assays, appeared to be delayed with respect to the production of ROS—these latter EPR measurements being assessed by a mini-invasive absolute quantitative method. Lastly, the subjective evaluation of general physical conditions revealed a number of moderate-intensity discomforts described by most of the subjects, excluding nausea and headache. These findings seem overall to suggest that the experimental design proposed here can be considered a suitable model for use in future research studies. In fact, the altitude and time of exposure chosen tended to simulate the conditions experienced by mountain lovers during a single-day trip in alpine environments. Moreover, the study might help to highlight some key elements in acclimatization, as well as being of help for all those people who work at high altitudes without sufficient time to acclimatize, such as mountain rescue personnel/teams operating on helicopters during emergency medical operations (i.e., pilots, mountain rescuers and medical doctors) [43]. Finally, our EPR methods could be applied as a standard procedure in mountain medicine for studying changes induced by hypoxia due to acute and chronic high altitude stays.

Author Contributions: All authors listed have made a substantial, direct and intellectual contribution to the work, and have approved it for publication: Conceptualization: S.M.-S., M.M. (Mauro Marzorati), S.P. and A.V.; Investigation: S.M.-S., A.V., C.L. and S.P.; Writing: S.M.-S., M.G., M.M. (Mauro Marzorati), and C.L.; G.B., CB. and A.V. revised the manuscript critically; Data Analysis: S.M.-S., M.G., M.M. (Michela Montorsi), A.V., G.B. and C.B. All authors have read and agreed to the published version of the manuscript.

Funding: This research received no external funding.

Institutional Review Board Statement: Ethics Committee approval from Local Bio-Ethical Committee, Milan, Italy (BESTA/IBFM, Report #27, 9 March 2016).

Informed Consent Statement: Informed consent was obtained from all subjects involved in the study.

Data Availability Statement: Data are available at request from the authors.

Acknowledgments: We are grateful to Dott. Claudio Marconi for their critical reading and suggestions. The authors are grateful to all the volunteer participants.

Conflicts of Interest: The authors declare no conflict of interest.

Abbreviations

AMS	Acute Mountain Sickness
BL	Baseline
EPR	Electron Paramagnetic Resonance
NH	Normobaric Hypoxia
OxS	Oxidative Stress
8-OH-dG	8-OH-2-deoxyguanosine
8-iso-PGF2α	8-Isoprostane
PC	Protein Carbonyl
ROS	Reactive Oxygen Species
TAC	Total Antioxidant Capacity
TBARS	Thiobarbituric Acid Reactive Substance
VAS	Visual Analog Scale

References

1. Connett, R.J.; Honig, C.R.; Gayeski, T.E.; Brooks, G.A. Defining hypoxia: A systems view of VO$_2$, glycolysis, energetics, and intracellular PO$_2$. *J. Appl. Physiol.* **1990**, *68*, 833–842. [CrossRef]
2. Bugger, H.; Pfeil, K. Mitochondrial ROS in myocardial ischemia reperfusion and remodeling. *Biochim. Biophys. Acta Mol. Basis Dis.* **2020**, *1866*, 165768. [CrossRef] [PubMed]
3. Sies, H.; Jones, D.P. Reactive oxygen species (ROS) as pleiotropic physiological signalling agents. *Nat. Rev. Mol. Cell Biol.* **2020**, *21*, 363–383. [CrossRef]
4. Joanny, P.; Steinberg, J.; Robach, P.; Richalet, J.P.; Gortam, C.; Gardeytye, B.; Jammes, Y. Operation Everest III (Comex'97): The effect of simulated sever hypobaric hypoxia on lipid peroxidation and antioxidant defence systems in human blood at rest and after maximal exercise. *Resuscitation* **2001**, *49*, 307–314. [CrossRef] [PubMed]
5. Smidt, M.C.; Askew, E.W.; Roberts, D.E.-; Prior, R.L.; Ensign, W.Y., Jr.; Hesslink, R.E., Jr. Oxidative stress in humans training in a cold, moderate altitude environment and their response to a phytochemical antioxidant supplement. *Wilderness Environ. Med.* **2002**, *13*, 94–105. [CrossRef]
6. Araneda, O.F.; García, C.; Lagos, N.; Quiroga, G.; Cajigal, J.; Salazar, M.P.; Behn, C. Lung oxidative stress as related to exercise and altitude. Lipid peroxidation evidence in exhaled breath condensate: A possible predictor of acute mountain sickness. *Eur. J. Appl. Physiol.* **2005**, *95*, 383–390. [CrossRef]
7. Møller, P.; Loft, S.; Lundby, C.; Olsen, N.V. Acute hypoxia and hypoxic exercise induce DNA strand breaks and oxidative DNA damage in humans. *Faseb J.* **2001**, *15*, 1181–1186. [CrossRef] [PubMed]
8. Jefferson, J.A.; Simoni, J.; Escudero, E.; Hurtado, M.; Swenson, E.R.; Wesson, D.E.; Schreiner, G.F.; Schoene, R.; Johnson, R.J.; Hurtado, A. Increased oxidative stress following acute and chronic high-altitude exposure. *High Alt. Med. Biol.* **2004**, *5*, 61–69. [CrossRef] [PubMed]
9. Strapazzon, G.; Malacrida, S.; Vezzoli, A.; Dal Cappello, T.; Falla, M.; Lochner, P.; Moretti, S.; Procter, E.; Brugger, H.; Mrakic-Sposta, S. Oxidative stress response to acute hypobaric hypoxia and its association with indirect measurement of increased intracranial pressure: A field study. *Sci. Rep.* **2016**, *6*, 32426. [CrossRef]
10. Malacrida, S.; Giannella, A.; Ceolotto, G.; Reggiani, C.; Vezzoli, A.; Mrakic-Sposta, S.; Moretti, S.; Turner, R.; Falla, M.; Brugger, H.; et al. Transcription factors regulation in human peripheral white blood cells during hypobaric hypoxia exposure: An in-vivo experimental study. *Sci. Rep.* **2019**, *9*, 9901. [CrossRef] [PubMed]
11. Irarrázaval, S.; Allard, C.; Campodónico, J.; Pérez, D.; Strobel, P.; Vásquez, L.; Urquiaga, I.; Echeverría, G.; Leighton, F. Oxidative stress in acute hypobaric hypoxia. *High Alt. Med. Biol.* **2017**, *18*, 128–134. [CrossRef] [PubMed]
12. Verratti, V.; Mrakic-Sposta, S.; Moriggi, M.; Tonacci, A.; Bhandari, S.; Migliorelli, D.; Bajracharya, A.; Bondi, D.; Agrò, E.F.; Cerretelli, P. Urinary physiology and hypoxia: A pilot study of moderate-altitude trekking effects on urodynamic indexes. *Am. J. Physiol. Ren. Physiol.* **2019**, *317*, F1081–F1086. [CrossRef] [PubMed]
13. Rasica, L.; Porcelli, S.; Limper, U.; Mrakic-Sposta, S.; Mazzolari, R.; Gelmini, F.; Beretta, G.; Marzorati, M. Beet on Alps: Time-course changes of plasma nitrate and nitrite concentrations during acclimatization to high-altitude. *Nitric Oxide* **2021**, *107*, 66–72. [CrossRef]
14. Mrakic-Sposta, S.; Gussoni, M.; Dellanoce, C.; Marzorati, M.; Montorsi, M.; Rasica, L.; Pratali, L.; D'Angelo, G.; Martinelli, M.; Bastiani, L.; et al. Effects of acute and sub-acute hypobaric hypoxia on oxidative stress: A field study in the Alps. *Eur. J. Appl. Physiol.* **2021**, *121*, 297–306. [CrossRef] [PubMed]

15. Mrakic-Sposta, S.; Biagini, D.; Bondi, D.; Pietrangelo, T.; Vezzoli, A.; Lomonaco, T.; Di Francesco, F.; Verratti, V. OxInflammation at High Altitudes: A Proof of Concept from the Himalayas. *Antioxidants* **2022**, *11*, 368. [CrossRef]
16. Mrakic Sposta, S.; Montorsi, M.; Porcelli, S.; Marzorati, M.; Healey, B.; Dellanoce, C.; Vezzoli, A. Effects of Prolonged Exposure to Hypobaric Hypoxia on Oxidative Stress: Overwintering in Antarctic Concordia Station. *Oxid. Med. Cell Longev.* **2022**, *2022*, 4430032. [CrossRef]
17. Miller, L.E.; McGinnis, G.R.; Kliszczewicz, B.; Slivka, D.; Hailes, W.; Cuddy, J.; Dumke, C.; Ruby, B.; Quindry, J.C. Blood oxidative-stress markers during a high-altitude trek. *Int. J. Sport Nutr. Exerc. Metab.* **2013**, *23*, 65–72. [CrossRef]
18. Shi, Q.H.; Wei, W.; Ran, J.H.; Wang, S.Y.; Liu, Z.X.; Di, G.; Chen, P.; Fu, J.F. Hydrogen Therapy Reduces Oxidative Stress-associated Risks Following Acute and Chronic Exposure to High-altitude Environment. *Biomed. Environ. Sci.* **2015**, *28*, 239–241.
19. Magalhaes, J.; Ascensao, A.; Viscor, G.; Soares, J.; Oliveira, J.; Marques, F.; Duarte, J. Oxidative stress in humans during and after 4 hours of hypoxia at a simulated altitude of 5500 m. *Aviat. Space Environ. Med.* **2004**, *75*, 16–22.
20. Bailey, D.M.; Ainslie, P.N.; Jackson, S.K.; Richardson, R.S.; Ghatei, M. Evidence against redox regulation of energy homoeostasis in humans at high altitude. *Clin. Sci.* **2004**, *107*, 589–600. [CrossRef]
21. Coppel, J.; Hennis, P.; Gilbert-Kawa, I.E.; Grocott, M.P.W. The physiological effects of hypobaric hypoxia versus normobaric hypoxia: A systematic review of crossover trials. *Extrem. Physiol. Med.* **2015**, *4*, 2. [CrossRef] [PubMed]
22. Bailey, D.M.; Taudorf, S.; Berg, R.M.; Lundby, C.; McEneny, J.; Young, I.S.; Evans, K.A.; James, P.E.; Shore, A.; Hullin, D.A.; et al. Increased cerebral output of free radicals during hypoxia: Implications for acute mountain sickness? *Am. J. Physiol. Regul. Integr. Comp. Physiol.* **2009**, *297*, R1283–R1292. [CrossRef] [PubMed]
23. Mrakic-Sposta, S.; Gussoni, M.; Montorsi, M.; Porcelli, S.; Vezzoli, A. Assessment of a standardized ROS production profile in humans by electron paramagnetic resonance. *Oxid. Med. Cell. Longev.* **2012**, *2012*, 973927. [CrossRef] [PubMed]
24. Mrakic-Sposta, S.; Gussoni, M.; Montorsi, M.; Porcelli, S.; Vezzoli, A. A quantitative method to monitor reactive oxygen species production by electron paramagnetic resonance in physiological and pathological conditions. *Oxid. Med. Cell. Longev.* **2014**, *2014*, 306179. [CrossRef]
25. Mrakic-Sposta, S.; Gussoni, M.; Porcelli, S.; Pugliese, L.; Pavei, G.; Bellistri, G.; Montorsi, M.; Tacchini, P.; Vezzoli, A. Training effects on ROS production determined by electron paramagnetic resonance in master swimmers. *Oxid. Med. Cell. Longev.* **2015**, *2015*, 804794. [CrossRef]
26. Mrakic-Sposta, S.; Gussoni, M.; Moretti, S.; Pratali, L.; Giardini, G.; Tacchini, P.; Dellanoce, C.; Tonacci, A.; Mastrorci, F.; Borghini, A.; et al. Effects of mountain ultra-marathon running on ROS production and oxidative damage by micro-invasive analytic techniques. *PLoS ONE* **2015**, *10*, e0141780. [CrossRef]
27. Mrakic-Sposta, S.; Vezzoli, A.; Malacrida, S.; Falla, M.; Strapazzon, G. "Direct" and "indirect" methods to detect oxidative stress during acute or chronic high-altitude exposure. *High Alt. Med. Biol.* **2017**, *18*, 303–304. [CrossRef]
28. Mrakic-Sposta, S.; Vezzoli, A.; Maderna, L.; Gregorini, F.; Montorsi, M.; Moretti, S.; Greco, F.; Cova, M.; Gussoni, M. R(+)-Thioctic Acid Effects on Oxidative Stress and Peripheral Neuropathy in Type II Diabetic Patients: Preliminary Results by Electron Paramagnetic Resonance and Electroneurography. *Oxid. Med. Cell. Longev.* **2018**, *2018*, 1767265. [CrossRef]
29. Mrakic-Sposta, S.; Vezzoli, A.; D'Alessandro, F.; Paganini, M.; Dellanoce, C.; Cialoni, D.; Bosco, G. Change in Oxidative Stress Biomarkers During 30 Days in Saturation Dive: A Pilot Study. *Int. J. Environ. Res. Public Health* **2020**, *17*, 7118. [CrossRef]
30. Bosco, G.; Giacon, T.A.; Paolocci, N.; Vezzoli, A.; Noce, C.D.; Paganini, M.; Agrimi, J.; Garetto, G.; Cialoni, D.; D'Alessandro, N.; et al. Dopamine/BDNF loss underscores narcosis cognitive impairment in divers: A proof of concept in a dry condition. *Eur. J. Appl. Physiol.* **2022**, *123*, 143–158. [CrossRef]
31. Colombo, E.; Marconi, C.; Taddeo, A.; Cappelletti, M.; Villa, M.L.; Marzorati, M.; Porcelli, S.; Vezzoli, A.; Bella, S.D. Fast reduction of peripheral blood endothelial progenitor cells in healthy humans exposed to acute systemic hypoxia. *J. Physiol.* **2012**, *590*, 519–532. [CrossRef] [PubMed]
32. Millet, P.M.; Faiss, R.; Pialoux, V. Point: Hypobaric hypoxia induces different physiological responses from normobaric hypoxia. *J. Appl. Physiol.* **2012**, *112*, 1783–1787. [CrossRef]
33. Ribon, A.; Pialoux, V.; Saugy, J.J.; Rupp, T.; Faiss, R.; Debevec, T.; Millet, G.P. Exposure to hypobaric hypoxia results in higher oxidative stress compared to normobaric hypoxia. *J. Respir. Physiol. Neurobiol.* **2016**, *223*, 23–27. [CrossRef] [PubMed]
34. Steiner, D.R.; Gonzalez, N.C.; Wood, J.G. Interaction between reactive oxygen species and nitric oxide in the microvascular response to systemic hypoxia. *J. Appl. Physiol.* **2001**, *93*, 1411–1418. [CrossRef] [PubMed]
35. Weissmann, N.; Sommer, N.; Schermuly, R.T.; Ghofrani, H.A.; Seeger, W.; Grimminger, F. Oxygen sensors in hypoxic pulmonary vasoconstriction. *Cardiovasc. Res.* **2006**, *71*, 620–629. [CrossRef]
36. Clanton, T.L. Hypoxia-induced reactive oxygen species formation in skeletal muscle. *J. Appl. Physiol.* **2007**, *102*, 2379–2388. [CrossRef]
37. Bailey, D.M.; Roukens, R.; Knauth, M.; Kallenberg, K.; Christ, S.; Mohr, A.; Genius, J.; Storch-Hagenlocher, B.; Meisel, F.; McEneny, J.; et al. Free radical-mediated damage to barrier function is not associated with altered brain morphology in high-altitude headache. *J. Cereb. Blood Flow Metab.* **2006**, *26*, 99–111. [CrossRef]
38. Wang, Y.X.; Zheng, Y.M. ROS-Dependent Signaling Mechanisms for Hypoxic Ca^{2+} Responses in Pulmonary Artery Myocytes. *Antioxid. Redox Signal* **2010**, *12*, 611–623. [CrossRef]

39. Balestra, C.; Arya, A.K.; Leveque, C.; Virgili, F.; Germonpré, P.; Lambrechts, K.; Lafère, P.; Thom, S.R. Varying Oxygen Partial Pressure Elicits Blood-Borne Microparticles Expressing Different Cell-Specific Proteins—Toward a Targeted Use of Oxygen? *Int. J. Mol. Sci.* **2012**, *23*, 7888. [CrossRef]
40. Rifkind, J.M.; Nagababu, E.; Ramasamy, S.; Ravi, L.B. Hemoglobin redox reactions and oxidative stress. *Redox Rep.* **2003**, *8*, 234–237. [CrossRef]
41. Abugo, O.O.; Rifkind, J.M. Oxidation of hemoglobin and the enhancement produced by nitroblue tetrazolium. *J. Biol. Chem.* **1994**, *269*, 24845–24853. [CrossRef] [PubMed]
42. Balagopalakrishna, C.; Manoharan, P.T.; Abugo, O.O.; Rifkind, J.M. Production of superoxide from hemoglobin-bound oxygen under hypoxic conditions. *Biochemistry* **1996**, *35*, 6393–6398. [CrossRef] [PubMed]
43. Theunissen, S.; Balestra, C.; Bolognési, S.; Borgers, G.; Vissenaeken, D.; Obeid, G.; Germonpré, P.; Honoré, P.M.; De Bels, D. Effects of Acute Hypobaric Hypoxia Exposure on Cardiovascular Function in Unacclimatized Healthy Subjects: A "Rapid Ascent" Hypobaric Chamber Study. *Int. J. Environ. Res. Public Health* **2022**, *19*, 5394. [CrossRef] [PubMed]
44. Murphy, M.P.; Bayir, H.; Belousov, V.; Chang, C.J.; Davies, K.J.A.; Davies, M.J.; Dick, T.P.; Finkel, T.; Forman, H.J.; Janssen-Heininger, Y.; et al. Guidelines for measuring reactive oxygen species and oxidative damage in cells and in vivo. *Nat. Metab.* **2022**, *4*, 651–662. [CrossRef] [PubMed]
45. Gallagher, E.J.; Bijur, P.E.; Latimer, C.; Silver, W. Reliability and validity of a visual analog scale for acute abdominal pain in the ED. *Am. J. Emerg. Med.* **2002**, *20*, 287–290. [CrossRef]
46. Serrano-Duenas, M. High altitude headache. A prospective study of its clinical characteristics. *Cephalalgia* **2005**, *25*, 1110–1116. [CrossRef]
47. Hendey, G.W.; Donner, N.F.; Fuller, K. Clinically significant changes in nausea as measured on a visual analog scale. *Ann. Emerg. Med.* **2005**, *45*, 77–81. [CrossRef]
48. Levy, O.; Amit-Vazina, M.; Segal, R.; Tishler, M. Visual Analogue Scales of Pain, Fatigue and Function in Patients with Various Rheumatic Disorders Receiving Standard Care. *Isr. Med. Assoc. J.* **2015**, *17*, 691–696.
49. Zisapel, N.; Nir, T. Determination of the minimal clinically significant difference on a patient visual analog sleep quality scale. *J. Sleep Res.* **2003**, *12*, 291–298. [CrossRef]
50. Savourey, G.; Guinet, A.; Besnard, Y.; Garcia, N.; Hanniquet, A.M.; Bittel, J. Evaluation of the Lake Louise acute mountain sickness scoring system in a hypobaric chamber. *Aviat. Space Environ. Med.* **1995**, *66*, 963–967.
51. Van Roo, J.D.; Lazio, M.P.; Pesce, C.; Malik, S.; Courtney, D.M. Visual analog scale (VAS) for assessment of acute mountain sickness (AMS) on Aconcagua. *Wilderness Environ. Med.* **2011**, *22*, 7–14. [CrossRef] [PubMed]
52. Wu, J.; Chen, Y.; Luo, Y. Evaluation of the Visual Analog Score (VAS) to Assess Acute Mountain Sickness (AMS) in a Hypobaric Chamber. *PLoS ONE* **2014**, *9*, e113376. [CrossRef] [PubMed]
53. Cialoni, D.; Brizzolari, A.; Samaja, M.; Bosco, G.; Paganini, M.; Pieri, M.; Lancellotti, V.; Marroni, A. Nitric Oxide and Oxidative Stress Changes at Depth in Breath-Hold Diving. *Front. Physiol.* **2001**, *11*, 609642. [CrossRef]
54. Grossini, E.; Garhwal, D.; Venkatesan, S.; Ferrante, D.; Mele, A.; Saraceno, M.; Scognamiglio, A.; Mandrioli, J.; Amedei, A.; De Marchi, F.; et al. The Potential Role of Peripheral Oxidative Stress on the Neurovascular Unit in Amyotrophic Lateral Sclerosis Pathogenesis: A Preliminary Report from Human and In Vitro Evaluations. *Biomedicines* **2022**, *10*, 691. [CrossRef]
55. Lorinczova, H.T.; Begum, G.; Temouri, L.; Renshaw, D.; Zariwala, M.G. Co-Administration of Iron and Bioavailable Curcumin Reduces Levels of Systemic Markers of Inflammation and Oxidative Stress in a Placebo-Controlled Randomised Study. *Nutrients* **2022**, *14*, 712. [CrossRef]
56. World Medical Association. World Medical Association Declaration of Helsinki: Ethical principles for medical research involving human subjects. *JAMA* **2013**, *310*, 2191–2194. [CrossRef] [PubMed]
57. Llorente-Cantarero, F.J.; Aguilar-Gómez, F.J.; Leis, R.; Bueno, G.; Rupérez, A.I.; Anguita-Ruiz, A.; Vázquez-Cobela, R.; Mesa, M.D.; Moreno, L.A.; Gil, A.; et al. Relationship between Physical Activity, Oxidative Stress, and Total Plasma Antioxidant Capacity in Spanish Children from the GENOBOX Study. *Antioxidants* **2021**, *10*, 320. [CrossRef]
58. Falone, S.; Mirabilio, A.; Pennelli, A.; Cacchio, M.; Di Baldassarre, A.; Gallina, S.; Amicarelli, F. Differential Impact of Acute Bout of Exercise on Redox- and Oxidative Damage-Related Profiles Between Untrained Subjects and Amateur Runners. *Physiol. Res.* **2010**, *59*, 953–961. [CrossRef]
59. Zanolin, M.E.; Girardi, P.; Degan, P.; Rava, M.; Olivieri, M.; DiGennaro, G.; Nicolis, M.; De Marco, R. Measurement of a urinary marker (8-hydroxydeoxy-guanosine, 8-OHdG) of DNA oxidative stress in epidemiological surveys: A pilot study. *Int. J. Biol. Markers* **2015**, *30*, e341–e345. [CrossRef]
60. Baillie, J.K.; Thompson, A.A.; Irving, J.B.; Bates, M.G.D.; Sutherland, A.I.; Macnee, W.; Maxwell, S.R.J.; Webb, D.J. Oral antioxidant supplementation does not prevent acute mountain sickness: Double blind, randomized placebo-controlled trial. *Eur. J. Nutr.* **2009**, *54*, 251–263. [CrossRef]
61. Faul, F.; Erdfelder, E.; Lang, A.G.; Buchner, A. G*Power 3: A flexible statis- tical power analysis program for the social, behavioral, and bio- medical sciences. *Behav. Res. Methods* **2007**, *39*, 175–191. [CrossRef] [PubMed]

Disclaimer/Publisher's Note: The statements, opinions and data contained in all publications are solely those of the individual author(s) and contributor(s) and not of MDPI and/or the editor(s). MDPI and/or the editor(s) disclaim responsibility for any injury to people or property resulting from any ideas, methods, instructions or products referred to in the content.

Article

Oxidative Stress Response Kinetics after 60 Minutes at Different Levels (10% or 15%) of Normobaric Hypoxia Exposure

Clément Leveque [1,2], Simona Mrakic Sposta [3], Sigrid Theunissen [1,*], Peter Germonpré [4,5], Kate Lambrechts [1], Alessandra Vezzoli [3], Maristella Gussoni [6], Morgan Levenez [1], Pierre Lafère [1,4], François Guerrero [2] and Costantino Balestra [1,4,7,8,*]

[1] Environmental, Occupational, Aging (Integrative) Physiology Laboratory, Haute Ecole Bruxelles-Brabant (HE2B), 1160 Brussels, Belgium; c.leveque.research@gmail.com (C.L.); klambrechts@he2b.be (K.L.); morganlevenez@gmail.com (M.L.); plafere@he2b.be (P.L.)
[2] Laboratoire ORPHY, Université de Bretagne Occidentale, UFR Sciences et Techniques, 93837 Brest, France; francois.guerrero@univ-brest.fr
[3] Institute of Clinical Physiology, National Research Council (CNR), 20162 Milan, Italy; simona.mrakicsposta@cnr.it (S.M.S.); alessandra.vezzoli@cnr.it (A.V.)
[4] DAN Europe Research Division (Roseto-Brussels), 1160 Brussels, Belgium; pgermonpre@gmail.com
[5] Hyperbaric Centre, Queen Astrid Military Hospital, 1120 Brussels, Belgium
[6] Institute of Chemical Sciences and Technologies "G. Natta", National Research Council (SCITEC-CNR), 20133 Milan, Italy; maristella.gussoni@unimi.it
[7] Anatomical Research and Clinical Studies, Vrije Universiteit Brussels (VUB), 1090 Brussels, Belgium
[8] Motor Sciences Department, Physical Activity Teaching Unit, Université Libre de Bruxelles (ULB), 1050 Brussels, Belgium
* Correspondence: sigtheunissen@gmail.com (S.T.); costantino.balestra@ulb.be (C.B.)

Abstract: In this study, the metabolic responses of hypoxic breathing for 1 h to inspired fractions of 10% and 15% oxygen were investigated. To this end, 14 healthy nonsmoking subjects (6 females and 8 males, age: 32.2 ± 13.3 years old (mean ± SD), height: 169.1 ± 9.9 cm, and weight: 61.6 ± 16.2 kg) volunteered for the study. Blood samples were taken before, and at 30 min, 2 h, 8 h, 24 h, and 48 h after a 1 h hypoxic exposure. The level of oxidative stress was evaluated by considering reactive oxygen species (ROS), nitric oxide metabolites (NOx), lipid peroxidation, and immune-inflammation by interleukin-6 (IL-6) and neopterin, while antioxidant systems were observed in terms of the total antioxidant capacity (TAC) and urates. Hypoxia abruptly and rapidly increased ROS, while TAC showed a U-shape pattern, with a nadir between 30 min and 2 h. The regulation of ROS and NOx could be explained by the antioxidant action of uric acid and creatinine. The kinetics of ROS allowed for the stimulation of the immune system translated by an increase in neopterin, IL-6, and NOx. This study provides insights into the mechanisms through which acute hypoxia affects various bodily functions and how the body sets up the protective mechanisms to maintain redox homeostasis in response to oxidative stress.

Keywords: hypoxia; oxygen biology; cellular reactions; human; oxygen therapy; human performance; decompression

1. Introduction

Acute hypoxia (AH) is an environmental condition that is regularly encountered, for example, by mine workers or telescope operators going to high altitudes, or by pilots flying at high altitudes [1]. Intermittent acute hypoxia is also a therapeutic approach that is of growing interest in scientific research because of its (often unrecognized) beneficial effects, as well as its adverse effects. Indeed, low-dose repetitive AH protocols have demonstrated numerous benefits, such as reducing hypertension [2], reducing inflammation [3], improving aerobic capacity [4], increasing bone mineral density [5], and improving memory [6–9] and cardiovascular function [10,11]. Furthermore, the positive effects of low-dose AH do not seem to be associated with detectable negative effects, such as systemic inflammation [12]. However, in order to optimize the use of AH as a therapeutic approach, it is important to maximize its benefits while avoiding any adverse effects. Hypoxia can have deleterious effects during stroke or cancer [13] and may negatively affect vascular function [14] or even cause altitude sickness in healthy mountaineers [15]. Of course, these harmful effects generally result from oxygen deprivation at lower oxygen fractions or for longer periods [16].

At the same time, it has been shown that intermittent variations in the inspired oxygen level, whether to hypoxia or hyperoxia, can also lead to multiple effects such as an increase in hemoglobin [17] or the stimulation of hypoxia-inducible factor 1-alpha, inflammatory markers such as nuclear factor kappa B and interleukin-6 (IL-6), antioxidant proteins as nuclear factor erythroid-2-related factor 2 (NRF2) and micro-RNAs [18].

Some authors have attempted to use hypoxia during training sessions to achieve an increased training benefit [19,20] by coupling high-intensity exercise sessions with simulated altitude. However, incorporating hypoxia into all high-intensity interval sessions had little effect on performance compared with normoxia training [21,22]. Other studies suggest that short-term exposure to hypoxic air during intense training can favorably remodel skeletal muscle [23–25]. However, there is no visible benefit to endurance performance, particularly in well-trained athletes [26].

It is known that reactive oxygen species (ROS) and the cellular redox state play a major role in modulating many signaling pathways. In moderate amounts, ROS are important for physiological processes, leading to positive cellular adaptive responses, while large amounts of ROS can damage lipids, proteins, and DNA, and lead to pathological responses [18]. Therefore, the exposure of healthy individuals or patients to severe hypoxia could potentially generate high levels of ROS and facilitate disease progression [27]. In contrast, a training program consisting of 15 to 24 sessions of intermittent exposure to severe hypoxia has gained popularity as a treatment in patients with a variety of chronic conditions [28–30]. Currently, the best protocol for acute exposure to severe hypoxia (in combination with normoxia or hyperoxia) to reach the best outcomes associated with a beneficial change in the redox status is not known [16,31,32]. Depending on the duration and severity of the hypoxia exposure, the effects on the different cellular functions can be positive or deleterious. It is therefore important to understand its kinetics after a single exposure before implementing intermittent hypoxia sessions for patient treatment or for training reasons, since the time between sessions is crucial to achieve optimal outcomes and different cell reactions could be targeted depending on the dose and repetitions [33,34]. The objective of this study is thus to observe the effects of oxy-inflammation over time in response to a single exposure to normobaric hypoxia at two different inspired fractions of oxygen (FiO_2): 10% and 15%.

2. Results

2.1. ROS and NOx Rate, Antioxidant Response (TAC), and 8-Isoprostane (8-iso-PGF2α) Levels after One Hour of Oxygen Exposure at an FiO_2 of 10% and 15%

Both levels of oxygen exposure, severe (10%) and mild (15%), elicited a significant increase in plasmatic ROS production rate, with a steeper increase and slower reduction for severe exposure (Figure 1A). Exposure to severe hypoxia produced more ROS than mild exposure and showed a pattern characterized by a significant increase, with a peak after 30 min for both 10% hypoxia (0.32 ± 0.03 µmol·min^{-1} compared with baseline; $p = 0.0015$; size effect = 0.16) and 15% hypoxia (0.27 ± 0.02 µmol·min^{-1}; $p < 0.001$; size effect = 0.24). This peak plateaus for about 2 h quantity of ROS decreases slowly until 48 h. The difference between the two levels of exposure disappeared after 24 h ($p = 0.87$). The antioxidants (TAC) (Figure 1B) decreased, with a nadir at 30 min for the 10% FiO_2 group (1.52 ± 0.22 mM; $p = 0.0017$; size effect = 0.50) and at 2 h for the 15% FiO_2 group (1.70 ± 0.20 mM; $p = 0.0010$; effect size = 0.2496). Antioxidants decreased more rapidly after severe hypoxia than after mild hypoxia ($p = 0.0191$). Notably, 8-isoprostane (pg/mg creatinine) (Figure 1C) followed the exact same trend for both levels of oxygen exposure, with a peak at 2 h (553 ± 199 pg·mg^{-1} creatinine after 10% hypoxia; p = 0.0461; size effect = 0.64 vs. 489 ± 161 pg·mg^{-1} creatinine after 15% hypoxia; p = 0.0046; size effect = 0.35). After 48 h, the values returned to baseline for both levels of exposure (10%: 259 ± 91 pg·mg^{-1} creatinine; p = 0.4499 and 15%: 325 ± 103 pg·mg^{-1} creatinine; p > 0.9999). Nitric oxide metabolites (Figure 1D) showed a peak 2 h after acute exposure to 10% oxygen compared with baseline (516 ± 132 µM; p = 0.013; size effect = 0.51), while no significant difference was observed after exposure to 15% oxygen (p = 0.1303; size effect = 0.27).

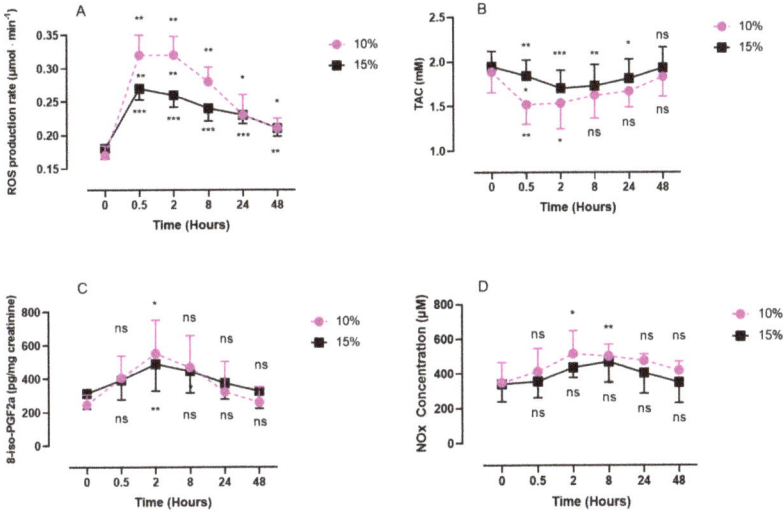

Figure 1. Evolution of ROS production rate (**A**), antioxidant response (TAC) (**B**), 8-iso-PGF2a (**C**), and NOx (**D**) after 60 min of mild (15%, n = 8) or severe hypoxia (10%, n = 6). Results are expressed as mean ± SD. T0 represents the pre-exposure baseline. Intra-group comparisons between results at T0 and each other time point are represented above and below the respective curves. Inter-group comparisons between 10% and 15% of oxygen exposure when significant are shown between the two curves (ns: not significant; *: $p < 0.05$, **: $p < 0.01$, ***: $p < 0.001$).

2.2. Inflammatory Response (IL-6, Neopterin, Creatinine, and Uric Acid) after One Hour of Oxygen Exposure at an FiO$_2$ of 10% or 15%

Interleukin 6 (IL-6) was measured in plasma samples while neopterin, creatinine, and urates were obtained from urine samples (Figures 2 and 3).

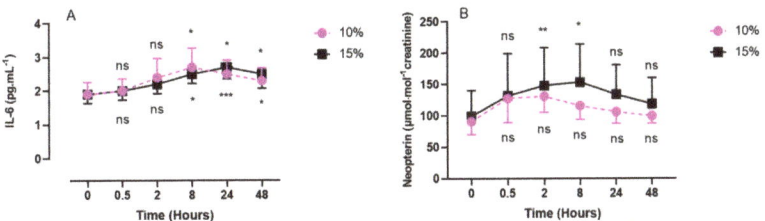

Figure 2. Evolution of the inflammatory response after 60 min of mild (15%, n = 8) or severe hypoxia (10%, n = 6) for interleukin-6 (IL-6) (**A**) and neopterin (**B**). Results are expressed as mean ± SD. T0 represents pre-exposure values. Intra-group comparisons between results at T0 and each other time point are represented above and below the respective curves. (ns: not significant; *: $p < 0.05$; **: $p < 0.01$; ***: $p < 0.001$).

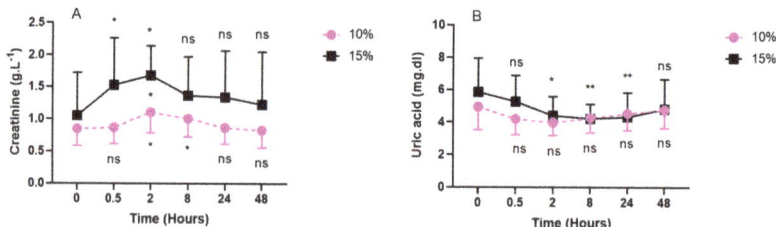

Figure 3. Evolution of urinary markers after 60 min of mild (15%, n = 8) or severe hypoxia (10%, n = 6) for creatinine (**A**) and uric Acid (**B**). Results are expressed as mean ± SD. T0 represents pre-exposure values. Intra-group comparisons between results at T0 and each other time point are represented above and below the respective curves. Inter-group comparisons between 10% and 15% of oxygen exposure when significant are shown between the two curves (ns: not significant; *: $p < 0.05$, **: $p < 0.01$; intragroup: Friedman; intergroup: unpaired t-test).

IL-6 showed a significant increase compared with the baseline, until reaching its peak at 8 h for the 10% group (2.7 ± 0.57 pg/mL; p = 0.0203; effect size = 0.72). Contrary to severe hypoxia, mild hypoxia (15%) showed a significant increase from 8 h post-exposure (2.5 ± 0.28 pg/mL; p = 0.0179), with a peak at 24 h (2.7 ± 0.34 pg/mL; p = 0.0001), and slowly decreased until 48 h.

Neopterin showed a similar trend during the first 30 min for mild (15%) and severe (10%) hypoxia and reached its peak at 2 h for severe hypoxia (130.6 ± 25.6 μmol/mol creatinine; p = 0.1475; effect size = 0.52) and at 8 h for mild hypoxia (153.0 ± 61.1 μmol/mol creatinine; p = 0.0441; effect size = 0.13). The values returned to baseline after 48 h for the two levels of hypoxia.

Compared with the baseline, creatinine and urates in urine exhibited an opposite U-shaped response, with creatinine's acme at 2 h post-exposure (10%: 1.11 ± 0.32 g/L; p = 0.0192; effect size = 0.17 vs. 15%: 1.68 ± 0.47 g/L; p = 0.0488; effect size = 0.10) and urates' nadir between 30 min and 2 h for severe hypoxia (10%) (30 min: 4.22 ± 0.96 mg/dL; p = 0.3312; 2 h: 4.0 ± 0.78 mg/dL; 0.3427; effect size = 0.13) and between 8 h and 24 h for mild hypoxia (15%) (8 h: 4.23 ± 0.89 mg/dL; p = 0.0041; 24 h: 4.33 ± 1.5 mg/dL; p = 0.0084; size effect = 0.18) (Figure 3).

2.3. Discomfort Perceived—Visual Analog Scale (VAS)

No subject developed malaise, tiredness, headaches, sleepiness, or nausea upon exposure to one hour of hypoxia, neither with 10% nor with 15% exposure. However, hypoxia at 10% (equivalent to an altitude of approximately 5700 m) was felt to be less comfortable than that at 15% (roughly 2500 m altitude) (81.0 ± 10.6% of declared discomfort vs. 12.9 ± 5.4% of declared discomfort, respectively; $p > 0.001$).

3. Discussion

The presented data confirm the results of previous studies by highlighting a significant increase in ROS production [35–38] during a short period of moderate or extreme hypoxia. We observed a faster and larger increase in ROS production as hypoxia increased. However, after 48 h of recovery, ROS levels returned close to the baseline. It is known that the mitochondrial complex I is inhibited by intermittent hypoxia through the activation of NOx (NADPH oxidase), thereby increasing the production of ROS [39]. In various situations, electrons escaping from enzymatic and nonenzymatic reactions initiate the production of ROS, represented by superoxide anion ($O_2^{\bullet-}$), hydrogen peroxide (H_2O_2), and hydroxide ($HO^{\bullet}$) [40]. In an aqueous solution, $O_2^{\bullet-}$ has a half-life of approximately 4 μsec, which gives it the ability to scatter over a distance ranging from 150 to 220 nm [41,42]. Thus, $O_2^{\bullet-}$ can react at various locations beyond where it is generated and, as a result, can affect surrounding molecules and organelles more extensively than $HO^{\bullet}$. However, this distance is insufficient for extracellularly produced $O_2^{\bullet-}$ to move within a cell. Therefore, $O_2^{\bullet-}$

generated inside the cell has the ability to damage various cellular components, including DNA, organelles, and cellular membranes' phospholipids. Our results are in agreement with this assumption since we observed an increase in 8-iso-PGF2α 2 h after the two levels of exposure, slightly delayed after the increase in ROS occurring 30 min after exposure.

It has been demonstrated that acute hypoxic conditions induce mitochondrial fission [43]. This reduction in mitochondrial fusion is further described in hypoxia-reoxygenation situations and is caused by decreased ATP production [44]. This adaptation appears to be a countermeasure to maintaining mitochondrial ROS production at a balanced level [45]. Furthermore, we observed an increase in NOx production, with a peak after 2 h and still significant after 8 h. Due to its radical nature, the reaction between superoxide and NO proceeds in a limited manner through diffusion (with a rate constant of k = 1.9 × 1010 $M^{-1}s^{-1}$) [46], which is faster than the SOD-catalyzed dismutation of superoxide. The advantage of trapping superoxide ions is to eliminate the radical electrons at an early stage, thereby halting subsequent radical chain reactions [40]. Indeed, our results suggest that the peak of NOx at 2 h occurring after the peak of ROS (30 min) indicates an early activity of NO as a ROS scavenger. This is further confirmed by the nonsignificant changes in NOx during normobaric hypoxia. This is consistent with previous findings [35], where the activity of GPX and SOD was not significantly increased after normobaric hypoxia [47]. Considering the abundant production of NO, the ability of NO to scavenge superoxide appears to be comparable to the activity of intracellular SOD and may even be more effective. However, the resulting ONOO- produced from this reaction is a powerful oxidant and is toxic to cells when produced in excess beyond the antioxidant capacity [48]. However, currently, new lines of evidence suggest a beneficial action of ONOO-. In the vascular system, for instance, moderate levels of ONOO- appear to stimulate prostaglandin synthesis and play a role in cellular signal transduction reactions [49]. Furthermore, under inflammatory conditions, the simultaneous production of NO and ONOO- suggests that the detoxification of superoxide by NO exceeds the cytotoxic action of ONOO- [50].

Although H_2O_2 was not directly measured, we hypothesize that the increase in NOx, in particular NO_2, may reflect the onset of an adaptive activity by angiogenesis [51].

In this study, we observed a decrease in urinary uric acid (UA) excretion, more clearly expressed after 15% of oxygen breathing. This suggests a consumption of uric acid as an antioxidant.

In fact, an evolutionary advantage of UA has been proposed by demonstrating its strong capacity to eliminate free radicals, making it an excellent scavenger [52]. Studies have shown that UA contributes up to 60% to the elimination of free radicals in human serum [53]. Furthermore, the systemic administration of UA has been associated with an increase in plasma antioxidant capacity, both at rest and after exercise, in healthy subjects [54,55]. Interestingly, after 48 h, we observed a return to baseline levels, suggesting that UA plays an antioxidant role without shifting to its function as a pro-oxidant [56].

Moreover, we observed an increase in urinary creatinine excretion, with a zenith 2 h after exposure to 10% and 15% hypoxia. This suggests an increase in creatine catabolism. Although the antioxidant mechanism of creatine is not yet fully understood, it has been shown to contribute to cellular homeostasis, particularly as a mitochondrial protector [57].

In our experimental setting, no muscular activity was present. Therefore, we believe creatinine excretion is a marker of its antioxidant activity. In fact, it is known that, in response to acute high-altitude exposures with muscular activity, hyperventilation causes alkalosis. The kidneys compensate for this alkalosis by excreting excess bicarbonate and retaining hydrogen ions to reduce respiratory alkalosis [58]. Our results are then in agreement with the putative (not yet fully known) mechanism of action of creatine as an antioxidant. However, it has been shown to increase the activity of antioxidant enzymes and the capability to eliminate ROS and reactive nitrogen species [59–61]. We indeed found a globally symmetrical reaction to creatinine on ROS production, NOx, neopterin, and 8-iso-PGF2α.

Interestingly, we observed an increase in the initiation of 8-iso-PGF2α, which is a marker of lipid peroxidation by ROS [62,63], at 2 h post-exposure. Lipid peroxidation has its peak between 2 and 8 h; this relatively late reaction may be understood because of creatin action (cf. supra).

Our study also showed an immune system stimulation. Indeed, the increasing concentration of neopterin can be monitored in medicine to evaluate the level of clinical inflammation resulting from physical trauma, cardiovascular diseases, cancer, and bacterial, parasitic, and/or viral infections [64–68]. A rapid increase in neopterin was also observed (after 2 h) following the ROS peak without pathological reasons since the hypoxic stimulus was of short duration and no other harmful situations (trauma, cardiovascular diseases, etc.) were present. This rapid reaction is of interest, as it would counteract the inflammasome complex favoring the NRF2 pathway, as already shown following mild "oxy-inflammation" of 60 min [69]. This result is very interesting in the context of preconditioning protocols with the aim of inhibiting inflammasomes [70].

Interestingly, neopterin modulation is inversely proportional to the importance of hypoxia. Indeed, we observed a greater increase in neopterin after exposure to 15% oxygen than after exposure to 10% oxygen. We speculate that a higher hyperoxia-induced increase in ROS production could contribute to this difference, as already recently shown in moderate hyperoxia compared with hypoxia (oxy-inflammation) [14].

All the renal countermeasures described seem to have an efficient antioxidant role in these short hypoxic exposures together with significant TAC variations. This was not found during longer hypoxic exposures [71].

Acute hypoxia stimulates the production of IL-6 and the polarization of M1 macrophages. IL-6 is increased via the induction of antioxidant response element and nuclear factor kappa B (NF-κB) [72]. Furthermore, IL-6 (staying significantly high for 48 h) activates the NRF2 signaling pathway, which allows for the expression of antioxidant genes and maintains redox homeostasis [73]. Furthermore, it has recently been shown that NRF2 plays a key role in providing the preconditions for normobaric hypoxia to enhance exercise endurance [74].

4. Limitations

Strengths:
- This study is, to our knowledge, one of the first to tackle the kinetic responses to a single short normobaric oxygen exposure at 10% and 15% of FiO_2;
- The measurements were taken until 48 h post-exposure and putatively open the avenue to new possible applications for hypoxic protocols;
- The electron paramagnetic resonance (EPR) method used for ROS analysis is the actual gold standard.

Weaknesses:
- The number of subjects was limited, but the sample can be considered homogenous since all were healthy participants;
- The analysis was not carried out in the nucleus of the cells but in the plasma. This could be considered a weakness for some, but it would need a thoroughly different experimental setting.

5. Materials and Methods

5.1. Experimental Protocol

After written informed consent, 48 healthy nonsmoking Caucasian subjects (32 males and 16 females) volunteered for this study. None of them had a history of previous cardiac abnormalities or were under any cardio- or vasoactive medication.

All experimental procedures were conducted in accordance with the Declaration of Helsinki [75] and approved by the Ethics Committee approval from the Bio-Ethical Committee for Research and Higher Education, Brussels (No. B200-2020-088).

After medical screening to exclude any latent morbidity, participants were prospectively randomized into six groups of 6–8 persons each. These groups were divided into hypoxia (10% and 15% of FiO_2), normobaric hyperoxia (30% and 100% of FiO_2 [34], and hyperbaric hyperoxia (1.4 ATA and 2.5 ATA) groups. All participants were asked to refrain from strenuous exercise for 48 h before the tests. No antioxidant nutrients, i.e., dark chocolate, red wine, or green tea, were permitted 8 h preceding and during the study. The subjects were also asked not to dive 48 h before the experiment and not to fly within 72 h before the experiment.

Fourteen participants were subjected to mild hypoxia (15%, n = 8) and extreme hypoxia (10%, n = 6) protocols. As far as age (10%: 34.0 ± 13.7 years old (mean ± SD) vs. 15%: 30.9 ± 13.8 years old; $p > 0.05$), height (10%: 168.2 ± 11.0 cm vs. 15%: 169.9 ± 9.8 cm; $p > 0.05$), weight (10%: 58.7 ± 21.3 kg vs. 15%: 63.8 ± 12.2 kg; $p > 0.05$), gender ratio, and health status are concerned, groups were comparable.

Oxygen-depleted air (oxygen partial pressure: 0.1 bar; 100 hPa, n = 6 and 0.15 bar; 150 hPa, n = 8) was administered for 1 h by means of an orofacial nonrebreather mask with a reservoir bag, care being taken to fit and tighten the mask on the subject's face.

Hypoxic gas at the two levels (10% and 15%) was supplied using a hypoxia generator and set to reach the chosen level of oxygen (HYP 123, Hypoxico–Hypoxico Europe GmbH, Bickenbach, Germany). Both levels of exposure flow were calibrated by means of an oximeter (Solo-O_2 Divesoft, Halkova, Czech Republic) in the mask used by the subject to ascertain that the desired oxygen level was reached [34].

Blood and urine samples were obtained before exposure (T0) and 30 min, 2 h, 8 h, 24 h, and 48 h after the end of oxygen administration (Figure 4). Previous experiments have shown that cellular responses after different oxidative exposures may take up to 24 h or even more. Therefore, we decided to take blood samples up to 48 h [14,18,69,76].

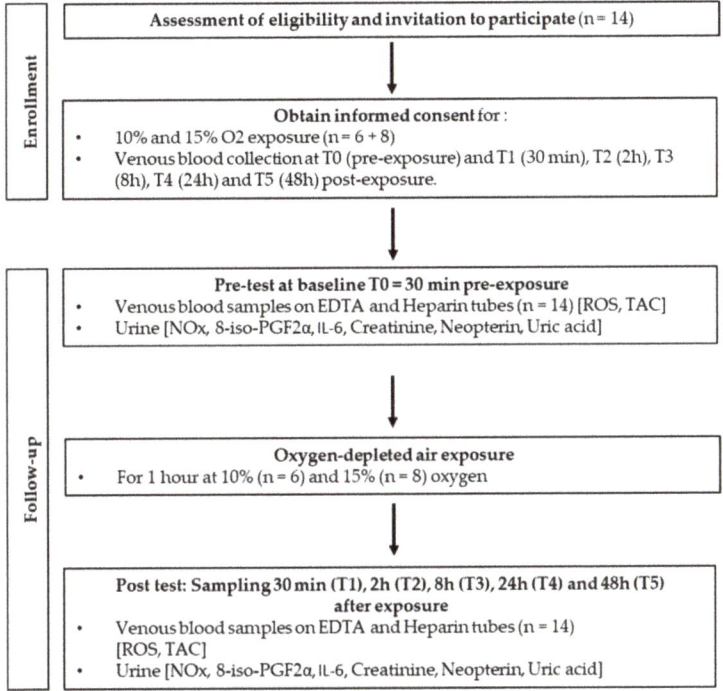

Figure 4. Experimental flowchart.

Each blood sample consisted of approximately 15 mL of venous human blood collected in lithium heparin and EDTA tubes (Vacutainer, BD Diagnostic, Becton Dickinson, Italia S.p.a., Florence, Italy). Plasma and red blood cells (RBCs) were separated via centrifugation (Eppendorf Centrifuge 5702R, Darmstadt Germany) at 1000× g at 4 °C for 10 min. The samples were then stored in multiple aliquots at −80 °C until assayed; analysis was performed within one month of sample collection.

Urine was collected by voluntary voiding in a sterile container and stored in multiple aliquots at −20 °C until assayed and thawed only before analysis.

5.2. Blood Sample Analysis

5.2.1. Determination of ROS Using Electron Paramagnetic Resonance (EPR)

An electron paramagnetic resonance instrument (E-Scan—Bruker BioSpin, GmbH, Rheinstetten, Germany) X-band, with a controller temperature at 37 °C interfaced to the spectrometer, was adopted for ROS production rate, as already performed by some of the authors [77–80]. EPR measurements are highly reproducible, as previously demonstrated [81]. EPR is the only noninvasive technique suitable for the direct and quantitative measurement of ROS. In particular, the spectroscopic technique (EPRS) is used in many fields of application, including biomedicine [82]. The reliability and reproducibility of EPR data obtained using the micro-invasive EPR method adopted in this study have already been reported previously [83].

Briefly, for ROS detection, 50 µL of plasma was treated with an equal volume of CMH (1-hydroxy-3-methoxycarbonyl-2,2,5,5-tetramethylpyrrolidine), and then 50 µL of this solution was placed inside a glass EPR capillary tube in the spectrometer cavity for data acquisition. A stable radical CP (3-Carboxy-2,2,5,5-tetramethyl-1-pyrrolidinyloxy) was used as an external reference to convert the obtained ROS values into absolute quantitative values (µmol/min). All EPR spectra were generated by adopting the same protocol and obtained by using a standard software program supplied by Bruker (Billerica, MA, USA) (version 2.11, WinEPR System).

5.2.2. Total Antioxidant Capacity (TAC)

The 6-hydroxy-2,5,7,8-tetramethylchroman-2-carboxylic acid (Trolox)-equivalent antioxidant capacity assay, a widely used kit-based commercial method, was used. Briefly, 10 uL of plasma was added in duplicate to 10 µL of metmyoglobin and 150 µL of the chromogen solution; then, reactions were initiated through the addition of 40 µL of H_2O_2, as indicated by the instructions (No. 709001, Cayman Chemical, Ann Arbor, MI, USA). Reaction mixtures were incubated at room temperature for 3 min and then read by measuring the absorbance signal at 750 nm using an Infinite M200 microplate reader spectrophotometer (Tecan, Grödig, Austria). A linear calibration curve was computed from pure Trolox-containing reactions.

5.3. Urine Sample Analysis

5.3.1. Nitric Oxide Metabolites (NO_2+NO_3)

NOx (NO_2+NO_3) concentrations were determined in urine via a colorimetric method based on the Griess reaction, using a commercial kit (Cayman Chemical, Ann Arbor, MI, USA), as previously described [84]. Samples were spectrophotometrically read at 545 nm.

5.3.2. 8-Isoprostane (8-iso-PGF2α)

Levels of 8-iso-PGF2α were measured using an immunoassay EIA kit (Cayman Chemical, Ann Arbor, MI, USA) in urine. This is a biomarker for lipid peroxidation and damage assessment. Samples and standards were spectrophotometrically read at 412 nm. Results were normalized using urine creatinine values.

5.3.3. Interleukin-6

IL-6 levels were determined using an ELISA assay kit (ThermoFisher Scientific, Waltham, MA, USA), based on the double-antibody "sandwich" technique in accordance with the manufacturer's instructions.

All the above samples and standards were read using a microplate reader spectrophotometer (Infinite M200, Tecan Group Ltd., Männedorf, Switzerland). The obtained values were assessed in duplicate, and the inter-assay coefficient of variation was in the range indicated by the manufacturer.

5.3.4. Creatinine, Neopterin, and Uric Acid Concentrations

Urinary creatinine, neopterin, interleukin 6 (IL-6), and uric acid concentrations were measured via high-pressure liquid chromatography (HPLC), as previously described [18], using a Varian instrument (pump 240, autosampler ProStar 410, SpectraLab Scientific Inc., Markham, ON, Canada) coupled to a UV–VIS detector (Shimadzu SPD 10-AV, λ = 240 nm, SpectraLab Scientific Inc., for creatinine and uric acid; and JASCO FP-1520, λ_{ex} = 355 nm and at λ_{em} = 450 nm, SpectraLab Scientific Inc., for neopterin).

After the urine centrifugation of 1500× g at 4 °C for 5 min, analytic separation procedures were performed at 50 °C on a 5 µm Discovery C18 analytical column (250 × 4.6 mm I.D., Supelco, Sigma-Aldrich, Merck Life Science S.r.l., Milano, Italy) at a flow rate of 0.9 mL/min. The calibration curves were linear over the range of 0.125–1 µmol/L, 0.625–20 mmol/L, and 1.25–10 mmol/L for neopterin, uric acid, and creatinine levels, respectively. The inter-assay and intra-assay coefficients of variation were <5%.

5.4. Visual Analog Scale (VAS)

Subjective mood, general wellness/malaise, restfulness/tiredness, headaches, sleepiness, and nausea were evaluated using a 0–100 mm visual analog scale (VAS). This scoring system was previously suggested for assessing discomfort and/or general malaise [85]. Based on its usefulness in performing other clinical evaluations, VAS was considered suitable to test the subjective perception of normobaric hypoxia effects [37,86].

5.5. Statistical Analysis

The normality of the results was verified using the Shapiro–Wilk test. Comparisons between results at different times and the baseline were carried out using repeated-measure one-way ANOVA tests when the results had a Gaussian distribution. Otherwise, a Friedman test was applied. Comparisons between the 10% and 15% exposure groups were performed using an unpaired t-test (parametric) or Mann–Whitney (nonparametric) test. All data are presented as mean ± standard deviation (SD). All statistical tests were performed using a standard computer statistical package, GraphPad Prism version 9.5.1., for PC (GraphPad Software, San Diego, CA, USA). A threshold of $p < 0.05$ was considered statistically significant. The sample size required for a repeated-measure analysis of variance (Friedman) was calculated using G*power calculator 3.1.9.7 software (Heinrich-Heine-Universität, Düsseldorf, Germany) (effect size = 0.65, alpha error = 0.05, power = 0.80), and the requisite number of participants for this study was six in each group, which parallels previous studies [87].

6. Conclusions

A short duration (60 min) of extreme and moderate hypoxia led to a significant increase in the production of reactive oxygen species (ROS), peaking 30 min after exposure and slowly recovering after 48 h.

Renal function was astonishingly quickly activated to counteract such hypoxic stimuli, using the antioxidant action of uric acid and creatinine to counteract ROS and NOx, together with TAC significant variations.

We also found an increase in lipid peroxidation caused by ROS, starting at 2 h post-exposure.

Finally, we observed an immune system stimulation through increasing concentrations of neopterin. The rapid increase in neopterin following the ROS peak suggests a counteraction to the inflammasome complex, favoring the NRF2 pathway. Interestingly, neopterin modulation is inversely proportional to the importance of hypoxia. These small variations are very interesting as preconditioning tools.

Overall, this study provides insights into the mechanisms through which acute hypoxia affects various bodily functions and how the body responds to hypoxia-induced oxidative stress. It also highlights the protective mechanisms that humans have in place to maintain redox homeostasis in response to environmental stressors.

Author Contributions: All authors listed have made a substantial, direct, and intellectual contribution to the work, and approved it for publication. Conceptualization, C.B., P.L., P.G., C.L., S.T., K.L., M.L., S.M.S., A.V., M.G. and F.G.; investigation, P.L., C.L., M.L., S.T., C.B., K.L., P.G., S.M.S., A.V. and M.G.; writing, C.L., S.T., C.B., P.G., P.L., S.M.S. and F.G.; funding, C.B., K.L. and S.T.; data analysis, C.L., S.M.S., A.V., M.G., C.B., S.T., K.L., M.L., P.L., F.G. and P.G. All authors have read and agreed to the published version of the manuscript.

Funding: This manuscript is part of the DELTO$_2$X Project is funded by WBE (Wallonia-Brussels Education), Belgium, to the Environmental, Occupational, and Aging (Integrative) Physiology Laboratory, Haute Ecole Bruxelles-Brabant (HE2B), Belgium. The sponsors had no role in the design and conduct of the study; collection, management, analysis, and interpretation of the data; preparation, review, or approval of the manuscript; or the decision to submit the manuscript for publication.

Institutional Review Board Statement: Ethics Committee approval was obtained from the Bio-Ethical Committee for Research and Higher Education, Brussels (No. B 200-2020-088).

Informed Consent Statement: Informed consent was obtained from all subjects involved in the study.

Data Availability Statement: Data are available at request from the authors.

Acknowledgments: Authors are grateful to all volunteer participants, especially students of the Haute Ecole Bruxelles-Brabant (Belgium), Motor Sciences Department (Physiotherapy).

Conflicts of Interest: The authors declare no conflict of interest.

Abbreviations

8-iso-PGF2α	8-Isoprostane
AH	Acute hypoxia
EPR	Electron paramagnetic resonance
FiO$_2$	Inspired fraction of oxygen
HO$^\bullet$	Hydroxide
H$_2$O$_2$	Hydrogen peroxide
IL-6	Interleukin-6
NOx	Nitric oxide metabolites
NRF2	Nuclear factor erythroid-2-related Factor 2
O$_2^{\bullet-}$ ONOO-	Superoxide anionPeroxynitrite
ROS	Reactive oxygen species
TAC	Total antioxidant capacity
UA	Uric acid
VAS	Visual analog scale

References

1. Cable, G.G. In-flight hypoxia incidents in military aircraft: Causes and implications for training. *Aviat. Space Environ. Med.* **2003**, *74*, 169–172. [PubMed]
2. Serebrovskaya, T.V.; Manukhina, E.B.; Smith, M.L.; Downey, H.F.; Mallet, R.T. Intermittent hypoxia: Cause of or therapy for systemic hypertension? *Exp. Biol. Med.* **2008**, *233*, 627–650. [CrossRef] [PubMed]
3. Serebrovskaya, T.V.; Nikolsky, I.S.; Nikolska, V.V.; Mallet, R.T.; Ishchuk, V.A. Intermittent hypoxia mobilizes hematopoietic progenitors and augments cellular and humoral elements of innate immunity in adult men. *High Alt. Med. Biol.* **2011**, *12*, 243–252. [CrossRef] [PubMed]
4. Urdampilleta, A.; González-Muniesa, P.; Portillo, M.P.; Martínez, J.A. Usefulness of combining intermittent hypoxia and physical exercise in the treatment of obesity. *J. Physiol. Biochem.* **2012**, *68*, 289–304. [CrossRef]
5. Guner, I.; Uzun, D.D.; Yaman, M.O.; Genc, H.; Gelisgen, R.; Korkmaz, G.G.; Hallac, M.; Yelmen, N.; Sahin, G.; Karter, Y.; et al. The effect of chronic long-term intermittent hypobaric hypoxia on bone mineral density in rats: Role of nitric oxide. *Biol. Trace Elem. Res.* **2013**, *154*, 262–267. [CrossRef]

6. Lu, X.J.; Chen, X.Q.; Weng, J.; Zhang, H.Y.; Pak, D.T.; Luo, J.H.; Du, J.Z. Hippocampal spine-associated Rap-specific GTPase-activating protein induces enhancement of learning and memory in postnatally hypoxia-exposed mice. *Neuroscience* 2009, *162*, 404–414. [CrossRef]
7. Zhang, J.X.; Chen, X.Q.; Du, J.Z.; Chen, Q.M.; Zhu, C.Y. Neonatal exposure to intermittent hypoxia enhances mice performance in water maze and 8-arm radial maze tasks. *J. Neurobiol.* 2005, *65*, 72–84. [CrossRef]
8. Tsai, Y.W.; Yang, Y.R.; Sun, S.H.; Liang, K.C.; Wang, R.Y. Post ischemia intermittent hypoxia induces hippocampal neurogenesis and synaptic alterations and alleviates long-term memory impairment. *J. Cereb. Blood Flow Metab.* 2013, *33*, 764–773. [CrossRef]
9. Tsai, Y.W.; Yang, Y.R.; Wang, P.S.; Wang, R.Y. Intermittent hypoxia after transient focal ischemia induces hippocampal neurogenesis and c-Fos expression and reverses spatial memory deficits in rats. *PLoS ONE* 2011, *6*, e24001. [CrossRef]
10. Haider, T.; Casucci, G.; Linser, T.; Faulhaber, M.; Gatterer, H.; Ott, G.; Linser, A.; Ehrenbourg, I.; Tkatchouk, E.; Burtscher, M.; et al. Interval hypoxic training improves autonomic cardiovascular and respiratory control in patients with mild chronic obstructive pulmonary disease. *J. Hypertens.* 2009, *27*, 1648–1654. [CrossRef]
11. Wang, Z.-H.; Chen, Y.-X.; Zhang, C.-M.; Wu, L.; Yu, Z.; Cai, X.-L.; Guan, Y.; Zhou, Z.-N.; Yang, H.-T. Intermittent hypobaric hypoxia improves postischemic recovery of myocardial contractile function via redox signaling during early reperfusion. *Am. J. Physiol.-Heart Circ. Physiol.* 2011, *301*, H1695–H1705. [CrossRef]
12. Querido, J.S.; Sheel, A.W.; Cheema, R.; Van Eeden, S.; Mulgrew, A.T.; Ayas, N.T. Effects of 10 days of modest intermittent hypoxia on circulating measures of inflammation in healthy humans. *Sleep Breath.* 2012, *16*, 657–662. [CrossRef]
13. De Bels, D.; Corazza, F.; Germonpre, P.; Balestra, C. The normobaric oxygen paradox: A novel way to administer oxygen as an adjuvant treatment for cancer? *Med. Hypotheses* 2010, *76*, 467–470. [CrossRef]
14. Balestra, C.; Lambrechts, K.; Mrakic-Sposta, S.; Vezzoli, A.; Levenez, M.; Germonpre, P.; Virgili, F.; Bosco, G.; Lafere, P. Hypoxic and Hyperoxic Breathing as a Complement to Low-Intensity Physical Exercise Programs: A Proof-of-Principle Study. *Int. J. Mol. Sci.* 2021, *22*, 9600. [CrossRef]
15. Clarke, C. Acute mountain sickness: Medical problems associated with acute and subacute exposure to hypobaric hypoxia. *Postgrad. Med. J.* 2006, *82*, 748–753. [CrossRef]
16. Puri, S.; Panza, G.; Mateika, J.H. A comprehensive review of respiratory, autonomic and cardiovascular responses to intermittent hypoxia in humans. *Exp. Neurol.* 2021, *341*, 113709. [CrossRef]
17. De Bels, D.; Theunissen, S.; Devriendt, J.; Germonpre, P.; Lafere, P.; Valsamis, J.; Snoeck, T.; Meeus, P.; Balestra, C. The 'normobaric oxygen paradox': Does it increase haemoglobin? *Diving Hyperb. Med.* 2012, *42*, 67–71.
18. Bosco, G.; Paganini, M.; Giacon, T.A.; Oppio, A.; Vezzoli, A.; Dellanoce, C.; Moro, T.; Paoli, A.; Zanotti, F.; Zavan, B.; et al. Oxidative Stress and Inflammation, MicroRNA, and Hemoglobin Variations after Administration of Oxygen at Different Pressures and Concentrations: A Randomized Trial. *Int. J. Environ. Res. Public Health* 2021, *18*, 9755. [CrossRef]
19. Hamlin, M.J.; Marshall, H.C.; Hellemans, J.; Ainslie, P.N. Effect of intermittent hypoxia on muscle and cerebral oxygenation during a 20-km time trial in elite athletes: A preliminary report. *Appl. Physiol. Nutr. Metab.* 2010, *35*, 548–559. [CrossRef]
20. Ventura, N.; Hoppeler, H.; Seiler, R.; Binggeli, A.; Mullis, P.; Vogt, M. The response of trained athletes to six weeks of endurance training in hypoxia or normoxia. *Int. J. Sports Med.* 2003, *24*, 166–172. [CrossRef]
21. Morton, J.P.; Cable, N.T. Effects of intermittent hypoxic training on aerobic and anaerobic performance. *Ergonomics* 2005, *48*, 1535–1546. [CrossRef] [PubMed]
22. Truijens, M.J.; Toussaint, H.M.; Dow, J.; Levine, B.D. Effect of high-intensity hypoxic training on sea-level swimming performances. *J. Appl. Physiol.* 2003, *94*, 733–743. [CrossRef] [PubMed]
23. De Smet, S.; Van Thienen, R.; Deldicque, L.; James, R.; Sale, C.; Bishop, D.J.; Hespel, P. Nitrate Intake Promotes Shift in Muscle Fiber Type Composition during Sprint Interval Training in Hypoxia. *Front. Physiol.* 2016, *7*, 233. [CrossRef] [PubMed]
24. Hoppeler, H.; Kleinert, E.; Schlegel, C.; Claassen, H.; Howald, H.; Kayar, S.R.; Cerretelli, P. Morphological adaptations of human skeletal muscle to chronic hypoxia. *Int. J. Sports Med.* 1990, *11* (Suppl. S1), S3–S9. [CrossRef]
25. Millet, G.P.; Girard, O. Editorial: High-Intensity Exercise in Hypoxia: Beneficial Aspects and Potential Drawbacks. *Front. Physiol.* 2017, *8*, 1017. [CrossRef]
26. Lundby, C.; Millet, G.P.; Calbet, J.A.; Bärtsch, P.; Subudhi, A.W. Does 'altitude training' increase exercise performance in elite athletes? *Br. J. Sports Med.* 2012, *46*, 792–795. [CrossRef]
27. Luo, Z.; Tian, M.; Yang, G.; Tan, Q.; Chen, Y.; Li, G.; Zhang, Q.; Li, Y.; Wan, P.; Wu, J. Hypoxia signaling in human health and diseases: Implications and prospects for therapeutics. *Signal Transduct. Target. Ther.* 2022, *7*, 218. [CrossRef]
28. Burtscher, M.; Pachinger, O.; Ehrenbourg, I.; Mitterbauer, G.; Faulhaber, M.; Pühringer, R.; Tkatchouk, E. Intermittent hypoxia increases exercise tolerance in elderly men with and without coronary artery disease. *Int. J. Cardiol.* 2004, *96*, 247–254. [CrossRef]
29. Bayer, U.; Likar, R.; Pinter, G.; Stettner, H.; Demschar, S.; Trummer, B.; Neuwersch, S.; Glazachev, O.; Burtscher, M. Intermittent hypoxic-hyperoxic training on cognitive performance in geriatric patients. *Alzheimers Dement.* 2017, *3*, 114–122. [CrossRef]
30. Dudnik, E.; Zagaynaya, E.; Glazachev, O.S.; Susta, D. Intermittent Hypoxia-Hyperoxia Conditioning Improves Cardiorespiratory Fitness in Older Comorbid Cardiac Outpatients Without Hematological Changes: A Randomized Controlled Trial. *High Alt. Med. Biol.* 2018, *19*, 339–343. [CrossRef]
31. Camacho-Cardenosa, A.; Burtscher, J.; Burtscher, M.; Camacho-Cardenosa, M. Editorial: Hypoxia as a therapeutic tool in search of healthy aging. *Front. Physiol.* 2023, *13*, 1112129. [CrossRef]

32. Mrakic-Sposta, S.; Gussoni, M.; Dellanoce, C.; Marzorati, M.; Montorsi, M.; Rasica, L.; Pratali, L.; D'Angelo, G.; Martinelli, M.; Bastiani, L.; et al. Effects of acute and sub-acute hypobaric hypoxia on oxidative stress: A field study in the Alps. *Eur. J. Appl. Physiol.* **2021**, *121*, 297–306. [CrossRef]
33. De Bels, D.; Tillmans, F.; Corazza, F.; Bizzari, M.; Germonpre, P.; Radermacher, P.; Orman, K.G.; Balestra, C. Hyperoxia Alters Ultrastructure and Induces Apoptosis in Leukemia Cell Lines. *Biomolecules* **2020**, *10*, 282. [CrossRef]
34. Balestra, C.; Arya, A.K.; Leveque, C.; Virgili, F.; Germonpre, P.; Lambrechts, K.; Lafere, P.; Thom, S.R. Varying Oxygen Partial Pressure Elicits Blood-Borne Microparticles Expressing Different Cell-Specific Proteins-Toward a Targeted Use of Oxygen? *Int. J. Mol. Sci.* **2022**, *23*, 7888. [CrossRef]
35. Mrakic-Sposta, S.; Gussoni, M.; Marzorati, M.; Porcelli, S.; Bosco, G.; Balestra, C.; Montorsi, M.; Lafortuna, C.; Vezzoli, A. The "ON-OFF" Switching Response of Reactive Oxygen Species in Acute Normobaric Hypoxia: Preliminary Outcome. *Int. J. Mol. Sci.* **2023**, *24*, 4012. [CrossRef]
36. Magalhães, J.; Ascensão, A.; Viscor, G.; Soares, J.; Oliveira, J.; Marques, F.; Duarte, J. Oxidative stress in humans during and after 4 h of hypoxia at a simulated altitude of 5500 m. *Aviat. Space Environ. Med.* **2004**, *75*, 16–22. [PubMed]
37. Bailey, D.M.; Ainslie, P.N.; Jackson, S.K.; Richardson, R.S.; Ghatei, M. Evidence against redox regulation of energy homoeostasis in humans at high altitude. *Clin. Sci.* **2004**, *107*, 589–600. [CrossRef]
38. Coppel, J.; Hennis, P.; Gilbert-Kawai, E.; Grocott, M.P. The physiological effects of hypobaric hypoxia versus normobaric hypoxia: A systematic review of crossover trials. *Extrem. Physiol. Med.* **2015**, *4*, 2. [CrossRef]
39. Khan, S.A.; Nanduri, J.; Yuan, G.; Kinsman, B.; Kumar, G.K.; Joseph, J.; Kalyanaraman, B.; Prabhakar, N.R. NADPH oxidase 2 mediates intermittent hypoxia-induced mitochondrial complex I inhibition: Relevance to blood pressure changes in rats. *Antioxid. Redox Signal.* **2011**, *14*, 533–542. [CrossRef]
40. Fridovich, I. Superoxide Radical And Superoxide Dismutases. *Annu. Rev. Biochem.* **1995**, *64*, 97–112. [CrossRef]
41. Jiménez-Banzo, A.; Sagristà, M.L.; Mora, M.; Nonell, S. Kinetics of singlet oxygen photosensitization in human skin fibroblasts. *Free. Radic. Biol. Med.* **2008**, *44*, 1926–1934. [CrossRef] [PubMed]
42. Redmond, R.W.; Kochevar, I.E. Spatially resolved cellular responses to singlet oxygen. *Photochem. Photobiol.* **2006**, *82*, 1178–1186. [CrossRef] [PubMed]
43. Kim, H.; Scimia, M.C.; Wilkinson, D.; Trelles, R.D.; Wood, M.R.; Bowtell, D.; Dillin, A.; Mercola, M.; Ronai, Z.A. Fine-Tuning of Drp1/Fis1 Availability by AKAP121/Siah2 Regulates Mitochondrial Adaptation to Hypoxia. *Mol. Cell* **2011**, *44*, 532–544. [CrossRef] [PubMed]
44. Liu, X.; Hajnóczky, G. Altered fusion dynamics underlie unique morphological changes in mitochondria during hypoxia–reoxygenation stress. *Cell Death Differ.* **2011**, *18*, 1561–1572. [CrossRef]
45. Fuhrmann, D.C.; Brüne, B. Mitochondrial composition and function under the control of hypoxia. *Redox Biol.* **2017**, *12*, 208–215. [CrossRef]
46. Huie, R.E.; Padmaja, S. The Reaction of no With Superoxide. *Free Radic. Res. Commun.* **1993**, *18*, 195–199. [CrossRef]
47. Ribon, A.; Pialoux, V.; Saugy, J.J.; Rupp, T.; Faiss, R.; Debevec, T.; Millet, G.P. Exposure to hypobaric hypoxia results in higher oxidative stress compared to normobaric hypoxia. *Respir. Physiol. Neurobiol.* **2016**, *223*, 23–27. [CrossRef]
48. Radi, R. Oxygen radicals, nitric oxide, and peroxynitrite: Redox pathways in molecular medicine. *Proc. Natl. Acad. Sci. USA* **2018**, *115*, 5839–5848. [CrossRef]
49. Schildknecht, S.; Ullrich, V. Peroxynitrite as regulator of vascular prostanoid synthesis. *Arch. Biochem. Biophys.* **2009**, *484*, 183–189. [CrossRef]
50. Fujii, J.; Homma, T.; Osaki, T. Superoxide Radicals in the Execution of Cell Death. *Antioxidants* **2022**, *11*, 501. [CrossRef]
51. Vermot, A.; Petit-Härtlein, I.; Smith, S.M.E.; Fieschi, F. NADPH Oxidases (NOX): An Overview from Discovery, Molecular Mechanisms to Physiology and Pathology. *Antioxidants* **2021**, *10*, 890. [CrossRef]
52. Ames, B.N.; Cathcart, R.; Schwiers, E.; Hochstein, P. Uric acid provides an antioxidant defense in humans against oxidant- and radical-caused aging and cancer: A hypothesis. *Proc. Natl. Acad. Sci. USA* **1981**, *78*, 6858–6862. [CrossRef]
53. Maxwell, S.R.; Thomason, H.; Sandler, D.; Leguen, C.; Baxter, M.A.; Thorpe, G.H.; Jones, A.F.; Barnett, A.H. Antioxidant status in patients with uncomplicated insulin-dependent and non-insulin-dependent diabetes mellitus. *Eur. J. Clin. Investig.* **1997**, *27*, 484–490. [CrossRef]
54. Waring, W.S.; Webb, D.J.; Maxwell, S.R. Systemic uric acid administration increases serum antioxidant capacity in healthy volunteers. *J. Cardiovasc. Pharmacol.* **2001**, *38*, 365–371. [CrossRef]
55. Waring, W.S.; Convery, A.; Mishra, V.; Shenkin, A.; Webb, D.J.; Maxwell, S.R.J. Uric acid reduces exercise-induced oxidative stress in healthy adults. *Clin. Sci.* **2003**, *105*, 425–430. [CrossRef]
56. Kang, D.-H.; Ha, S.-K. Uric Acid Puzzle: Dual Role as Anti-oxidant and Pro-oxidant. *Electrolyte Blood Press.* **2014**, *12*, 1–6. [CrossRef]
57. Arazi, H.; Eghbali, E.; Suzuki, K. Creatine Supplementation, Physical Exercise and Oxidative Stress Markers: A Review of the Mechanisms and Effectiveness. *Nutrients* **2021**, *13*, 869. [CrossRef]
58. Luks, A.M.; Johnson, R.J.; Swenson, E.R. Chronic kidney disease at high altitude. *J. Am. Soc. Nephrol.* **2008**, *19*, 2262–2271. [CrossRef]
59. Matthews, R.T.; Yang, L.; Jenkins, B.G.; Ferrante, R.J.; Rosen, B.R.; Kaddurah-Daouk, R.; Beal, M.F. Neuroprotective effects of creatine and cyclocreatine in animal models of Huntington's disease. *J. Neurosci.* **1998**, *18*, 156–163. [CrossRef]

60. Lawler, J.M.; Barnes, W.S.; Wu, G.; Song, W.; Demaree, S. Direct antioxidant properties of creatine. *Biochem. Biophys. Res. Commun.* **2002**, *290*, 47–52. [CrossRef]
61. Sestili, P.; Martinelli, C.; Bravi, G.; Piccoli, G.; Curci, R.; Battistelli, M.; Falcieri, E.; Agostini, D.; Gioacchini, A.M.; Stocchi, V. Creatine supplementation affords cytoprotection in oxidatively injured cultured mammalian cells via direct antioxidant activity. *Free Radic. Biol. Med.* **2006**, *40*, 837–849. [CrossRef] [PubMed]
62. Beckman, K.B.; Ames, B.N. Oxidative decay of DNA. *J. Biol. Chem.* **1997**, *272*, 19633–19636. [CrossRef]
63. Kasai, H. Analysis of a form of oxidative DNA damage, 8-hydroxy-2′-deoxyguanosine, as a marker of cellular oxidative stress during carcinogenesis. *Mutat. Res.* **1997**, *387*, 147–163. [CrossRef] [PubMed]
64. Pedersen, E.R.; Midttun, Ø.; Ueland, P.M.; Schartum-Hansen, H.; Seifert, R.; Igland, J.; Nordrehaug, J.E.; Ebbing, M.; Svingen, G.; Bleie, Ø.; et al. Systemic markers of interferon-γ-mediated immune activation and long-term prognosis in patients with stable coronary artery disease. *Arterioscler. Thromb. Vasc. Biol.* **2011**, *31*, 698–704. [CrossRef] [PubMed]
65. Melichar, B.; Spisarová, M.; Bartoušková, M.; Krčmová, L.K.; Javorská, L.; Študentová, H. Neopterin as a biomarker of immune response in cancer patients. *Ann. Transl. Med.* **2017**, *5*, 280. [CrossRef] [PubMed]
66. Baydar, T.; Yuksel, O.; Sahin, T.T.; Dikmen, K.; Girgin, G.; Sipahi, H.; Kurukahvecioglu, O.; Bostanci, H.; Sare, M. Neopterin as a prognostic biomarker in intensive care unit patients. *J. Crit. Care* **2009**, *24*, 318–321. [CrossRef]
67. Eisenhut, M. Neopterin in Diagnosis and Monitoring of Infectious Diseases. *J. Biomark.* **2013**, *2013*, 196432. [CrossRef]
68. Signorelli, S.S.; Anzaldi, M.; Fiore, V.; Candido, S.; Di Marco, R.; Mangano, K.; Quattrocchi, C.; Neri, S. Neopterin: A potential marker in chronic peripheral arterial disease. *Mol. Med. Rep.* **2013**, *7*, 1855–1858. [CrossRef]
69. Fratantonio, D.; Virgili, F.; Zucchi, A.; Lambrechts, K.; Latronico, T.; Lafere, P.; Germonpre, P.; Balestra, C. Increasing Oxygen Partial Pressures Induce a Distinct Transcriptional Response in Human PBMC: A Pilot Study on the "Normobaric Oxygen Paradox". *Int. J. Mol. Sci.* **2021**, *22*, 458. [CrossRef]
70. De Paula Martins, R.; Ghisoni, K.; Lim, C.K.; Aguiar, A.S.; Guillemin, G.J.; Latini, A. Neopterin preconditioning prevents inflammasome activation in mammalian astrocytes. *Free Radic. Biol. Med.* **2018**, *115*, 371–382. [CrossRef]
71. Mrakic-Sposta, S.; Montorsi, M.; Porcelli, S.; Marzorati, M.; Healey, B.; Dellanoce, C.; Vezzoli, A. Effects of Prolonged Exposure to Hypobaric Hypoxia on Oxidative Stress: Overwintering in Antarctic Concordia Station. *Oxid. Med. Cell. Longev.* **2022**, *2022*, 4430032. [CrossRef]
72. Schaefer, E.; Wu, W.; Mark, C.; Yang, A.; Digiacomo, E.; Carlton-Smith, C.; Salloum, S.; Brisac, C.; Lin, W.; Corey, K.E.; et al. Intermittent hypoxia is a proinflammatory stimulus resulting in IL-6 expression and M1 macrophage polarization. *Hepatol. Commun.* **2017**, *1*, 326–337. [CrossRef]
73. Peng, Y.; Yang, Q.; Gao, S.; Liu, Z.; Kong, W.; Bian, X.; Li, Z.; Ye, J. IL-6 protects cardiomyocytes from oxidative stress at the early stage of LPS-induced sepsis. *Biochem. Biophys. Res. Commun.* **2022**, *603*, 144–152. [CrossRef]
74. Wang, L.; Yang, S.; Yan, L.; Wei, H.; Wang, J.; Yu, S.; Kong, A.T.; Zhang, Y. Hypoxia preconditioning promotes endurance exercise capacity of mice by activating skeletal muscle Nrf2. *J. Appl. Physiol.* **2019**, *127*, 1267–1277. [CrossRef]
75. World Medical, A. World Medical Association Declaration of Helsinki: Ethical principles for medical research involving human subjects. *JAMA* **2013**, *310*, 2191–2194. [CrossRef]
76. Cimino, F.; Balestra, C.; Germonpre, P.; De Bels, D.; Tillmans, F.; Saija, A.; Speciale, A.; Virgili, F. Pulsed high oxygen induces a hypoxic-like response in human umbilical endothelial cells and in humans. *J. Appl. Physiol.* **2012**, *113*, 1684–1689. [CrossRef]
77. Mrakic-Sposta, S.; Vezzoli, A.; D'Alessandro, F.; Paganini, M.; Dellanoce, C.; Cialoni, D.; Bosco, G. Change in Oxidative Stress Biomarkers During 30 Days in Saturation Dive: A Pilot Study. *Int. J. Environ. Res. Public Health* **2020**, *17*, 7118. [CrossRef]
78. Moretti, S.; Mrakic-Sposta, S.; Roncoroni, L.; Vezzoli, A.; Dellanoce, C.; Monguzzi, E.; Branchi, F.; Ferretti, F.; Lombardo, V.; Doneda, L.; et al. Oxidative stress as a biomarker for monitoring treated celiac disease. *Clin. Transl. Gastroenterol.* **2018**, *9*, 157. [CrossRef]
79. Mrakic-Sposta, S.; Vezzoli, A.; Rizzato, A.; Della Noce, C.; Malacrida, S.; Montorsi, M.; Paganini, M.; Cancellara, P.; Bosco, G. Oxidative stress assessment in breath-hold diving. *Eur. J. Appl. Physiol.* **2019**, *119*, 2449–2456. [CrossRef]
80. Bosco, G.; Rizzato, A.; Quartesan, S.; Camporesi, E.; Mrakic-Sposta, S.; Moretti, S.; Balestra, C.; Rubini, A. Spirometry and oxidative stress after rebreather diving in warm water. *Undersea Hyperb. Med.* **2018**, *45*, 191–198. [CrossRef]
81. Mrakic-Sposta, S.; Gussoni, M.; Montorsi, M.; Porcelli, S.; Vezzoli, A. A quantitative method to monitor reactive oxygen species production by electron paramagnetic resonance in physiological and pathological conditions. *Oxid. Med. Cell. Longev.* **2014**, *2014*, 306179. [CrossRef] [PubMed]
82. Menzel, A.; Samouda, H.; Dohet, F.; Loap, S.; Ellulu, M.S.; Bohn, T. Common and Novel Markers for Measuring Inflammation and Oxidative Stress Ex Vivo in Research and Clinical Practice—Which to Use Regarding Disease Outcomes? *Antioxidants* **2021**, *10*, 836. [CrossRef] [PubMed]
83. Mrakic-Sposta, S.; Gussoni, M.; Montorsi, M.; Porcelli, S.; Vezzoli, A. Assessment of a standardized ROS production profile in humans by electron paramagnetic resonance. *Oxid. Med. Cell. Longev.* **2012**, *2012*, 973927. [CrossRef] [PubMed]
84. Ciccone, M.M.; Bilianou, E.; Balbarini, A.; Gesualdo, M.; Ghiadoni, L.; Metra, M.; Palmiero, P.; Pedrinelli, R.; Salvetti, M.; Scicchitano, P.; et al. Task force on: 'Early markers of atherosclerosis: Influence of age and sex'. *J. Cardiovasc. Med.* **2013**, *14*, 757–766. [CrossRef]
85. Wu, J.; Chen, Y.; Luo, Y. Evaluation of the visual analog score (VAS) to assess acute mountain sickness (AMS) in a hypobaric chamber. *PLoS ONE* **2014**, *9*, e113376. [CrossRef]

86. Bailey, D.M.; Bain, A.R.; Hoiland, R.L.; Barak, O.F.; Drvis, I.; Hirtz, C.; Lehmann, S.; Marchi, N.; Janigro, D.; MacLeod, D.B.; et al. Hypoxemia increases blood-brain barrier permeability during extreme apnea in humans. *J. Cereb. Blood Flow Metab.* **2022**, *42*, 1120–1135. [CrossRef]
87. Leveque, C.; Mrakic-Sposta, S.; Lafère, P.; Vezzoli, A.; Germonpré, P.; Beer, A.; Mievis, S.; Virgili, F.; Lambrechts, K.; Theunissen, S.; et al. Oxidative Stress Response's Kinetics after 60 Minutes at Different (30% or 100%) Normobaric Hyperoxia Exposures. *Int. J. Mol. Sci.* **2022**, *24*, 664. [CrossRef]

Disclaimer/Publisher's Note: The statements, opinions and data contained in all publications are solely those of the individual author(s) and contributor(s) and not of MDPI and/or the editor(s). MDPI and/or the editor(s) disclaim responsibility for any injury to people or property resulting from any ideas, methods, instructions or products referred to in the content.

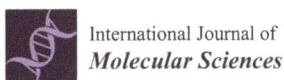

Article

Proteomic Analysis Reveals That Mitochondria Dominate the Hippocampal Hypoxic Response in Mice

Qianqian Shao [1,†], Jia Liu [1,†], Gaifen Li [1,2], Yakun Gu [1], Mengyuan Guo [1], Yuying Guan [1,2], Zhengming Tian [1], Wei Ma [1], Chaoyu Wang [1] and Xunming Ji [1,2,*]

1. Laboratory of Brain Disorders, Beijing Institute of Brain Disorders, Ministry of Science and Technology, Collaborative Innovation Center for Brain Disorders, Beijing Advanced Innovation Center for Big Data-Based Precision Medicine, Capital Medical University, Beijing 100069, China
2. Department of Neurosurgery, Xuanwu Hospital, Capital Medical University, Beijing 100053, China
* Correspondence: jixm@ccmu.edu.cn; Tel.: +86-139-1107-7166
† These authors contributed equally to this work.

Abstract: Hypoxic stress occurs in various physiological and pathological states, such as aging, disease, or high-altitude exposure, all of which pose a challenge to many organs in the body, necessitating adaptation. However, the exact mechanisms by which hypoxia affects advanced brain function (learning and memory skills in particular) remain unclear. In this study, we investigated the effects of hypoxic stress on hippocampal function. Specifically, we studied the effects of the dysfunction of mitochondrial oxidative phosphorylation using global proteomics. First, we found that hypoxic stress impaired cognitive and motor abilities, whereas it caused no substantial changes in the brain morphology or structure of mice. Second, bioinformatics analysis indicated that hypoxia affected the expression of 516 proteins, of which 71.1% were upregulated and 28.5% were downregulated. We demonstrated that mitochondrial function was altered and manifested as a decrease in NADH dehydrogenase (ubiquinone) 1 alpha subcomplex 4 expression, accompanied by increased reactive oxygen species generation, resulting in further neuronal injury. These results may provide some new insights into how hypoxic stress alters hippocampal function via the dysfunction of mitochondrial oxidative phosphorylation.

Keywords: hippocampus; hypoxia; mitochondrial oxidative phosphorylation; CIV activity; NADH dehydrogenase (ubiquinone) 1 alpha subcomplex 4

Citation: Shao, Q.; Liu, J.; Li, G.; Gu, Y.; Guo, M.; Guan, Y.; Tian, Z.; Ma, W.; Wang, C.; Ji, X. Proteomic Analysis Reveals That Mitochondria Dominate the Hippocampal Hypoxic Response in Mice. *Int. J. Mol. Sci.* **2022**, *23*, 14094. https://doi.org/10.3390/ijms232214094

Academic Editors: Fabio Virgili, Simona Mrakic-Sposta and Costantino Balestra

Received: 9 September 2022
Accepted: 13 November 2022
Published: 15 November 2022

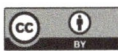

Copyright: © 2022 by the authors. Licensee MDPI, Basel, Switzerland. This article is an open access article distributed under the terms and conditions of the Creative Commons Attribution (CC BY) license (https://creativecommons.org/licenses/by/4.0/).

1. Introduction

Hypoxia is one of the most common and severe stressors to an organism's homeostasis, which enables cells and organs insufficient energy supply, and occurs in various physiological and pathological states. It has become increasingly clear that hypoxia contributes to the pathological development of a number of diseases, such as stroke, obstructive sleep apnea (OSA) [1], and neurodegenerative diseases ((Parkinson's disease (PD) [2] and Alzheimer's disease (AD)) [3]. Sever hypobaric hypoxia-induced detrimental effects on cognitive function in humans, such as cerebral edema, mood disturbances, cognitive impairment, or verbal memory [4,5]. Moreover, as compared with low altitude, young adult (20–24 years old) residents living in Lhasa, Tibet (3650 m) were impaired in verbal and spatial working memory [4]. Tesler et al. [6] demonstrated that a hypoxic environment has negative consequences on sleep-dependent memory performance associated with memory consolidation by a reduction in slow waves. Additionally, Hota et al. showed that acclimatized lowlanders staying at altitudes 4300 m increased the prevalence of mild cognitive impairment [7]. Yet, the mechanism by which hypoxia affects advanced brain function (learning and memory skills in particular) has yet to be fully uncovered.

Adaptation to low-oxygen environments is primarily mediated by the hypoxia-inducible factor (HIF) transcription factor family. Under normoxia, HIFα subunits are polyubiquitylated by prolyl hydroxylases (PHDs) and subsequently degraded [8]. In the presence of hypoxic pressure, PHDs are inactivated via oxidation, which inhibits HIFα polyubiquitylation, causing it to dimerize with HIF1β to form transcriptionally active complexes [9]. As a result, HIFs can regulate a variety of downstream response elements in response to hypoxic challenges. These findings opened new avenues for the discoveries of how cells perceive and adapt to oxygen availability, and the researchers who discovered this mechanism received the Nobel Prize in Physiology or Medicine in 2019 [9]. However, the critical molecule and complex networks that respond to decreased oxygen levels have yet to be fully elucidated.

It is well known that mitochondrial-mediated oxidation via glucose yields up to 30–38 ATP/glucose; however, when there is an inadequate supply of oxygen, glycolysis produces only two ATP/glucose, which fails to meet the cellular demand. Each process can be complementary to the other [10–12]. Aragones and colleagues found that when oxygen levels are insufficient, mitochondrial oxidative phosphorylation (OXPHOS) is reduced [13]; however, to satisfy the cellular demand, cells continue to consume oxygen. As a result, OXPHOS generates by-product reactive oxygen species (ROS) continuously. After an extended time of oxygen deficiency, ROS-induced oxidative stress causes tricarboxylic acid cycle (TCA) and electron transfer chain (ETC)-related enzyme inactivation, resulting in irreversible mitochondrial structural and functional damage. As a result, mitochondrial oxidative metabolism is completely interrupted [13]. Anaerobic glycolysis cannot fully compensate for the ATP loss caused by the cessation of oxidative metabolism, which eventually leads to cell energy depletion and cell death [12]. Hypoxia is known to induce ETC dysfunction; however, existing studies lack reports at the proteomic level.

Mitochondria are the major oxygen-consuming organelles of the cell and therefore oxidative phosphorylation of mitochondria is affected by oxygen deficiency [14]. Oxidative phosphorylation occurs via electron transfer in the electron transport chain and ATP synthesis. The ETC consists of three proton pumps, NADH dehydrogenase (complex I, CI), bc1-complex (complex III, CIII), and cytochrome c oxidase (COX; complex IV, CIV) [15]. In addition, the ETC contains succinate dehydrogenase (complex II, CII), which feeds electrons from succinate into the ETC but does not pump protons, as well as the small electron carrier's cytochrome c and ubiquinone. CIV is the terminal of the ETC and therefore the rate-limiting step. CIV has a high affinity for O_2 and plays a central role in catalyzing molecular oxygen to generate water [16]. However, the regulation mechanism of hypoxia on CIV is unclear.

Here, we perform proteomics to study how the hippocampus initiates the adaptation mechanism to cope with the impact of oxygen deficiency under hypoxia stress. We found that under hypoxic stress, although the morphology and structure of neurons were not significantly altered, the cognitive and motor abilities of mice were impaired. Proteomics analysis showed that mitochondrial function was altered, which manifested as a decrease in NDUFA4 expression, indicating that CIV activity and oxygen utilization were decreased, and normal mitochondrial membrane potential was severely impaired. As a result, mitochondria were not able to meet the high energy consumption demand of hippocampal neurons, which resulted in increased ROS generation. In addition, although the protein expression of mitochondrial complexes I, III, and IV was upregulated, we believe that this may be an ineffective feedback response under hypoxic stress, resulting in further neuronal injury.

2. Results

2.1. Hypoxic Stress Impaired Cognitive and Motor Function but Did Not Alter the Morphology or Structure of Hippocampal Neurons

To explore the effect of short-term hypoxia on the hippocampus, we simulated the altitude of Lhasa and provided mice with 13% oxygen (hypoxic conditions) for 1 or 3 days (H1D and H3D, respectively). The latest research shows that 3.65 days in the lifetime of a mouse is equivalent to one human year [17]. Compared with the control group, hypoxia

H1D or H3D had no significant effect on the body weight of mice (Figure 1A). Unexpectedly, the new object recognition experiment showed that the cognitive ability of mice was significantly impaired after H1D or H3D compared with the control group (CON, Figure 1B). The rotarod test showed that the motor function of mice was significantly reduced after H1D and H3D compared with the CON (Figure 1B). It is well known that the cognitive ability of mice is closely related to the morphological and structural integrity of hippocampal neurons [18]. Therefore, hematoxylin and eosin (HE), and Nissl staining were performed to identify the morphological and structural changes in the hippocampus. Compared with the control group, we observed that hippocampal tissue was undamaged and neither hippocampal nor cortical neurons showed morphological and structural abnormalities in the hippocampus and cortex after H1D and H3D (Figure 1C). Nissl staining results also showed that short-term hypoxia did not result in significant damage to hippocampal or cortical neurons compared with the CON (Figure 1D). In summary, we believe that although short-term hypoxia does not cause changes in neuronal morphology and structure, it may lead to functional alterations, manifested as cognitive and motor impairment in mice.

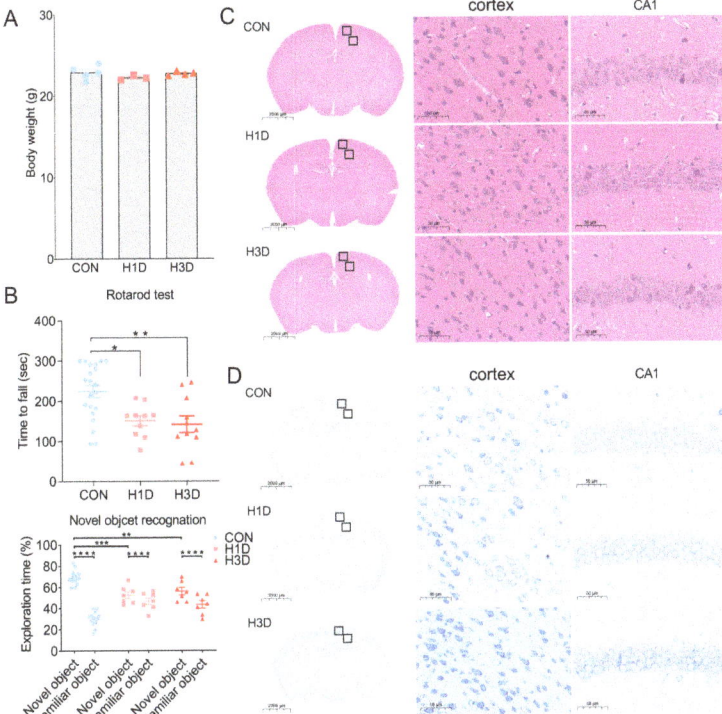

Figure 1. Hypoxic stress impaired cognitive and motor function but did not alter the morphology or structure of hippocampal neurons. (**A**) During hypoxia, body weight did not change. Data are presented as mean ± SEM (one-way ANOVA), n = 3–5 biological replicates per condition. (**B**) The rotarod test showed the mobility of mice was significantly reduced compared with the CON. Data are expressed as the mean ± SEM (one-way ANOVA). * $p < 0.05$ H1D vs. CON, ** $p < 0.01$ H3D vs. CON (n = 7–14). The new object recognition experiment showed that the cognitive ability of mice was significantly decreased after hypoxia compared with the control group (CON). Data are expressed as the means ± SEM (two-way ANOVA). **** $p < 0.0001$ vs. familiar object, ** $p < 0.01$ and *** $p < 0.001$ vs. CON (n = 7–14). (**C,D**) Hippocampal and cortical tissues were undamaged, and neurons showed no morphological or structural abnormalities in the hippocampus and cortex under H1D and H3D by HE staining (**C**) and Nissl staining (**D**).

2.2. Global Proteomic Signatures of the Hippocampus under Hypoxic Stress

To evaluate whether the impairment caused by hypoxia on cognition and behavior originated from alterations in neuronal function, we performed global proteomics to conduct an overall analysis of the hippocampus of mice in the subacute phases of hypoxia. A database search using spectra from each tandem mass tag (TMT) run separately identified 4355 proteins across all the time points (Supplemental Table S1). As shown in Figure 2A, each variety presented a characteristic concentration profile, with red, green, and white boxes representing upregulated, downregulated, and unchanged expression proteins, respectively. The results showed that the protein expression of H1D mice was similar, while that of H3D mice was altered, compared with the CON (Figure 2A). Specifically, compared with the control group, 71 proteins were upregulated and 51 downregulated in H1D mice. By contrast, in H3D mice, 332 proteins were upregulated and 106 downregulated (fold change (FC) $\geq$ 1.2 or $\leq$ 0.67, $p \leq 0.05$; Figure 2B). Venn analysis of the above differential proteins showed that 42 proteins had the same expression trend in H1D and H3D, of which 34 proteins showed an upward trend and eight showed a downward trend. Only two proteins showed an opposite expression trend in H1D and H3D (Figure 2C). A volcano map shows the expression of proteins with significant differences in the H1D and H3D mice more intuitively (Figure 2D). To further identify the differentially expressed proteins, we screened out the 20 proteins with the highest differential expression changes between H1D mice and the CON and H3D mice and CON. Among the proteins, fourteen proteins in H1D mice were located in mitochondria, six of which were upregulated proteins (including Atp5fc1, Pam16, Fdx1, Etfdh, Ndufc2, Pdpr) and eight downregulated (Sfxn1, Cs, Atp5f1d, Nrgn, Sncb, Hagh, Vdac3, Cyb5b) (Figure 2E); whereas in H3D mice, five proteins were located in the mitochondria, three of which were upregulated (Maob, Ndufaf3, Rhoa) and two downregulated (Rida, Agps) (Figure 2F).

To further assess the effect of hypoxia on hippocampal signaling pathways, we performed Gene Ontology (GO) enrichment and Kyoto Encyclopedia of Genes and Genomes pathway (KEGG) analyses. GO-enriched pathways in H1D mice included DNA process, IMP-induced process, negative regulation of hydrogen peroxide–neuron death, AMP deaminase activity, and isocitrate dehydrogenase (NAD$^+$) activity. Interestingly, the enriched pathways also had a significant influence on mitochondrial function, mainly related to the reduction of mitochondrial inner membrane components. In addition, glucose aerobic metabolism was downregulated. That is, isocitrate metabolic and ATP metabolic processes were reduced and NAD$^+$ activity decreased (Supplementary Figure S1A). Furthermore, KEGG enrichment results demonstrated that hypoxia mainly affected Parkinson's disease, Huntington's disease, oxidative phosphorylation, African trypanosomiasis, and the citrate cycle pathway. In addition, the pathways of oxidative phosphorylation and the TCA cycle were lowered (Supplementary Figure S1B).

GO-enriched pathways in H3D mice included Gamma-aminobutyric acid receptor clustering, proton-transporting ATP synthase complex, neuron maturation, temperature homeostasis, regulation of cell motility, and protein maturation by iron–sulfur cluster transfer (Supplementary Figure S1C). The KEGG enrichment results showed that the main influencing pathways were taurine and hypotaurine metabolism and salivary secretion (Supplementary Figure S1D). In summary, the damage of short-term hypoxia on cognitive and behavioral abilities in mice is mainly due to changes in neuronal function, which may be mainly manifest as mitochondrial dysfunction.

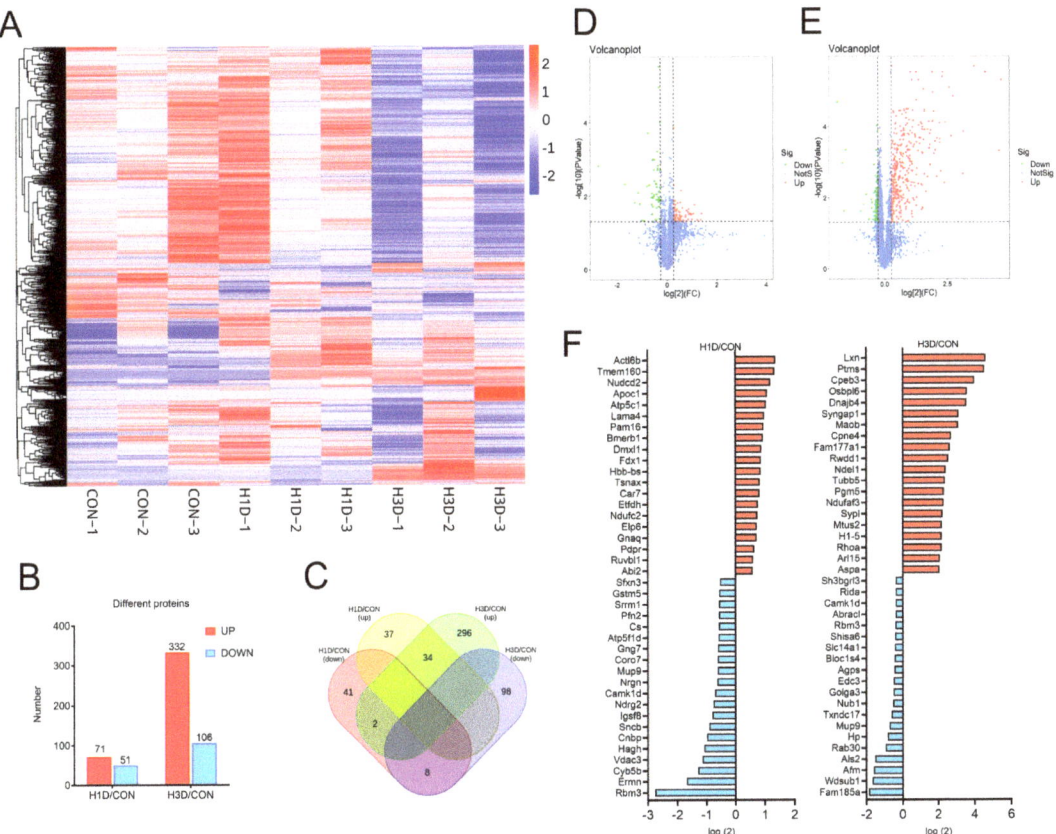

Figure 2. Global proteomic signatures of the hippocampus under hypoxic stress. (**A**) Heat map presenting a respective characteristic concentration profile. (**B**) The proteins were considered significantly regulated at $p \leq 0.05$ and a fold change (FC) ≥ 1.2 or ≤ 0.67. (**C**) Venn diagram of the identified significantly regulated proteins with different time duration exposures to hypoxia. (**D**,**E**) Volcano map showing the expression of proteins with significant differences more intuitively. (**F**) Top 20 proteins with the most prominent differences between H1D or H3D mice and CON mice. The red represents upregulation, the blue downregulation.

2.3. Hippocampal Proteome Dynamic Alterations Induced by Hypoxic Stress

Next, we estimated the effects of hypoxia on hippocampal protein expression and found that 4355 proteins were clustered by non-biased expression pattern clustering. This analysis co-polymerized six clusters with specific expression patterns, in which hypoxia led to upregulation in the first (n = 426) and sixth clusters (n = 592), downregulation in the second cluster (n = 819) and third (n = 1554) clusters, and an initial increase followed by a return to physiological levels in the fourth (n = 329) and fifth (n = 635) clusters (Figure 3A). We further explored whether proteins in different clusters had specific functions to cope with hypoxia. It was found that many proteins in a specific cluster shared cellular components, molecular functions, or acted on the same biological processes. The complete GO entries for each cluster can be found in the Appendix (Supplemental Table S2).

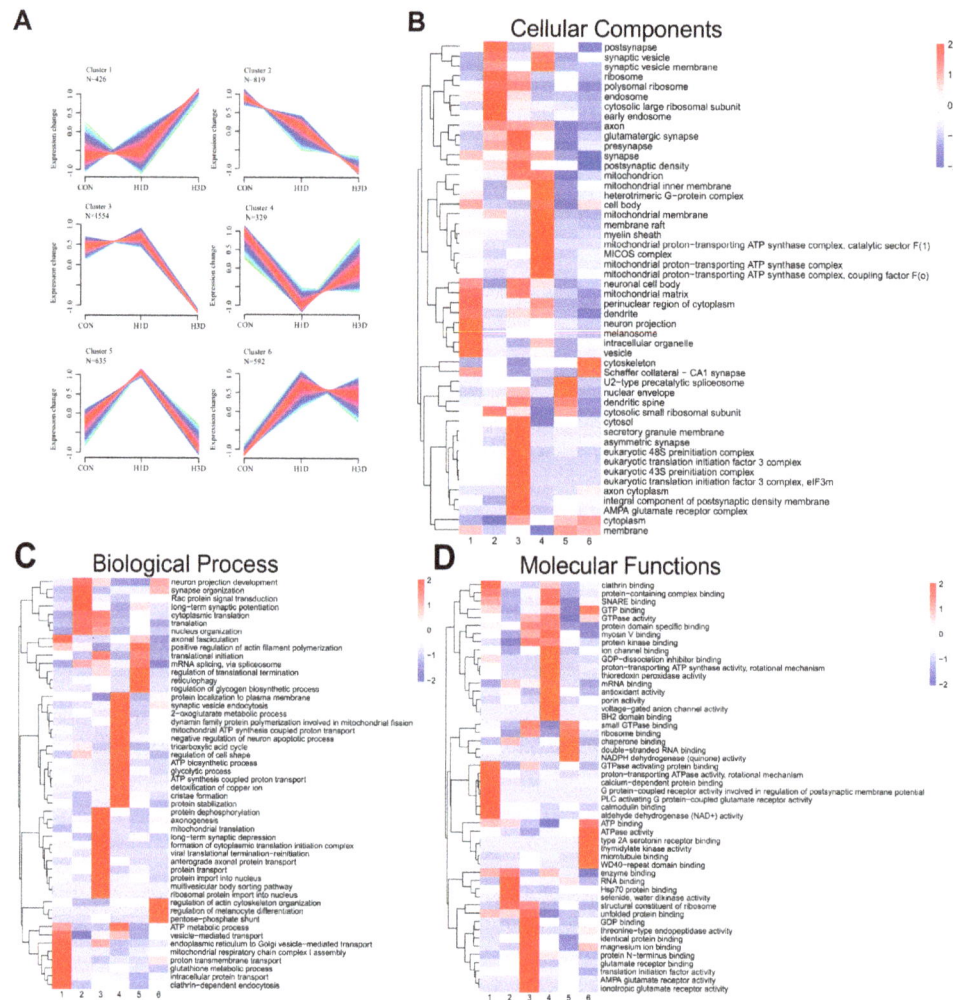

Figure 3. Temporal analysis of hippocampal proteome dynamic alterations induced by hypoxic stress. (**A**) Unsupervised clustering of proteome dynamics revealed six clusters with distinct protein expression profiles: n represents the number of proteins per cluster. The color represents memberships. The red represents more memberships, the blue and green low memberships. (**B**–**D**) GO enrichment analysis of each cluster was performed using Fisher's exact test ($p < 0.05$). Biological processes (BP) (**B**), molecular functions (MF) (**C**), and cellular components (CC) (**D**) of the clusters are visualized.

The relative expression level of cluster 1 proteins continued to increase from H1D to H3D. This expression pattern corresponds to the body's adaptation to chronic hypoxia. Specifically, cluster 1 contained a total of 426 proteins, and the enriched biological processes included intracellular protein transport, organelles to Golgi vesicle-mediated transport, glutathione metabolism, mitochondrial respiratory chain complex I assembly, and ATP metabolism (Figure 3B).

Molecular functions included GTP binding, proton-transporting ATPase activity, protein-containing complex binding, GTPase activating protein binding, and calcium-dependent protein binding (Figure 3D). Cluster 6 contained 592 proteins, and compared with the CON, the expression of H1D proteins dramatically increased, and remained at an increased level throughout the experiment. Enriched biological processes included actin cytoskeleton organization (Rhof, Rhob) and neuronal projection development (Mrtfb, Lgi1) (Figure 3B). Molecular function mainly involved GTP binding and GTPase activity (Figure 3D). Cluster 3 contained 1554 proteins, showing a sharp decrease in protein expression from H1D to H3D. Biological processes mainly involved protein transport (Arf2, Rab4b) (Figure 3B), while the molecular function was mainly identical to protein binding (Acacb) (Figure 3D). Cluster 2 contained 819 proteins, all of which were downregulated under hypoxic stress. The related biological processes comprised translation and neuronal projection development (Figure 3B). Molecular functions included the structural component of the ribosome and RNA binding (Figure 3D). Cluster 4 consisted of 1554 proteins and compared with the CON, the expression of H1D proteins decreased; however, the expression levels returned to physiological levels at H3D. The GO biological processes mainly included mitochondrial ATP synthesis coupled proton transport (Atp5f1d), the TCA cycle (Idh3g, Cs), synaptic vesicle endocytosis (Sncb), glycolysis (Tpi1), and cristae formation (Chchd6) (Figure 3B). Molecular functions involved GTP binding and GTPase activity (Septin7) and protein-containing complex binding (Park7, Ndufa4, Atp5f1d, Ywhaz) (Figure 3D). Cluster 5 contained 635 proteins, and compared with the CON, the expression of H1D proteins increased; however, the expression levels returned to physiological levels at H3D. Interestingly, GO analysis results indicated that almost all the biological processes and molecular functions were associated with mitochondrial functions. Moreover, it is worth noting that GO cellular components analysis showed that all the clusters were enriched in proteins related to mitochondrial components (Figure 3C). Overall, our present temporal hypoxia proteomics study also confirmed that the short-term hypoxic exposure altered distinct biological processes and signaling pathways in the hippocampus region in a temporal-dependent manner. Therefore, we further analyzed mitochondrial-related proteins.

2.4. Hypoxic Stress Mainly Caused Mitochondrial Dysfunction

To demonstrate the expression levels and functional changes in mitochondrial-related proteins, we used protein component analysis to filter mitochondrial-related proteins. The UniProtKB mouse protein database was used to screen all mitochondrial-related proteins, including reported proteins located in mitochondria under physiological or pathological states. In summary, 787 mitochondrial-related proteins were extracted from the total protein list (Supplemental Table S3). Similarly, compared with the CON, only 4.8% of mitochondrial proteins showed significant changes after H1D, of which 24 proteins were downregulated and 14 upregulated. At H3D, 9.3% of mitochondrial proteins showed significant changes, of which 14 were downregulated and 59 upregulated (Figure 4A–C).

Similarly, we also clustered the expression patterns of mitochondrial proteins, including six cluster-specific expression patterns. Clusters 2 and 5 showed a decreasing trend in protein expression, in which cluster 2 contained 269 proteins and cluster 5 contained 145 proteins (Figure 4D). Clusters 3 and 4 showed an increasing trend in protein expression, in which cluster 3 contained 111 proteins and cluster 4 contained 86 proteins (Figure 4D). Cluster 1 contained 85 proteins, which initially showed a decreasing trend in expression, but returned to physiological levels at H3D. Cluster 6 contained 91 proteins, which showed the opposite trend to that of Cluster 5, with initially increased expression followed by a return to physiological levels at H3D (Figure 4D).

GO biological processes results indicated that the biological processes of cluster 1 included mitochondrial ATP synthesis coupled proton transport, 2-oxoglutarate metabolic, ATP, cristae formation, and ATP synthesis coupled proton transport. The biological processes of Cluster 2 involved migration organization, mitochondrial translation, mitochondrial electron transport, NADH to ubiquinone, and mitochondrial ATP synthesis coupled electron transport. The biological processes of Cluster 3 included mitochondrial acetyl-CoA adduct from pyruvate and dTDP adduct. Fatty acid beta-oxidation uses acyl-CoA dehydrogenase and mitochondrial organization. Cluster 4 biological processes included aerobic respiration, negative regulation of cell death, ATP metabolism, oxidative stress, and chaperone-mediated protein complex assembly. Cluster 5 biological processes included neuronal death and apoptosis. The biological processes of the neuronal apoptosis process and activation of cysteine-type endopeptidase activity are involved in the neuronal apoptosis process. Cluster 6 biological processes were associated with 10-formyltetrahydrofolate acidification, mitochondrial transport, mitochondrial calcium ion transmembrane transport, regulation of cellular hyperosmotic salinity, and heme biosynthesis. It is noteworthy that all clusters were related to mitochondrial respiratory chain complex I assembly (Supplementary Figure S2). Clusters 1–5 were correlated with the TCA cycle and clusters 2–5 with fatty acid beta-oxidation (Supplementary Figure S2). Supplementary Figure S2 showed the top 20 biological processes of each cluster.

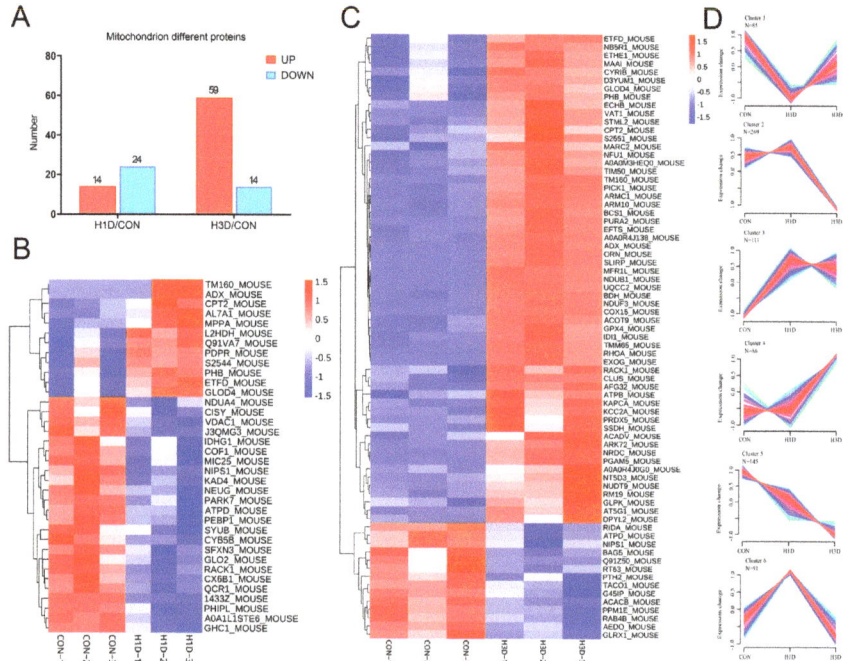

Figure 4. Hypoxic stress mainly caused mitochondrial dysfunction. (**A**) Mitochondrial proteins of interest were considered significantly regulated at $p \leq 0.05$ and a fold change ≥ 1.2 or ≤ 0.67. (**B**,**C**) Heat map showing the prominent different mitochondrial proteins in H1D (**B**) and H3D (**C**) mice compared with the CON. (**D**) Unsupervised clustering of proteome dynamics revealed six clusters with mitochondrial protein expression profiles: n represents the number of proteins per cluster. The color represents memberships. The red represents more memberships, the blue and green low memberships.

2.5. Hypoxic Stress Impaired Mitochondrial Oxidative Phosphorylation by Suppressing Mitochondrial Complex IV

It is well known that the main functions of mitochondria are directly related to the TCA cycle and oxidative phosphorylation. The above results demonstrated that hypoxic stress could cause mitochondrial dysfunction, while the segment of mitochondrial function was affected by hypoxia. Therefore, we further analyzed the differentially expressed mitochondrial-related proteins (FC ≥ 1.2 or ≤ 0.67 and $p \leq 0.05$) and constructed a multi-protein interaction network using the STRING database (http://string-db.org (accessed on 14 January 2022)) [19]. Compared with the CON, the interaction networks of H1D mice were significantly different and were related to the TCA cycle, oxidative phosphorylation, and fatty acid beta-oxidation (Figure 5A). Similarly, compared with the CON, interaction networks in H3D mice were significantly different and included fatty acid beta-oxidation, oxidative phosphorylation, and oxidative stress reaction (Figure 5B). Mitochondrial oxidative phosphorylation is the main process to utilize oxygen; therefore, we next determined if mitochondrial oxidative phosphorylation was affected under hypoxia by exploring mitochondrial electron transport chain complexes.

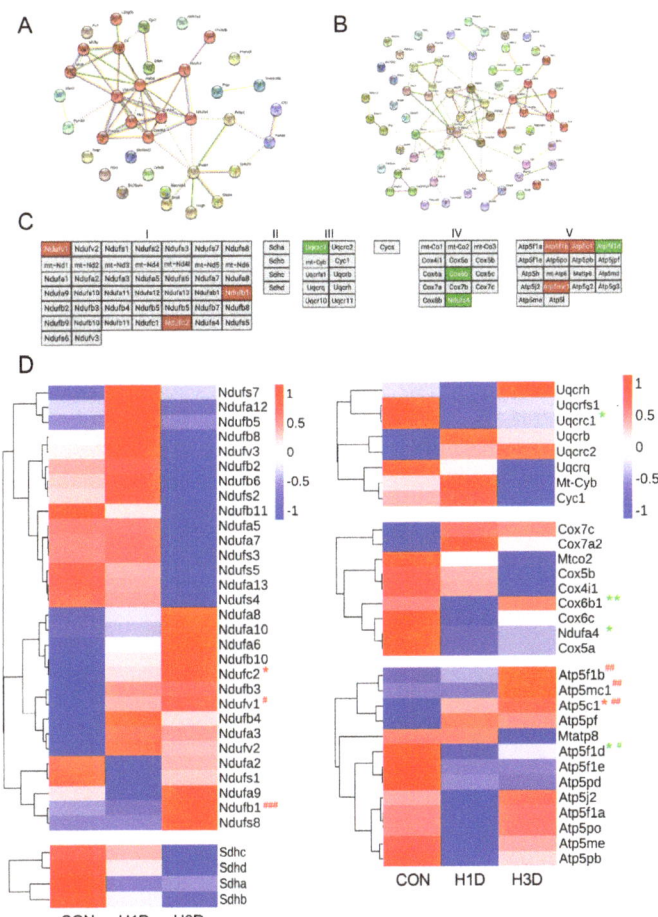

Figure 5. Hypoxic stress impaired mitochondrial oxidative phosphorylation by suppressing mitochondrial complex IV. (**A**,**B**) The differentially expressed mitochondrial-related proteins compared with the CON had a multiprotein interaction network constructed by the STRING Database in H1D (**A**) and H3D (**B**) mice. (**C**) The newly reported mitochondrial electron transport chain complex proteins. The red represents upregulation, the green downregulation, and the gray no change or unidentified. (**D**) The list of mitochondrial oxidative phosphorylation proteins. The red represents upregulation (FC ≥ 1.2, * $p < 0.05$ H1D vs. CON, # $p < 0.05$, ## $p < 0.01$, ### $p < 0.001$ H3D vs. CON), green downregulation (FC ≤ 0.67, * $p < 0.05$, ** $p < 0.01$ H1D vs. CON, # $p < 0.05$ H3D vs. CON).

The newly reported mitochondrial electron transport chain complex proteins are shown in Figure 5C [15]. Combined with our proteomic results, 60 mitochondrial electron transport chain proteins and 15 ATP synthase-related proteins were identified. Among them, the upregulated proteins included three complex I proteins (Ndufv1, Ndufb1) and three complex V proteins (Atp5f1b, Atp5c1, Atp5mc1); whereas, the downregulated proteins included one complex III protein (Uqcrc1), two complex IV proteins (Ndufa4, Cox6b) and one complex V protein (Atp5f1d) (Figure 5C,D). Previous studies have shown that complex IV is the main oxygen consumption site of oxidative phosphorylation and is the rate-limiting step of oxidative phosphorylation [16]. Therefore, we believe that hypoxia impeded the utilization of oxygen in mitochondrial complex IV.

2.6. Hypoxic Stress Caused Mitochondrial Complex IV Dysfunction by Downregulating NDUFA4 Expression

To further verify the effect of hypoxia on mitochondrial, we used immunofluorescence to detect NDUFA4 expression. The results showed that, compared with the CON, the expression of NDUFA4 in the hippocampal CA1 area was significantly decreased at H3D, while the proportion of NDUFA4-positive cells in the CA1 area did not change significantly (Figure 6A–C). In the hippocampal CA3 area, compared with the CON, the expression of NDUFA4 was significantly decreased at H1D and H3D, whereas the proportion of NDUFA4-positive cells was significant only at H3D (Figure 6A–C). In the RAD and DG regions of the hippocampus, the expression of NDUFA4 and the proportion of positive cells did not change significantly (Figure 6A–C). Interestingly, in the cortex, we found a similar situation, where at H3D there was increased NDUFA4 expression and the proportion of NDUFA4-positive cells was obviously decreased (Figure 6A–C). It is well known that ROS generation is closely related to mitochondrial respiration activity. Therefore, we further verified the production of ROS in the experimental mice. The results showed that, compared with the CON, hypoxia significantly increased ROS production in the hippocampal CA1 area at H1D and H3D, with no significant changes in other hippocampal regions, (CA-3, RAD, and DG) (Figure 6D,E). Furthermore, the production of ROS in the cortex also increased significantly (Figure 6D,E). In summary, we established that hypoxia could reduce the expression of NDUFA4, reduce the activity of CIV, hinder the utilization of charged ions and oxygen, and increase the level of ROS.

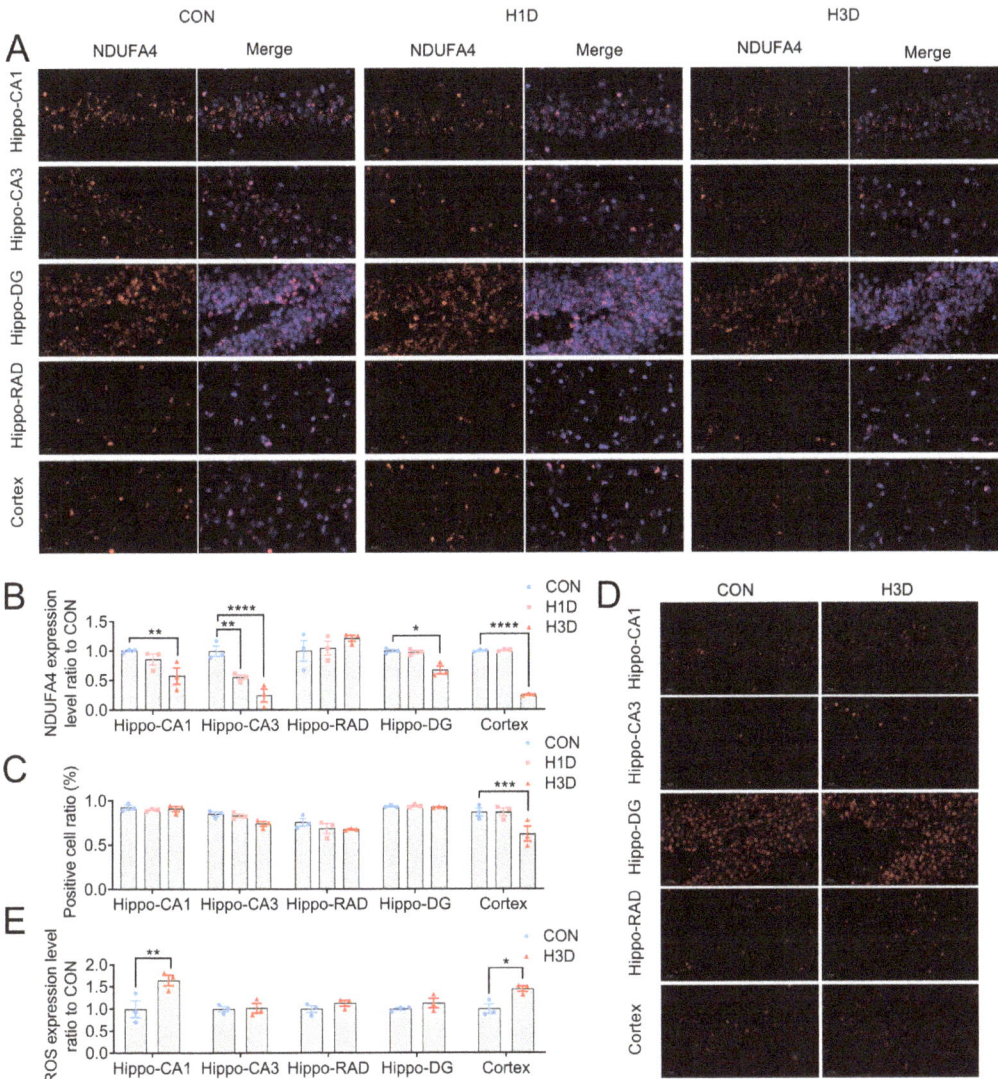

Figure 6. Hypoxic stress caused mitochondrial complex IV dysfunction by downregulating NDUFA4 expression. (**A**) Representative immunofluorescence images of NDUFA4 (red) in the hippocampus (CA-1, CA-3, DG, RAD) and cortex of the different groups. Nuclei are stained in blue (DAPI). (**B**) Quantification of the NDUFA4-positive area based on immunofluorescence staining sections by ImageJ Pro Plus 6.0 software. Statistical analysis of the fluorescence intensity of NDUFA4 was conducted on three slices from three animals per group. Data are expressed as the means ± SEM (two-way ANOVA). ** $p < 0.01$ H1D vs. CON, *$p < 0.05$, ** $p < 0.01$, **** $p < 0.0001$ H3D vs. CON (n = 3). (**C**) The ratio of positive cells based on immunofluorescence staining sections by ImageJ software. Data are expressed as the means ± SEM (two-way ANOVA). *** $p < 0.001$ H3D vs. CON (n = 3). (**D**) Representative immunofluorescence images of ROS (red) in the hippocampus (CA1, CA3, DG, RAD) and cortex of the different groups. Nuclei are stained in blue (DAPI). (**E**) Quantification of the ROS-positive area based on immunofluorescence staining sections by ImageJ Pro Plus software. Data are expressed as the means ± SEM (two-way ANOVA). * $p < 0.05$, ** $p < 0.01$ H3D vs. CON (n = 3).

3. Discussion

In this study, we investigated the effects of hypoxia stress on the hippocampus of mice using the global proteome approach. First, we found that hypoxia did not cause substantial changes in the morphology and structure of the brain but resulted in impaired cognitive and motor abilities in mice. Second, bioinformatics analysis indicated that hypoxia affected the expression of 516 proteins, of which 71.1% were found to be upregulated proteins and 28.5% downregulated. GO and KEGG analysis showed that short-term chronic hypoxia mainly disturbed mitochondrial function. Intriguingly, we found that the expression levels of CIV-related proteins (Ndufa4 and Cox6b) were downregulated. Based on the structure-related studies of Ndufa4, it was found that Ndufa4 exists as CIV monomers, which inhibit the dimerization of CIV and maintain CIV in its active form [20]. In summary, we believe that hypoxia leads to decreased CIV activity and impaired electronic respiratory chain productivity.

Mitochondria consume 85–90% of the oxygen in the body, whereas oxidative phosphorylation generates 90% of the ATP used in the body [21]. It is conceivable that the change in oxygen concentration initially affects the mitochondrial electron transport chain. Hypoxia impacts mitochondrial function in a variety of ways, including altering the manner in which the TCA cycle and electron transport chain complexes [22] consume NADH and FADH2, which in turn generates ROS. Hypoxia limits the entry of pyruvate into the TCA cycle, reduces PHDs enzymatic activity [23], and stabilizes the expression of HIFs. Next, HIFs induce the expression of lactate dehydrogenase A (LDHA) and pyruvate dehydrogenase kinase 1 (PDK1) [11,24]. LDHA then converts pyruvate into lactate and reduces pyruvate entering the mitochondrial matrix. In addition, PDK1 phosphorylates pyruvate dehydrogenase, preventing pyruvate conversion into acetyl-CoA [9], thus inhibiting the TCA cycle. Second, hypoxia affects the activity of the electron transport chain. It has been reported that hypoxia can enhance the activity of CIV in two ways.

First, HIFs induce the expression of nuclear-encoded subunit COX4 subtype 2 and mitochondrial protein LON, so that COX4 subtype 1 is degraded by proteasomes, thereby improving the efficiency of the electron transport [25]. Second, HIFs induce hypoxia-inducible gene domain family member 1A expression and enhance CIV activity by yet-unknown mechanisms [26]. In contrast to hypoxia-induced increases in CIV activity, CI, CII, and CIII activities have been shown to be decreased under hypoxic conditions [9]. Indeed, HIFs were shown to attenuate CI activity by inducing NADH dehydrogenase (ubiquinone) 1α subcomplex, 4-like 2 (NDUFA4L2) expression, by a yet-unknown mechanism [22].

It is not clear how hypoxia induces ROS production. Mitochondria are both the production and degradation sites of ROS. The balance between ROS generation and degradation depends on the ROS flux across the mitochondrial membrane [12]. Under normal physiological conditions, the ATP:ADP ratio is maintained, and the high level of ATP combined with CIV produces isomerization inhibition, which maintains CIV activity at a low level, thereby maintaining a low mitochondrial membrane potential and preventing excessive harmful ROS generation [27]. However, hypoxia can break this balance, causing increased CIV activity and mitochondrial membrane potential accompanied by excessive production of ROS [27]. Recent studies have shown that the ETC electron transport efficiency remains at a high level during acute hypoxia ($O_2 < 5\%$), resulting in an exponential increase in ROS generation rate [9]. Under chronic hypoxia, NDUFA4L2 expression is increased resulting in decreased CI activity [22], impaired ETC complex assembly, and reduced electron transfer efficiency. Therefore, CIII-mediated ROS production is reduced [9,28]. Our results showed that the enriched mitochondrial redox enzymes in the hippocampus (Gpx1, Gpx4, Prdx5, Txnrd2) hold the potential to be therapeutic targets against hypoxia-induced oxidative stress.

CIV, also known as cytochrome c oxidase, is the terminal of the electron transport chain and is therefore the rate-limiting enzyme of the electron transport chain. CIV has a high affinity for O_2, and is the main consumer of O_2, reducing it to H_2O [16,29]. This process is accompanied by proton pumping from the mitochondrial matrix to form a proton transmembrane gradient [30], which ATP synthase uses to produce ATP [31]. NDUFA4 was initially considered as the subunit CIV [32]. In recent years, research has indicated that NDUFA4 is the 14th subunit of CIV [33]. Interestingly, the expression of NDUFA4 was decreased in poor prognosis cancer patients [28,34,35]. In addition, studies have shown that NDUFA4 is essential for CIV biosynthesis and complex activity, and NDUFA4 structure-related studies have found that NDUFA4 exists between CIV monomers, thereby inhibiting the dimerization of CIV and maintaining CIV in its active state [20]. NDUFA4 has been closely linked to the enzyme complex. Specifically, NDUFA4 deletion or mutation causes CIV function inactivation, eventually leading to illness [33]. Our results showed that hypoxia caused the downregulation of NDUFA4 expression, a process that may be related to a decrease in CIV activity, which reduces oxygen consumption and ultimately ROS generation. Although we found that the decrease in NDUFA4 expression resulted in a decrease in CIV activity, we were surprised that our results suggested that the proteins related to mitochondrial complexes CI, CIII, and CV showed an increasing trend, which was contrary to previous results of hypoxia-induced decreases in CI, CII, and CIII activity [9]. Our explanation is that hypoxia leads to a decrease in CIV activity and oxygen utilization ability, resulting in an imbalance in the energy consumption of the hippocampus. Therefore, there may be ineffective feedback under stress, which further leads to neuronal functional damage by a yet unknown mechanism/pathway.

Collectively, our study suggested that hypoxic stress impaired the cognitive and motor abilities of mice, but the morphology and structure of neurons in did not change significantly under short-term hypoxic stimulation. Proteomics analysis demonstrated that mitochondrial function changed, which was manifested as a decrease in NDUFA4 expression. These results indicated that mitochondrial CIV activity and oxygen utilization ability were reduced, which resulted in impaired mitochondrial membrane potential and ultimately insufficient energy for hippocampal neurons. The importance of NDUFA4 is well-established and underscored by its association with hypoxia. Further investigations should be conducted to clarify the complicated relationship between hypoxia and mitochondrial function.

4. Materials and Methods

4.1. Animals

Male C57BL/6J mice (7–8 weeks old) were purchased from SPF Biotechnology Company (Beijing, China) and housed at room temperature (22–25 °C) under a 12:12 h light/dark cycle with free access to food and water. All procedures were approved by the Animal Care and Use Committee of the Institute of Animal Management, Capital Medical University, and conducted in accordance with ethical requirements.

4.2. Hypoxia Treatment

The mice were administered hypoxic treatment in a closed hypoxic camber (China Innovation Instrument Co., Ltd., Ningbo, China), which accurately set the desired hypoxic concentration and pattern. A total of 30 mice were randomly divided into three groups (10 mice in each): control (CON) and chronic hypoxia (continuously with 13% O_2 for 1 and 3 days (H1D and H3D), respectively. Among the ten animals in each group, three were used for HE staining and Nissl staining, three for proteomic analysis, and four for ROS fluorescence staining. To avoid the reoxygen starting, the behavioral test and the brain samples collected were processed at the same time once the hypoxic treatment finished.

4.3. Rotarod Test

The rotarod test was used to analyze motor function in mice as previously described [36]. Briefly, mice were trained on the Rota Rod (Panlab Rota Rod from Broad Institute, Cambridge, MA, USA) at a constant accelerated speed from 4 to 40 rpm for 300 s at least 5 days before competitive assessment. Each trial day consisted of five tests per mouse. The length of time that the mice remained on the rod on the five occasions was then averaged.

4.4. Novel Object Recognition

Mice were placed in an open-field apparatus for 30 min in the absence of objects before training, and locomotor behavior was recorded using a video-tracking system (SMART v3.0 from RDW Biotechnology Company, Shenzhen, China). Each mouse was then allowed to freely explore two simple identical objects placed at fixed different locations for 5 min as described previously [37]. After the familiarization phase, in the final test, where one familiar object A was replaced by another novel object B, mice were placed in the chamber again for 5 min with the procedure being video recorded. We used the exploration time (%) [ET, ET = TB/(TA + TB), TB = exploring time on B, TA = exploring time on A] to assess short-term memory.

4.5. HE and Nissl Staining

Mice were anesthetized with 1% chloral hydrate by intraperitoneal injection and sacrificed. To evaluate histological damage, mice in each group (n = 3) were sacrificed and transcardially perfused with 100 mL of saline and then 100 mL of a freshly prepared 4% w/v paraformaldehyde in 0.01M phosphate-buffered saline (PBS, pH 7.4). The brains were then removed and fixed in 4% paraformaldehyde for 24 h. The issue was dehydrated by a series of alcohol gradients and then embedded in wax. The wax was subsequently trimmed and sectioned coronally into 4μm slices for subsequent HE or Nissl staining.

4.5.1. HE Staining

The sections were dewaxed in xylene twice for 20 min, then successively dehydrated in 100% ethanol, 100% ethanol, and 75% ethanol, for 5 min each, and rinsed with tap water. The sections were then stained with hematoxylin solution (HE dye solution set, Servicebio, G1003, Wuhan, China) for 3–5min and rinsed with tap water. Next, the sections were treated with hematoxylin differentiation solution, rinsed with tap water, treated with hematoxylin Scott tap bluing, and rinsed with tap water. After, the sections were fixed with 85% ethanol and 95% ethanol for 5 min each, then stained with Eosin dye for 5 min. Finally, the sections were dehydrated with 100% ethanol three times for 5 min each, placed in xylene three times for 5 min each, and sealed with neutral gum.

4.5.2. Nissl Staining

The sections were dewaxed in xylene twice for 20 min, then successively dehydrated in 100% ethanol, 100% ethanol, and 75% ethanol, for 5 min each, and then rinsed with tap water. The sections were then stained with Nissl dye (Servicebio, G1036) for 3–5 min, rinsed with tap, immersed in 0.1% glacial acetic acid differentiation solution, and rinsed in tap water. Finally, the sections were sealed with neutral gum.

4.6. Immunofluorescence Staining for ROS Detection

As previously described, mice in each group (n = 3) were sacrificed and the brains were quickly removed and snap-frozen in liquid nitrogen to preserve ROS, after which they were sectioned (10μm). Frozen slides were then placed at room temperature to eliminate obvious liquid. After, the sections were incubated with spontaneous fluorescence quenching reagent (Servicebio, G1221) for 5 min, washed, and incubated in ROS staining solution (Sigma, D7008, 1:500, Saint Louis, MO, USA) for a further 30 min at 37 °C for 30 min away from light. After washing with PBS (pH 7.4), the sections were incubated with DAPI solution for 10 min at room temperature. Finally, after washing again in PBS (pH 7.4), the slices were sealed with anti-fade mounting medium. Fluorescent microscopy was then employed to visualize ROS-positive cells.

4.7. Immunofluorescence Labeling

As previously described, frozen sections were baked in an oven for 10–20 min at 37 °C to dry the moisture and fixed in paraformaldehyde for 30 min. After washing with PBS (pH 7.4), the slices were incubated in EDTA antigen retrieval buffer recovery (pH 8.0), washed three times with PBS (pH 7.4), and blocked in 3% bovine serum albumin or 10% donkey serum for 30 min, depending on the respective antibodies that were to be used. The slides were then incubated with primary antibody (Huabio, Hangzhou, China, anti-NDUFA4 antibody, ER64130, 1:100) overnight at 4 °C. After washing three times with PBS the sections were then incubated with secondary antibody (Servicebio, CY3 goat anti-rabbit, GB21303, 1:300) for 50 min at room temperature. Next, the sections were counterstained with DAPI for 10 min at room temperature to visualize the cell nuclei. Finally, the sections were washed, incubated with fluorescence quenching reagent (Servicebio, G1221) for 5 min, and then sealed with an anti-fade mounting medium. Fluorescent microscopy was used to visualize fluorescence staining.

4.8. Proteomic Analysis

4.8.1. Sample Preparation

Mice in each group (n = 3) were anesthetized with 1% chloral hydrate by intraperitoneal injection and then the brains were harvested immediately. Next, the hippocampus was separated, snap frozen in liquid nitrogen, and stored at −80 °C until use. The frozen tissue was homogenized in lysis buffer (7M urea (Bio-Rad), 2M thiourea (Sigma-Aldrich, Saint Louis, MO, USA), 0.1% CHAPS (Bio-Rad)), ground with three titanium dioxide abrasive beads (70 Hz, 120 s), and centrifuged for 5 min at $5000 \times g$ and 4 °C. The supernatant was then collected and centrifuged for 30 min at $15,000 \times g$ and 4 °C. The final supernatant was collected and stored at −80 °C until further use. The total protein concentration was measured by the Bradford protein assay and 200 μg of total protein was incubated with 5 μL of 200 mM reducing reagent for 1 h at 55 °C. Next, 5 μL of 375 mM iodoacetamide was added to the solution and allowed to incubate for 10 min at room temperature in the dark. Finally, 200 μL of 100 mM dissolution buffer (AB Sciex) was added and the solution was then centrifuged for 20 min at $12,000 \times g$. Finally, the solution was digested in trypsin for 14 h at room temperature, then lyophilized and redissolved with 100 mM dissolution buffer for labeling.

4.8.2. TMT Labeling

The TMT reagent (Thermofisher, 90111, Waltham, MA, USA) was incubated at room temperature, after which 41 μL of absolute ethyl alcohol was added to the TMT reagent (0.8 mg/tube) and mixed well. Next, 41 μL of TMT reagent was added to 100 μg of the hippocampal tissue homogenate and the mixture was oscillated, centrifuged, and incubated for 1 h at room temperature, after which 5% quenching reagent (8 μL) was added and let stand for 15 min to terminate the reaction. The samples were stored after lyophilization.

4.8.3. Peptide Identification by Nano UPLC-MS/MS

The acquired peptide fractions were suspended with 20 μL of buffer A (0.1% FA, 2% ACN) and centrifuged for 10 min at 12,000 rpm. Next, 10 μL of the supernatant was injected into the nano UPLC-MS/MS system consisting of a Nanoflow HPLC system (EASY-nLC 1000 system from Thermo Scientific, Waltham, MA, USA) and Orbitrap Fusion Lumos mass spectrometer (Thermo Scientific). The sample was loaded onto an Acclaim PepMap100 C18 column and then separated by an EASY-Spray C18 column. The mass spectrometer was operated in the positive ion mode (source voltage 2.1 KV) and full MS scans were performed with the Orbitrap over the range of 300–1500 m/z at a resolution of 120,000. For MS/MS scans, the 20 most abundant ions with multiple charge states were selected for higher energy collisional dissociation fragmentation following one MS full scan. The peptide false discovery rate (FDR) was determined based on PSMs when searched against the reverse, decoy database. Peptides assigned only to a given protein group were considered unique. The FDR was set to 0.01 for protein identifications.

The database used in this experiment is Uniprot_Mus_musculus (2020.8.13 Download) database. The resulting MS/MS data were processed using Proteome Discoverer 1.4.

4.8.4. Protein Identification

Protein identification was set as follows: precursor ion mass tolerance, ±15 ppm; fragment ion mass tolerance, ±20 mmu; max missed cleavages, 2; static modification, carboxy aminomethylation (57.021 Da) of Cys residues; dynamic modifications, oxidation modification (+15.995 Da) of Met residues.

4.8.5. Bioinformatic Analysis

Hierarchical clustering analysis was performed to evaluate the batch effects in the proteomic data regarding sample groups. Samples exhibited a high similarity within the same group, while different groups of samples were obviously different.

GO and KEGG (http://www.genome.jp/kegg (accessed on 17 January 2021)) analyses were conducted to analyze the protein families and pathways in each group. The probable interacting partners were predicted by the STRING database (http://string-db.org (accessed on 14 January 2022)).

4.9. Statistical Methods

According to the P-value of primary data, proteins with a $p \leq 0.05$ and FC ≥ 1.2 or ≤ 0.67 were considered statistically significant. The body weight and protein expression ratio analyses were performed using ordinary one-way ANOVA, followed by GraphPad Prism 9.0 software (GraphPad Software, San Diego, CA, USA). The normalized expression ratio for the CON was taken as 1. We also analyzed the cognitive and motor abilities of the mice by two-way ANOVA. Data are expressed as mean ± SEM for at least three independent experiments. Differences were considered significant at $p < 0.05$.

Supplementary Materials: The following supporting information can be downloaded at: https://www.mdpi.com/article/10.3390/ijms232214094/s1.

Author Contributions: Conceptualization, J.L. and X.J.; methodology, G.L.; validation, Y.G. (Yakun Gu), M.G., Y.G. (Yuying Guan), Z.T., W.M., C.W.; formal analysis, Q.S. and J.L.; resources, G.L.; data curation, Q.S.; writing—original draft preparation, Q.S. and J.L.; writing—review and editing, Q.S. and J.L.; visualization, Q.S. and J.L.; supervision, J.L. and X.J.; project administration, X.J.; funding acquisition, J.L. and X.J. All authors have read and agreed to the published version of the manuscript.

Funding: This research was funded by the National Natural Science Foundation of China (Grant numbers: 32100925, 82027802), the Beijing Nova Program (Grant number: Z211100002121038), the Beijing Hundred Thousand and Ten Thousand Talent Project (Grant number: 2019A36), and the Beijing Municipal Health Commission (Grant number: 303-01-005-0019).

Institutional Review Board Statement: The animal study protocol was approved by the Institutional Review Board (or Ethics Committee) of Capital Medical University (AEEI-2020-093)." for studies involving animals.

Informed Consent Statement: Not applicable.

Data Availability Statement: All data are displayed in the manuscript.

Conflicts of Interest: The authors declare no conflict of interest.

Abbreviations

CI	NADH dehydrogenase;
CII	Succinate dehydrogenase;
CIV	Mitochondrial complex IV;
CIII	Bc1-complex;
COX	Cytochrome c oxidase;
COX4I1	COX4 subtype 1;
COX4I2	COX4 subtype 2;
ETC	Electron transfer chain;
HIF	Hypoxia-inducible Factor;

GO	Gene Ontology;
KEGG	Kyoto Encyclopedia of Genes and Genomes;
LDHA	Lactate dehydrogenase A;
NDUFA4	NADH dehydrogenase (ubiquinone) 1 alpha subcomplex 4;
OXPHOS	Oxidative phosphorylation;
PDH	Pyruvate dehydrogenase;
PDK1	Pyruvate dehydrogenase kinase 1;
PHDS	Prolyl hydroxylases;
ROS	Reactive oxygen species;
TCA	Tricarboxylic acid cycle;

References

1. Trzepizur, W.; Blanchard, M.; Ganem, T.; Balusson, F.; Feuilloy, M.; Girault, J.M.; Meslier, N.; Oger, E.; Paris, A.; Pigeanne, T.; et al. Sleep Apnea-Specific Hypoxic Burden, Symptom Subtypes, and Risk of Cardiovascular Events and All-Cause Mortality. *Am. J. Respir. Crit. Care Med.* **2022**, *205*, 108–117. [CrossRef] [PubMed]
2. Kaczynska, K.; Orlowska, M.E.; Andrzejewski, K. Respiratory Abnormalities in Parkinson's Disease: What Do We Know from Studies in Humans and Animal Models? *Int. J. Mol. Sci.* **2022**, *23*, 3499. [CrossRef] [PubMed]
3. Kazim, S.F.; Sharma, A.; Saroja, S.R.; Seo, J.H.; Larson, C.S.; Ramakrishnan, A.; Wang, M.; Blitzer, R.D.; Shen, L.; Pena, C.J.; et al. Chronic Intermittent Hypoxia Enhances Pathological Tau Seeding, Propagation, and Accumulation and Exacerbates Alzheimer-like Memory and Synaptic Plasticity Deficits and Molecular Signatures. *Biol. Psychiatry* **2022**, *91*, 346–358. [CrossRef] [PubMed]
4. Curila, K.; Jurak, P.; Halamek, J.; Prinzen, F.; Waldauf, P.; Karch, J.; Stros, P.; Plesinger, F.; Mizner, J.; Susankova, M.; et al. Ventricular activation pattern assessment during right ventricular pacing: Ultra-high-frequency ECG study. *J. Cardiovasc. Electrophysiol.* **2021**, *32*, 1385–1394. [CrossRef]
5. Wilson, M.H.; Newman, S.; Imray, C.H. The cerebral effects of ascent to high altitudes. *Lancet Neurol.* **2009**, *8*, 175–191. [CrossRef]
6. Tesler, N.; Latshang, T.D.; Lo Cascio, C.M.; Stadelmann, K.; Stoewhas, A.C.; Kohler, M.; Bloch, K.E.; Achermann, P.; Huber, R. Ascent to moderate altitude impairs overnight memory improvements. *Physiol. Behav.* **2015**, *139*, 121–126. [CrossRef]
7. Hota, S.K.; Sharma, V.K.; Hota, K.; Das, S.; Dhar, P.; Mahapatra, B.B.; Srivastava, R.B.; Singh, S.B. Multi-domain cognitive screening test for neuropsychological assessment for cognitive decline in acclimatized lowlanders staying at high altitude. *Indian J. Med. Res.* **2012**, *136*, 411–420.
8. Markolovic, S.; Wilkins, S.E.; Schofield, C.J. Protein Hydroxylation Catalyzed by 2-Oxoglutarate-dependent Oxygenases. *J. Biol. Chem.* **2015**, *290*, 20712–20722. [CrossRef]
9. Lee, P.; Chandel, N.S.; Simon, M.C. Cellular adaptation to hypoxia through hypoxia inducible factors and beyond. *Nat. Rev. Mol. Cell Biol.* **2020**, *21*, 268–283. [CrossRef]
10. Mookerjee, S.A.; Gerencser, A.A.; Nicholls, D.G.; Brand, M.D. Quantifying intracellular rates of glycolytic and oxidative ATP production and consumption using extracellular flux measurements. *J. Biol. Chem.* **2017**, *292*, 7189–7207. [CrossRef]
11. Papandreou, I.; Cairns, R.A.; Fontana, L.; Lim, A.L.; Denko, N.C. HIF-1 mediates adaptation to hypoxia by actively downregulating mitochondrial oxygen consumption. *Cell Metab.* **2006**, *3*, 187–197. [CrossRef] [PubMed]
12. Liang, S.; Dong, S.; Liu, W.; Wang, M.; Tian, S.; Ai, Y.; Wang, H. Accumulated ROS Activates HIF-1alpha-Induced Glycolysis and Exerts a Protective Effect on Sensory Hair Cells Against Noise-Induced Damage. *Front. Mol. Biosci.* **2021**, *8*, 806650. [CrossRef] [PubMed]
13. Aragones, J.; Schneider, M.; Van Geyte, K.; Fraisl, P.; Dresselaers, T.; Mazzone, M.; Dirkx, R.; Zacchigna, S.; Lemieux, H.; Jeoung, N.H.; et al. Deficiency or inhibition of oxygen sensor Phd1 induces hypoxia tolerance by reprogramming basal metabolism. *Nat. Genet.* **2008**, *40*, 170–180. [CrossRef] [PubMed]
14. Scharping, N.E.; Rivadeneira, D.B.; Menk, A.V.; Vignali, P.D.A.; Ford, B.R.; Rittenhouse, N.L.; Peralta, R.; Wang, Y.; Wang, Y.; DePeaux, K.; et al. Mitochondrial stress induced by continuous stimulation under hypoxia rapidly drives T cell exhaustion. *Nat. Immunol.* **2021**, *22*, 205–215. [CrossRef]
15. Vercellino, I.; Sazanov, L.A. The assembly, regulation and function of the mitochondrial respiratory chain. *Nat. Rev. Mol. Cell Biol.* **2022**, *23*, 141–161. [CrossRef] [PubMed]
16. Kadenbach, B. Complex IV—The regulatory center of mitochondrial oxidative phosphorylation. *Mitochondrion* **2021**, *58*, 296–302. [CrossRef]
17. Dutta, S.; Sengupta, P. Men and mice: Relating their ages. *Life Sci.* **2016**, *152*, 244–248. [CrossRef]
18. Abrous, D.N.; Koehl, M.; Lemoine, M. A Baldwin interpretation of adult hippocampal neurogenesis: From functional relevance to physiopathology. *Mol. Psychiatry* **2022**, *27*, 383–402. [CrossRef]
19. Szklarczyk, D.; Gable, A.L.; Lyon, D.; Junge, A.; Wyder, S.; Huerta-Cepas, J.; Simonovic, M.; Doncheva, N.T.; Morris, J.H.; Bork, P.; et al. STRING v11: Protein-protein association networks with increased coverage, supporting functional discovery in genome-wide experimental datasets. *Nucleic Acids Res.* **2019**, *47*, D607–D613. [CrossRef]
20. Zong, S.; Wu, M.; Gu, J.; Liu, T.; Guo, R.; Yang, M. Structure of the intact 14-subunit human cytochrome c oxidase. *Cell Res.* **2018**, *28*, 1026–1034. [CrossRef]

21. Jain, I.H.; Zazzeron, L.; Goli, R.; Alexa, K.; Schatzman-Bone, S.; Dhillon, H.; Goldberger, O.; Peng, J.; Shalem, O.; Sanjana, N.E.; et al. Hypoxia as a therapy for mitochondrial disease. *Science* **2016**, *352*, 54–61. [CrossRef] [PubMed]
22. Tello, D.; Balsa, E.; Acosta-Iborra, B.; Fuertes-Yebra, E.; Elorza, A.; Ordonez, A.; Corral-Escariz, M.; Soro, I.; Lopez-Bernardo, E.; Perales-Clemente, E.; et al. Induction of the mitochondrial NDUFA4L2 protein by HIF-1alpha decreases oxygen consumption by inhibiting Complex I activity. *Cell Metab.* **2011**, *14*, 768–779. [CrossRef] [PubMed]
23. Kaelin, W.G., Jr.; Ratcliffe, P.J. Oxygen sensing by metazoans: The central role of the HIF hydroxylase pathway. *Mol. Cell* **2008**, *30*, 393–402. [CrossRef] [PubMed]
24. Kim, J.W.; Tchernyshyov, I.; Semenza, G.L.; Dang, C.V. HIF-1-mediated expression of pyruvate dehydrogenase kinase: A metabolic switch required for cellular adaptation to hypoxia. *Cell Metab.* **2006**, *3*, 177–185. [CrossRef]
25. Fukuda, R.; Zhang, H.; Kim, J.W.; Shimoda, L.; Dang, C.V.; Semenza, G.L. HIF-1 regulates cytochrome oxidase subunits to optimize efficiency of respiration in hypoxic cells. *Cell* **2007**, *129*, 111–122. [CrossRef]
26. Hayashi, T.; Asano, Y.; Shintani, Y.; Aoyama, H.; Kioka, H.; Tsukamoto, O.; Hikita, M.; Shinzawa-Itoh, K.; Takafuji, K.; Higo, S.; et al. Higd1a is a positive regulator of cytochrome c oxidase. *Proc. Natl. Acad. Sci. USA* **2015**, *112*, 1553–1558. [CrossRef]
27. Ramzan, R.; Vogt, S.; Kadenbach, B. Stress-mediated generation of deleterious ROS in healthy individuals—Role of cytochrome c oxidase. *J. Mol. Med.* **2020**, *98*, 651–657. [CrossRef]
28. Lai, R.K.; Xu, I.M.; Chiu, D.K.; Tse, A.P.; Wei, L.L.; Law, C.T.; Lee, D.; Wong, C.M.; Wong, M.P.; Ng, I.O.; et al. NDUFA4L2 Fine-tunes Oxidative Stress in Hepatocellular Carcinoma. *Clin. Cancer Res.* **2016**, *22*, 3105–3117. [CrossRef]
29. Spinelli, J.B.; Rosen, P.C.; Sprenger, H.G.; Puszynska, A.M.; Mann, J.L.; Roessler, J.M.; Cangelosi, A.L.; Henne, A.; Condon, K.J.; Zhang, T.; et al. Fumarate is a terminal electron acceptor in the mammalian electron transport chain. *Science* **2021**, *374*, 1227–1237. [CrossRef]
30. Yoshikawa, S.; Shimada, A. Reaction mechanism of cytochrome c oxidase. *Chem. Rev.* **2015**, *115*, 1936–1989. [CrossRef]
31. Ramzan, R.; Dolga, A.M.; Michels, S.; Weber, P.; Culmsee, C.; Rastan, A.J.; Vogt, S. Cytochrome c Oxidase Inhibition by ATP Decreases Mitochondrial ROS Production. *Cells* **2022**, *11*, 992. [CrossRef] [PubMed]
32. Pitceathly, R.D.S.; Taanman, J.W. NDUFA4 (Renamed COXFA4) Is a Cytochrome-c Oxidase Subunit. *Trends Endocrinol. Metab.* **2018**, *29*, 452–454. [CrossRef] [PubMed]
33. Clayton, S.A.; Daley, K.K.; MacDonald, L.; Fernandez-Vizarra, E.; Bottegoni, G.; O'Neil, J.D.; Major, T.; Griffin, D.; Zhuang, Q.; Adewoye, A.B.; et al. Inflammation causes remodeling of mitochondrial cytochrome c oxidase mediated by the bifunctional gene C15orf48. *Sci. Adv.* **2021**, *7*, eabl5182. [CrossRef] [PubMed]
34. Lv, Y.; Nie, S.L.; Zhou, J.M.; Liu, F.; Hu, Y.B.; Jiang, J.R.; Li, N.; Liu, J.S. Overexpression of NDUFA4L2 is associated with poor prognosis in patients with colorectal cancer. *ANZ J. Surg.* **2017**, *87*, E251–E255. [CrossRef]
35. Meng, L.; Yang, X.; Xie, X.; Wang, M. Mitochondrial NDUFA4L2 protein promotes the vitality of lung cancer cells by repressing oxidative stress. *Thorac. Cancer* **2019**, *10*, 676–685. [CrossRef] [PubMed]
36. Burberry, A.; Wells, M.F.; Limone, F.; Couto, A.; Smith, K.S.; Keaney, J.; Gillet, G.; van Gastel, N.; Wang, J.Y.; Pietilainen, O.; et al. C9orf72 suppresses systemic and neural inflammation induced by gut bacteria. *Nature* **2020**, *582*, 89–94. [CrossRef] [PubMed]
37. Hedayati Moghadam, M.; Rezaee, S.A.R.; Hosseini, M.; Niazmand, S.; Salmani, H.; Rafatpanah, H.; Asarzadegan Dezfuli, M.; Amel Zabihi, N.; Abareshi, A.; Mahmoudabady, M. HTLV-1 infection-induced motor dysfunction, memory impairment, depression, and brain tissues oxidative damage in female BALB/c mice. *Life Sci.* **2018**, *212*, 9–19. [CrossRef] [PubMed]

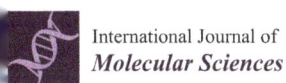

Article

Oxidative Stress Response Kinetics after 60 Minutes at Different (1.4 ATA and 2.5 ATA) Hyperbaric Hyperoxia Exposures

Clément Leveque [1,2], Simona Mrakic Sposta [3], Sigrid Theunissen [1,*], Peter Germonpré [4,5], Kate Lambrechts [1], Alessandra Vezzoli [3], Gerardo Bosco [6], Morgan Lévénez [1], Pierre Lafère [1,4], François Guerrero [2] and Costantino Balestra [1,4,7,8,*]

1. Environmental, Occupational, Aging (Integrative) Physiology Laboratory, Haute Ecole Bruxelles-Brabant (HE2B), 1160 Brussels, Belgium; cleveque@he2b.be (C.L.); klambrechts@he2b.be (K.L.); morganlevenez@gmail.com (M.L.); plafere@he2b.be (P.L.)
2. Laboratoire ORPHY, Université de Bretagne Occidentale, UFR Sciences et Techniques, 6 Avenue Le Gorgeu, 93837 Brest, France; francois.guerrero@univ-brest.fr
3. Institute of Clinical Physiology, National Research Council (CNR), 20162 Milan, Italy; simona.mrakicsposta@cnr.it (S.M.S.); alessandra.vezzoli@cnr.it (A.V.)
4. DAN Europe Research Division (Roseto-Brussels), 1160 Brussels, Belgium; pgermonpre@gmail.com
5. Hyperbaric Centre, Queen Astrid Military Hospital, 1120 Brussels, Belgium
6. Environmental Physiology & Medicine Lab, Department of Biomedical Sciences, University of Padova, 35131 Padova, Italy; gerardo.bosco@unipd.it
7. Anatomical Research and Clinical Studies, Vrije Universiteit Brussels (VUB), 1090 Brussels, Belgium
8. Physical Activity Teaching Unit, Motor Sciences Department, Université Libre de Bruxelles (ULB), 1050 Brussels, Belgium
* Correspondence: sigtheunissen@he2b.be (S.T.); costantino.balestra@ulb.be (C.B.)

Abstract: Hyperbaric oxygen therapy (HBOT) is a therapeutical approach based on exposure to pure oxygen in an augmented atmospheric pressure. Although it has been used for years, the exact kinetics of the reactive oxygen species (ROS) between different pressures of hyperbaric oxygen exposure are still not clearly evidenced. In this study, the metabolic responses of hyperbaric hyperoxia exposures for 1 h at 1.4 and 2.5 ATA were investigated. Fourteen healthy non-smoking subjects (2 females and 12 males, age: 37.3 ± 12.7 years old (mean ± SD), height: 176.3 ± 9.9 cm, and weight: 75.8 ± 17.7 kg) volunteered for this study. Blood samples were taken before and at 30 min, 2 h, 24 h, and 48 h after a 1 h hyperbaric hyperoxic exposure. The level of oxidation was evaluated by the rate of ROS production, nitric oxide metabolites (NOx), and the levels of isoprostane. Antioxidant reactions were assessed through measuring superoxide dismutase (SOD), catalase (CAT), cysteinylglycine, and glutathione (GSH). The inflammatory response was measured using interleukin-6, neopterin, and creatinine. A short (60 min) period of mild (1.4 ATA) and high (2.5 ATA) hyperbaric hyperoxia leads to a similar significant increase in the production of ROS and antioxidant reactions. Immunomodulation and inflammatory responses, on the contrary, respond proportionally to the hyperbaric oxygen dose. Further research is warranted on the dose and the inter-dose recovery time to optimize the potential therapeutic benefits of this promising intervention.

Keywords: oxygen biology; cellular reactions; human; oxygen therapy; human performance; hyperbaric oxygen therapy; oxygen dose

1. Introduction

Hyperbaric oxygen therapy (HBOT) is a therapeutical approach based on breathing pure oxygen (O_2) in an augmented atmospheric pressure. According to the Undersea and Hyperbaric Medical Society (UHMS), this pressure may equal or exceed 1.4 atmospheres (ATA). However, all current UHMS-approved indications require that patients breathe near 100% oxygen while enclosed in a chamber pressurized to a minimum of 2 ATA (https://www.uhms.org/resources/hbo-indications.html) (accessed on 30 June 2023).

Depending on the protocol, the duration of a single session varies from 1 to 1.5 h (without considering the time needed to reach the intended pressure, which may take up to 15 min for pressurization and 15 min for depressurization), the repetition of exposures varies from one to three times daily, with 20 to 60 therapeutical doses to be administered depending on the condition [1]. Frequently, this method utilizes pressures between 2 to 3 ATA. Nevertheless, promising results have also been obtained for certain conditions with pressures less than 2 ATA (1.5 ATA) [2,3], and in some studies, even 'hyperbaric air' seems to be of interest [4]. While some protocols accept the use of 6 ATA (e.g., for the treatment of gas embolism), little benefit is usually reported from pressures above 3 ATA as this may be associated with a plethora of adverse effects [5].

Although it has been used for years, the exact kinetics of the reactive oxygen species between different levels of hyperbaric oxygen exposure are still not clearly evidenced and, without much scientific evidence, it is common practice to apply HBOT sessions every 24 h [6]. The need for several sessions to reach a relevant effect is likewise commonly accepted; however, the optimal hyperbaric oxygen levels and the time needed between each session to optimize cellular responses—such as Hypoxia inducible factor (HIF-1α) or nuclear factor kappa β (NF-Kβ), erythroid related factor 2 (NRF2), cellular vesicles and microparticles, Caspase 3 [7–10]—are still debated and stand solely on observational clinical outcomes. Some recent experimental works have been evaluating the effects of different levels of oxygen on oxidative stress under hypoxic [11–14], normobaric hyperoxic [15–17], and hyperbaric hyperoxic [4,6–8] conditions. The encouraging, but also challenging, results lead even to question if some oxygen levels formerly considered as 'HBOT sham' [18] may be of therapeutic interest [4,7].

The purpose of this study was to investigate oxidative, inflammatory, and enzymatic reactions following exposures for 60 min at two different (mild or high) levels of hyperbaric oxygen, 1.4 ATA and 2.5 ATA.

The lower level (1.4 ATA) was chosen because it approaches the level of hyperoxia that may be reached during some underwater diving exposures but also because the therapeutical use of such lower oxygen pressures is being debated. The higher level of hyperbaric hyperoxia is the common average therapeutical exposure.

2. Results

2.1. ROS, NOx, and 8-Isoprostane (8-Iso-PGF2α) Levels after One Hour of Oxygen Exposure at 1.4 and 2.5 ATA

Both oxygen exposures, mild (1.4 ATA) and high (2.5 ATA), elicited a significant increase of plasmatic ROS production rate with a similar kinetic of rise and decrease. Both oxygen exposures induced a significant increase in ROS production with a peak after 2 h (0.408 ± 0.06 µmol·min^{-1} at 1.4 ATA compared to the baseline, $p < 0.001$; and 0.406 ± 0.06 µmol·min^{-1} at 2.5 ATA, $p < 0.01$). Two-way ANOVA (time post exposure x oxygen level) shows a non-significant difference between the two groups (F (4, 52) = 0.86; $p = 0.490$) (Figure 1A). This peak plateaus for about 2 h, and then the quantity of ROS decreases slowly until 48 h without returning to control levels.

Nitric oxide metabolites (Figure 1B) show changes characterized by a significant decrease; they are the lowest after 2 h for both 1.4 ATA (175.4 ± 45.62 µM, $p < 0.01$) and 2.5 ATA (235.1 ± 121 µM, $p < 0.001$). We observed a reactive increase of nitric oxide metabolites 24 h after 2.5 ATA exposure (496.9 ± 249 µM, $p < 0.001$). Two-way ANOVA (time post exposure x oxygen level) shows a non-significant difference between the two groups (F (4, 52) = 0.855; $p = 0.497$).

For 8-isoprostane (pg/mg creatinine) (Figure 1C), a faster increase after the 2.5 ATA exposure is present compared to the 1.4 ATA exposure. These changes reach a peak plateau 2 h after 2.5 ATA (541 ± 2 02 pg·mg^{-1} creatinine, $p < 0.01$) and around 24 h after 1.4 ATA (560.2 ± 2 09 pg·mg^{-1} creatinine, $p < 0.001$). Two-way ANOVA (time post exposure x oxygen level) shows a non-significant difference between the two groups (F (4, 52) = 0.905; $p = 0.468$).

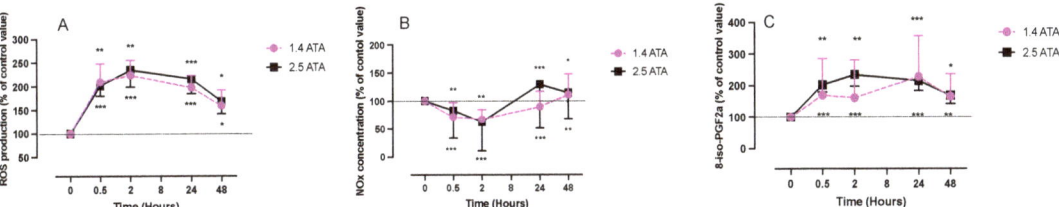

Figure 1. Evolution of ROS (plasma) production rate (**A**), NOx (urine) (**B**), and 8-iso-PGF2a (urine) (**C**) after 60 min of mild (1.4 ATA, n = 6) or high hyperbaric exposure (2.5 ATA, n = 8). Results are expressed as mean ± SD as a percentage of the control value. T0 represents pre-exposure baseline (ROS: 0.18 ± 0.016 µmol·min^{-1}) (Nox: 265.7 ± 43.76 µM) (8-iso-PGF2a: 286 ± 124). Intra-group comparisons between results at T0 and each other time point are represented above and below the respective curves. Inter-group comparisons between 1.4 and 2.5 ATA exposure when significant are shown between the 2 curves (*: $p < 0.05$, **: $p < 0.01$, ***: $p < 0.001$).

Unexpectedly, SOD concentration did not show any change during the 48 h following expositions (Figure 2A). Two-way ANOVA (time post exposure x oxygen level) shows a non-significant difference between the two groups (F (4, 56) = 0.0266; $p = 0.999$), contrary to the CAT levels that increase rapidly after both exposures (1.4 ATA after 30 min: 32.92 ± 11.04 µg/µml, $p < 0.05$; 2.5 ATA after 2 h: 32.62 ± 5.97, $p < 0.01$), whereas two-way ANOVA (time post exposure x oxygen level) shows again a non-significant difference between the two groups (F (4, 52) = 2.47; $p = 0.056$) (Figure 2B). This increase remained constant during the 48 h following both exposures.

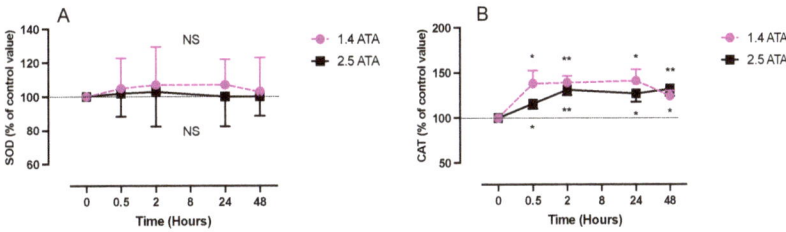

Figure 2. Evolution of SOD (plasma) (**A**) and CAT (**B**), after 60 min of mild (1.4 ATA, n = 6) or high hyperbaric exposure (2.5 ATA, n = 8). Results are expressed as mean ± SD as a percentage of the control value. T0 represents pre-exposure baseline (SOD: 3 ± 1.9 U/mL) (CAT: 24 ± 5.3 U/mL). Intra-group comparisons between results at T0 and each other time point are represented above and below the respective curves. Inter-group comparisons between 1.4 and 2.5 ATA exposure when significant are shown between the 2 curves (ns: not significant; *: $p < 0.05$, **: $p < 0.01$).

2.2. Inflammatory Response (IL-6, Neopterin and Creatinine) after One Hour of Oxygen Exposure at 1.4 and 2.5 ATA

Interleukin 6 (IL-6) was measured in plasma samples while neopterin and creatinine were obtained from urine (Figure 3A).

IL-6 shows a significant increase compared to the baseline, presenting its peak at 2 h for the 1.4 ATA group (3.82 ± 0.92 pg/mL; $p < 0.05$) as well as for the 2.5 ATA group (3.36 ± 2.31 pg/mL; $p < 0.01$). Two-way ANOVA (time post exposure x oxygen level) shows a non-significant difference between the two groups at any time (F (4, 48) = 0.390; $p = 0.815$).

Although neopterin rose in both groups, this increase was significantly more pronounced after the 2.5 ATA exposure with a peak at 2 h (83.58 ± 20 µmol/mol creatinine;

$p < 0.01$). This is confirmed by the two-way ANOVA (time exposure x oxygen level) of $F (4, 56) = 5.32; p = 0.001$. The plateau was also reached after 2 h in the 1.4 ATA group (57.28 ± 20.8 μmol/mol creatinine; $p < 0.01$). In both groups, values returned to normal after 48 h (Figure 3B).

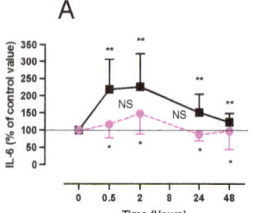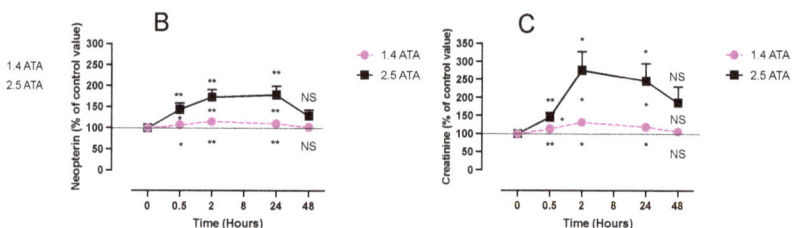

Figure 3. Evolution of the inflammatory response (urine) (IL-6 in (**A**), neopterin in (**B**), and creatinine in (**C**)) after 60 min of mild (1.4 ATA, n = 6) or high hyperbaric exposure (2.5 ATA, n = 8). Results are expressed as mean ± SD as a percentage of the control value. T0 represents pre-exposure baseline (IL-6: 2.818 ± 1.028 pg·mL^{-1}; neopterin: 49.62 ± 17.79 mol·mol^{-1}; creatinine: 1.1 ± 0.68 g·L^{-1}). Intra-group comparisons between results at T0 and each other time point are represented above and below the respective curves. Inter-group comparisons between 1.4 and 2.5 ATA exposure when significant are shown between the 2 curves (ns: not significant; *: $p < 0.05$, **: $p < 0.01$).

Similar to neopterin, creatinine (Figure 3C) increased in both groups with a significantly remarkable effect after the 2.5 ATA exposure (2 h post 1.4 ATA: 1.31 ± 0.66 g/L; $p < 0.01$ vs. 2 h at 2.5 ATA: 2.52 ± 0.67 g/L; $p < 0.01$), with a return to the baseline after 48 h. Two-way ANOVA (time post exposure x oxygen level) shows $F (4, 56) = 3.43; p = 0.014$.

Cysteinylglycine levels increased rapidly 2 h after 1.4 ATA exposure (11 ± 3.5 μmol·L^{-1}, $p < 0.05$) and 2.5 ATA (8.1 ± 3.8 μmol·L^{-1}, $p < 0.001$). Values returned to the baseline after 24 h in the 1.4 ATA group and later and after 48 h in the 2.5 ATA group (Figure 4A). We did not observe significant changes in both groups with two-way ANOVA (time post exposure x oxygen level): $F (4, 48) = 0.498; p = 0.737$.

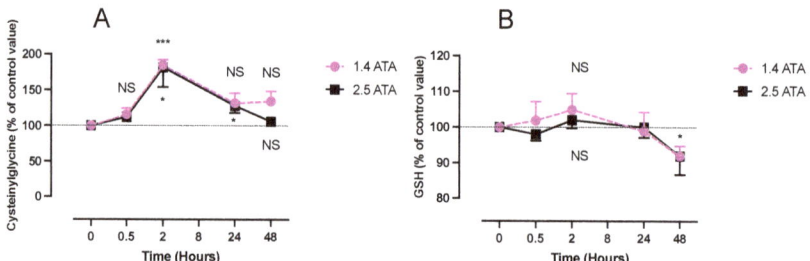

Figure 4. Evolution of cysteinylglycine (plasma) and glutathione (RBC) (GSH) after 60 min of mild (1.4 ATA, n = 6) or high hyperbaric hyperoxia (2.5 ATA, n = 8). Cysteinylglycine (**A**) and glutathione (GSH) (**B**). Results are expressed as mean ± SD. T0 represents baseline pre-exposure values (cysteinylglycine: 38.19 ± 5.715 μmol.L^{-1}; GSH: 894.7 ± 176.4 μM). Intra-group comparisons between results at T0 and each other time point are represented above and below the respective curves. Inter-group comparisons between 1.4 ATA and 2.5 ATA of oxygen exposure when significant are shown between the 2 curves (ns: not significant; *: $p < 0.05$, ***: $p < 0.001$).

We did not observe any significant changes of glutathione concentrations (GSH), except for a slight decrease 48 h after a 2.5 ATA exposure (918.5 ± 171 μmol·L^{-1}, $p < 0.05$), and this is confirmed by two-way ANOVA (time post exposure x oxygen level): $F (4, 48) = 0.268; p = 0.897$ (Figure 4B).

3. Discussion

Our study is, to the best of our knowledge, the first to compare the kinetics of a one-hour exposure to mild (1.4 ATA) and high (2.5 ATA) hyperbaric oxygen dose in healthy subjects.

Based on very recent data, we were motivated to explore a new perspective, which involves viewing oxygen not merely as a conventional drug but rather as a powerful trigger for complex molecular reactions [19]. Fundamentally, this process operates through the concepts of 'dose-response' and 'dose-time', inducing various effects such as oxidative stress, metabolic alterations, and inflammation [20], a phenomenon widely recognized in pathological conditions [21].

Just a decade ago, reactive oxygen species (ROS) were primarily believed to induce harmful effects and were only linked to various pathological conditions [22]. Over time, this perspective shifted, and it was recognized that the presence of reactive oxygen species (ROS) in cells suggests that their production may trigger specific beneficial effects [23]. Our results seem to confirm the reality of such effects at these levels of oxygen breathing.

Firstly, we observed a similar kinetic of plasma reactive oxygen species (ROS) at 1.4 ATA (140 kPa) and 2.5 ATA (250 kPa). The peak production is reached at around 2 h and remains above the baseline level for 48 h. This similar evolution of ROS between the two exposures is an intriguing observation, which suggests that despite the very different oxygen dose, comparable rates of ROS production occur (this is statistically confirmed by two-way ANOVA). Our results apparently contradict a recent study that assessed the effect of HBOT on oxidative markers and immune response [6]. Indeed, in this study, no significant modification of plasma ROS was found following a single HBOT session of 75 min of breathing 100% oxygen through a tight-fitting facemask at a pressure of 240 kPa (2.4 ATA) with two 5 min 'air-breaks' (breathing normal air) and a 10 min pressure reduction. Our protocol involved a 60 min exposure at 1.4 ATA and 2.5 ATA with 100% oxygen without any 'air-breaks'. Although slightly different, our protocol demonstrates a significant increase of ROS production already 30 min after the end of the exposure. While it may be possible that the 'air-breaks' that were performed (twice for 5 min) were sufficient to drastically reduce oxidative stress, our results are not able to confirm this hypothesis. More research with a different experimental setup would be needed to assess this difference [24].

Secondly, we observed an increase in creatinine levels; these may be due probably to the vasoconstriction of renal afferent arterioles caused by reactive oxygen species (ROS); this constriction is more pronounced (significant two-way ANOVA) for the higher oxygen exposure (2.5 ATA). The peak of the creatinine increase occurs when nitric oxide metabolite (NOx) levels are at their lowest (in both exposures). This suggests the following mechanism: during hyperoxic exposure, the induced vasoconstriction reduces renal or other organs' in-flow of blood. This decrease in blood in-flow reduces shear stress and, consequently, the production of nitric oxide (NO). Concomitantly, the bioavailability of NO is reduced by the presence of ROS that exert a scavenging action, given the fact that there are no enzymatic mechanisms for NO inactivation, while its biological life after synthesis in vessels depends on reactions with hemoglobin in the blood, tissue thiols, molecular oxygen, and the superoxide anion. In conditions of extreme hyperoxia, when there is a sharp increase in the production of superoxide anions, existing NO can be neutralized by $O_2^{\bullet-}$, leading to decreases in its tissue condition, a weakening of its basal vasorelaxing action, and thus to the development of vasoconstriction. Verification of this hypothesis was addressed some years ago by the Demchenko team by analyzing changes in brain blood flow in response to alterations in the balance between NO and $O_2^{\bullet-}$ in the brain using hyperbaric oxygenation, an intravenous administration of superoxide dismutase, and an inhibition of NO synthase. The vasodilatory effect of superoxide dismutase in hyperbaric oxygenation was not seen in animals given prior doses of the NO synthase inhibitor [25]. These results provide evidence that one mechanism for hyperoxic vasoconstriction in the brain consists of the inactivation of NO by superoxide anions, decreasing its basal vasorelaxing action.

In fact, during the hyperbaric sessions, without physical activity, only vasoconstriction is present, shear stress is reduced, and a laminar flow is favored.

Under fully developed laminar flow conditions, much of the released NO/nitrite remains concentrated in near-wall fluid laminae, in which nitrite levels can accumulate to vasoactive concentrations in downstream resistance vessels. This local synthesis and delivery minimizes the washout (wasting) of endogenous NO [26]. The resulting vasodilation lowers regional vascular resistance and, in turn, increases regional blood flow as well as wall shear stress in the parent branches, which finally creates a positive feedback effect that causes further local arterial NO release [27]. A certain quantity of NO would thus be 'non-circulating' during the HBOT session, explaining the NOx reduction measured directly after hyperbaric oxygen exposure.

We may then hypothesize that after the hyperbaric session, the locally present NO will be released in circulation because of the normal 'everyday-life' physical activity, and this could explain its rebound increase after 24 h, persisting up to 48 h. Our results confirm a previous study that did not find a systemic increase in NO during hyperbaric oxygen exposures [28].

The increase in reactive oxygen species (ROS) stimulates catalase (CAT) to initiate the breakdown of H_2O_2 into H_2O and O_2 [26]. In contrast to normobaric hyperoxia [17], our study highlights an increase in CAT production in response to oxidative stress. It is worth noting that CAT exhibits one of the highest turnover rates among known enzymes, with approximately 40,000,000 molecules per second [29,30]. Unlike other peroxidases, CAT does not generate free radicals. Paradoxically, oxidative stress induced by hypoxia appears to be more difficult to cope with than hyperoxia-induced oxidative stress [12].

Generally, as a response, an increased rate of radical production leads to an increment in the levels of antioxidant enzymes; in fact, CAT showed an increased activity very fast after the 1 h HBO exposure. SOD activity apparently remained unchanged at the end of the HBO session and for the next 48 h (no difference for the two-way ANOVA for time post exposure X oxygen level). Interestingly, at the time of the 15th treatment, a significant decrement in SOD and CAT activities (−20% each) was observed compared to the 1st HBO exposure [31]. Other authors found different results showing no variation even after the 20th hyperbaric session [32]. We do not have a definite explanation for this apparent contradiction, but it has been proposed that most likely, the species involved in SOD and CAT inactivation is singlet oxygen and that following several hyperbaric sessions, the protective reactions against this reactive species may vary.

This stress response includes the transcriptional activation of various genes encoding antioxidant and detoxification enzymes as an attempt to dampen the deleterious effects of increased ROS production. Neutrophils could release antioxidant enzymes and particularly CAT into the extracellular space in order to increase the antioxidant effect surrounding the neutrophil. This secretion could be important to avoid oxidative damage in tissues induced by neutrophil ROS generation. Previous studies showed that CAT is colocalized to the specific granules with peroxisomal and lysosomal proteins such as MPO, hydrolases, and peroxidases [33]. Sureda and coworkers [34] observed that the presence of CAT in these granules, in addition to the detected increase in extracellular CAT activity after neutrophil activation, agrees with the possible existence of antioxidant enzymes released from neutrophils.

This can explain the increase of plasmatic CAT, and this is further confirmed by other results showing an activation of the immune system with the significant increase of neopterin and creatinine. It is worth underlining that the two-way ANOVA calculations for the oxygen pressure exposure show a difference in both parameters. This seems to show that oxygen levels have a selective effect on the immune response, which could have been further confirmed if the CAT difference was significant for both exposures; but the two-way ANOVA did not quite reach a level of significance ($p = 0.056$).

If we consider other antioxidant actors, glutathione (GSH) evolution is somehow complex. Following one of its metabolites, cysteinylglycine (CYSGLY), we see a significant increase 2 h after exposure for both oxygen levels (though it is non-significant for oxygen pressure and time post exposure, according to the two-way ANOVA test). This increase is not paralleled by a GSH decrease. We understand this situation as a growing activity of GSH until 2 h post-oxygen. After this peak, a reduction of its metabolite (CYSGLY) is present until 48 h, where basal levels are again reached (both exposures). This decrease of GSH (48 h after exposure) can be interpreted either as a reduction of its production or as an inability of the GSH production to keep up with the ROS still present.

This latter explanation may be the reason behind the mitochondrial dysfunction present (at least) during the first hyperbaric exposures [35]. Indeed, animal studies show a reduction of the mitochondrial membrane rest potential during the first one to five treatments which stimulates the mitochondrial apoptotic pathway and stimulates reactive biogenesis during the following treatments [28,36].

Contrary to our previous results on normobaric hyperoxia, we observed a direct increase in IL-6, suggesting a stimulation of the NFR2/NF-Kβ pathway [37,38]. Additionally, we observe a simultaneous increase in neopterin production, indicating an immunomodulatory role of hyperbaric hyperoxia [39]. Neopterin is generated in response to a γ-interferon-mediated activation of monocytes and macrophages and thus is a direct product of immune system activation [40,41]. Neopterin has been shown to elicit a cytoprotective action of cerebral tissue [42]. This provides an additional argument regarding the effects of hyperbaric hyperoxia exposure on cognitive improvements [43], and remarkably, both exposure levels show a significant increase but with a higher effect for 2.5 ATA.

This fact seems to show a dose–response effect that will encourage further research on the targeted use of oxygen exposures since, for instance, in lower hyperoxia levels (30% and 100% of FiO_2), no such increase is observed [17], but it is present during moderate hypoxia (15% of FiO_2) [12]. One other factor to consider is that cellular responses to oxygen are not necessarily directly proportional to the inspired level of oxygen, as there is not a linear relationship between alveolar oxygen pressures and the quantity of molecular oxygen at the cellular (and mitochondrial) level [19]. Factors such as pulmonary gas transfer efficiency, arterial wall thickness and endothelial 'health', and capillary-to-cell distance (as with an increased extravascular fluid compartment, e.g., local oedema or lower capillary density in sclerotic tissue) will all play a role in determining how the inspired oxygen pressure 'translates' to an increased or decreased cellular presence of molecular oxygen. Even though the observed effects may not directly be extrapolated to non-healthy patients, our observations in young healthy volunteers offer a clue to the dynamic and kinetics of oxygen-mediated cellular reactions. They show that depending on the oxygen level breathed, some effects are similar while others are markedly different; each observed effect clearly has its own 'dose-dependent' kinetic.

Limitations

    Strengths:
- This study is, to our knowledge, one of the first to investigate the kinetics of responses to a single short hyperbaric oxygen exposure at 1.4 ATA and 2.5 ATA.
- The measurements were conducted until 48 h post-exposure and putatively open the avenue to new possible applications for hyperbaric oxygen breathing protocols.

    Weaknesses:
- The subject numbers are limited, but the sample can be considered as homogenous since all were healthy participants.
- The analysis was not made in the nucleus of the cells but in the plasma, red blood cells, or urine; this could be considered a weakness for some, but it would need a thoroughly different experimental setting.

4. Materials and Methods

4.1. Experimental Protocol

After written informed consent, 48 healthy non-smoking Caucasian subjects (32 males and 16 females) volunteered for this study. None of them had a history of previous cardiac abnormalities or were under any cardio or vaso-active medication.

All experimental procedures were conducted in accordance with the Declaration of Helsinki [44] and approved by the Ethics Committee approval from the Bio-Ethical Committee for Research and Higher Education, Brussels (N° B200-2020-088).

After medical screening to exclude any latent morbidity, participants were prospectively randomized into 6 groups of 6–8 persons each. These groups were divided into hypoxia (10% and 15% of FiO_2) [12], normobaric hyperoxia (30% and 100% of FiO_2) [7], and hyperbaric hyperoxia (1.4 ATA and 2.5 ATA). All participants were asked to refrain from strenuous exercise for 48 h before the tests. No antioxidant nutrients, i.e., dark chocolate, red wine, or green tea were permitted in the 8 h preceding and during the study. The subjects were also asked not to dive 48 h before the experiment and not to fly within 72 h before the experiment.

Fourteen participants completed the mild hyperbaric hyperoxia (1.4 ATA, n = 6) and high hyperbaric hyperoxia (2.5 ATA, n = 8) protocols. Age (1.4 ATA: 36.0 ± 12.3 years old (mean ± SD) vs. 2.5 ATA: 38.3 ± 13.6 years old; p = 0.75), height (1.4 ATA: 174.2 ± 13.4 cm vs. 2.5 ATA: 177.9 ± 6.9 cm; p = 0.51), and weight (1.4 ATA: 67.7 ± 13.0 kg vs. 2.5 ATA: 81.8 ± 19.0 kg; p = 0.14) were collected.

Hyperbaric oxygen (oxygen partial pressure: 1.4 ATA; 1400 hPa, n = 6, and 2.5 bar; 2500 hPa, n = 8) was administered for 1 h in a hyperbaric multiplace chamber (Haux-Starmed 2800, Haux-Life-Support GmbH, Karlsbad-Ittersbach, Germany) of the Military Hospital Brussels, Belgium, by means of a tight-fitting orofacial mask connected to the Haux-Oxymaster demand-valve system. A 60 min time was chosen to reduce the risk of oxygen toxicity.

Blood and urine samples were obtained before exposure (T0) and 30 min, 2 h, 24 h, and 48 h after the end of oxygen administration. The originally planned and accepted protocol included blood sampling 8 h after exposure (see experimental flowchart—Figure 5); for technical reasons, this could not be achieved, but to be consistent with our previous works and also to better depict the sampling duration, we kept this time point in the graphs' X-axis. Previous experiments have shown that cellular responses after different oxidative exposures may continue for 24 h and even more; we therefore decided to take blood samples up to 48 h [8,10,13,45].

Each blood sample consisted of approximately 15 mL of venous human blood collected in lithium heparin and EDTA tubes (Vacutainer, BD Diagnostic, Becton Dickinson, Italia S.p.A., Milan, Italy). Plasma and red blood cells (RBCs) were separated by centrifugation (Eppendorf Centrifuge 5702R, Darmstadt, Germany) at $1000\times g$ at 4 °C for 10 min. The samples of blood cells and plasma were then stored in multiple aliquots at −80 °C until assayed and thawed; an analysis was performed within one month from collection. Urine was collected by voluntary voiding in a sterile container and stored in multiple aliquots at −20 °C until assayed and thawed only before analysis.

4.2. Blood Sample Analysis

4.2.1. Determination of ROS by Electron Paramagnetic Resonance (EPR)

An electron paramagnetic resonance instrument (E-Scan—Bruker BioSpin, GmbH, Rheinstetten, Germany) X-band, with a controller temperature at 37 °C interfaced to the spectrometer, was adopted for the ROS production rate, as already performed by some of the authors herein [46–49]. The EPR measurements are highly reproducible, as previously demonstrated [50]. EPR is the only non-invasive technique suitable for a direct and quantitative measure of ROS. In particular, the spectroscopic technique (EPRS) finds many fields of application, among which is bio-medicine [51]. The reliability and reproducibility of EPR data obtained by the herein adopted micro-invasive EPR method has been already reported previously [52].

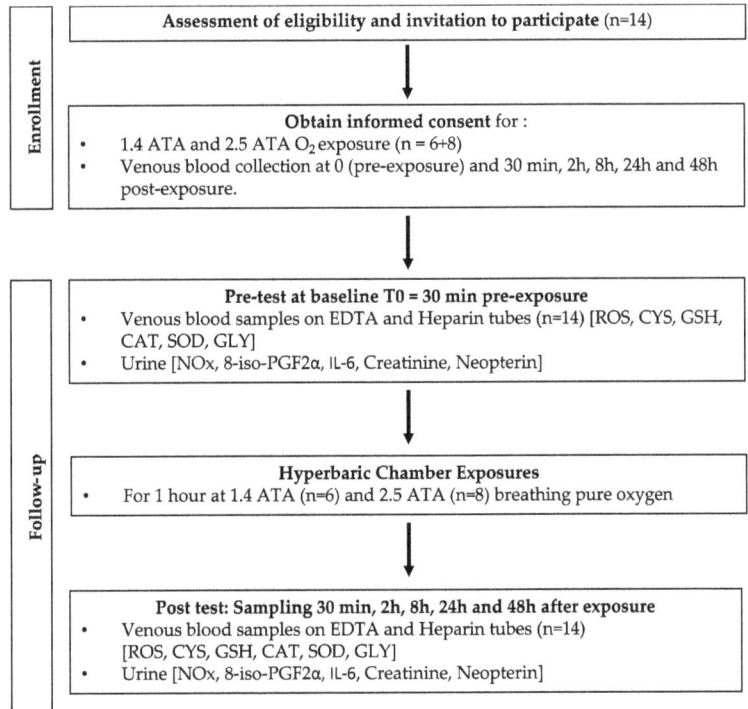

Figure 5. Experimental flowchart.

Briefly, for ROS detection, 50 µL of plasma were treated with an equal volume of CMH (1-hydroxy-3-methoxycarbonyl-2,2,5,5-tetramethylpyrrolidine), and then 1 mM of the CMH solution was prepared in a buffer (Krebs-Hepes buffer (KHB)) containing a 25 µM deferroxamine methane-sulfonate salt (DF) chelating agent and 5 µM sodium diethyldithio-carbamate trihydrate (DETC)) at pH 7.4. The plasma was incubated with CMH (1:1) for 60 s; 50 µL of this solution were placed inside a glass EPR capillary tube in the spectrometer cavity for data acquisition. A stable radical CP (3-Carboxy-2,2,5,5-tetramethyl-1-pyrrolidinyloxy) was used as an external reference to convert ROS determinations in absolute quantitative values (µmol/min). All EPR spectra were collected by adopting the same protocol and obtained by using software standardly supplied by Bruker (Billerica, MA, USA) (version 2.11, WinEPR System).

4.2.2. Superoxide Dismutase (SOD) and Catalase (CAT)

SOD and CAT plasmatic levels were measured by enzyme-linked immunosorbent assay (ELISA kits), according to the manufacturer's instructions. SOD activity was assessed by Cayman's SOD assay kit (706002) that utilizes a tetrazolium salt for the detection of superoxide radicals generated by xanthine oxidase and hypoxathine. One unit of SOD is defined as the amount of enzymes needed to exhibit 50% dismutation of the superoxide radical measured in changes in absorbance (450 nm) per minute at 25 °C and at pH 8.0. CAT activity was assessed by Cayman's assay kit (707002) that utilizes the peroxidic function of CAT. The method is based on the reaction of enzymes with methanol in the presence of an optimal concentration of H_2O_2. The formaldehyde produced is measured colorimetrically with Purpald (540 nm) as chromogen. One unit of CAT is defined as the amount of enzymes that will cause the formation of 1 nmol of formaldehyde per minute at 25 °C. All samples and standards were read by a microplate reader spectrophotometer (Infinite M200, Tecan Group Ltd., Männedorf, Switzerland). The determinations were assessed in duplicate, and the inter-assay coefficient of variation was in the range indicated by the manufacturer.

4.2.3. Total Aminothiols (CYS: Cysteine; CYSGLY: Cysteinylglycine and GSH: Glutathione)

Total and reduced aminothiols (CYS: cysteine; CYSGLY: cysteinylglycine; and GSH: glutathione) were measured in erythrocytes (for GSH) and plasma (for CYS and CYSGLY), according to previously validated methods [53,54], at room temperature by an isocratic HPLC analysis on a Discovery C-18 column (250 × 4.6 mm I.D, Supelco, Sigma-Aldrich, St. Louis, MO, USA), eluted with a solution of a 0.1 M acetate buffer, pH 4.0 methanol, 81:19 (v/v), at a flow rate of 1 mL/min. Fluorescence intensities were measured with an excitation wavelength at 390 nm and an emission wavelength at 510 nm, using a fluorescence spectrophotometer (Jasco, Tokyo, Japan). A standard calibration curve was used for the assayed samples.

4.3. Urine Sample Analysis

4.3.1. Nitric Oxide Metabolites ($NO_2 + NO_3$)

NOx ($NO_2 + NO_3$) concentrations were determined in urine via a colorimetric method based on the Griess reaction, using a commercial kit (Cayman Chemical, Ann Arbor, MI, USA), as previously described [55]. Samples were spectrophotometrically read at 545 nm.

4.3.2. 8-Isoprostane (8-Iso-PGF2α)

Levels of 8-iso-PGF2α were measured using an immunoassay EIA kit (Cayman Chemical, Ann Arbor, MI, USA) in urine. This is a biomarker for lipid peroxidation damage assessment. Samples and standards were spectrophotometrically read at 412 nm. Results were normalized by urine creatinine values.

4.3.3. Interleukin-6

IL-6 levels were determined using the ELISA assay kit (ThermoFisher Scientific, Waltham, MA, USA) based on the double-antibody "sandwich" technique, in accordance with the manufacturer's instructions.

All the above samples and standards were read by a microplate reader spectrophotometer (Infinite M200, Tecan Group Ltd., Männedorf, Switzerland). The determinations were assessed in duplicate, and the inter-assay coefficient of variation was in the range indicated by the manufacturer.

4.3.4. Creatinine and Neopterin Concentrations

Urinary creatinine and neopterin concentrations were measured by the high-pressure liquid chromatography (HPLC) method, as previously described [45], by the Varian instrument (pump 240, autosampler ProStar 410, SpectraLab Scientific Inc., Markham, ON, Canada) coupled to a UV-VIS detector (Shimadzu SPD 10-AV, λ = 240 nm, SpectraLab Scientific Inc. for creatinine; and JASCO FP-1520, λ_{ex} = 355 nm and at λ_{em} = 450 nm, SpectraLab Scientific Inc. for neopterin).

After urine centrifugation at 1500× g at 4 °C for 5 min, analytic separations were performed at 50 °C on a 5 μm Discovery C-18 analytical column (250 × 4.6 mm I.D., Supelco, Sigma-Aldrich, Merck Life Science S.r.l., Milano, Italy) at a flow rate of 0.9 mL/min. The calibration curves were linear over the range of 0.125–1 μmol/L and 1.25–10 mmol/L for the neopterin and creatinine levels, respectively. The inter-assay and intra-assay coefficients of variation were <5%.

4.4. Statistical Analysis

Statistical analyses were conducted using GraphPad Prism 10 for Mac (La Jolla, CA, USA). Data are given as a percentage of pre-exposure values. Taking the baseline measures as 100%, the percentage or fold changes were calculated for each measurement time, allowing an appreciation of the magnitude of change rather than the absolute values. The difference between the percentage of pre-exposure values and 100% was compared by a two-tailed one-sample t-test when normality of the sample was reached, as assessed by the d'Agostino and Pearson tests. Otherwise, the non-parametric Wilcoxon Rank Sum test was used. Comparisons between the 1.4 ATA and 2.5 ATA groups were performed using the unpaired t-test (parametric) or Mann–Whitney (non-parametric). In parallel, to assess differences in the baseline values between conditions, a two-way ANOVA was performed with oxygen pressure (1.4 ATA and 2.5 ATA) and time after exposure. When sphericity was not assumed, analysis of variance (ANOVA) main effects and interactions were interpreted with the Greenhouse–Geisser correction. Sidak-corrected multiple comparisons were used to analyze significant interactions and main effects. The alpha level was set at 0.05. Data are presented as mean (M) ± standard deviation (SD). The significance level was set at $p < 0.05$.

The sample size required for a repeated measures analysis of variance was calculated using the G*power calculator 3.1.9.7 software (Heinrich-Heine-Universität, Düsseldorf, Germany) (effect size = 0.65, alpha error = 0.05, Power = 0.80), and the requisite number of participants for this study was 6 in each group, which parallels previous studies [17].

5. Conclusions

A short term (60 min) period of mild (1.4 ATA) and high (2.5 ATA) hyperbaric hyperoxia leads to a similar significant increase in the production of reactive oxygen species (ROS), peaking 2 h after exposure and slowly recovering after 48 h, without yet reaching pre-exposure levels at that time.

Similar physiological reactions seem to be present for both very different oxygen doses (1.4 and 2.5 ATA) concerning antioxidant coping strategies. Immunomodulation and inflammatory responses, on the contrary, respond proportionally to the hyperbaric oxygen dose.

Overall, this study provides insights into the cellular effects of a single exposure of hyperbaric hyperoxia, which may either be similar for both doses studied or dose-dependent (such as the immune system response). A further study of the dynamics and kinetics of these effects may lead to new insights as to the optimal dose and administration schedule (inter-dose recovery time) to optimize the therapeutic benefits of intermittent oxygen therapy (either hyperbaric or normobaric). In fact, a more detailed understanding of these effects is paramount to advancing the clinical use of this promising treatment modality.

Author Contributions: Conceptualization: C.B., P.L., P.G., C.L., S.T., K.L., M.L., S.M.S., A.V., G.B. and F.G.; investigation: P.L., C.L., M.L., S.T., C.B., K.L., P.G., S.M.S., A.V. and G.B.; writing: C.L., S.T., C.B., P.G., P.L., S.M.S. and F.G.; funding: C.B., F.G., K.L., S.T. and G.B.; data analysis: C.L., S.M.S., A.V., C.B., S.T., K.L., M.L., P.L., F.G., P.G. and G.B. All authors have read and agreed to the published version of the manuscript.

Funding: This manuscript is part of the DELTO$_2$X Project that is funded by WBE (Wallonia-Brussels-Education) Belgium for the Environmental, Occupational, Aging (Integrative) Physiology Laboratory, Haute Ecole Bruxelles-Brabant (HE2B), Belgium. The sponsors had no role in the design and conduct of this study; the collection, management, analysis, and interpretation of the data; the preparation, review, or approval of this manuscript; and the decision to submit this manuscript for publication.

Institutional Review Board Statement: Ethics Committee approval was obtained from the Bio-Ethical Committee for Research and Higher Education, Brussels (N° B 200-2020-088).

Informed Consent Statement: Informed consent was obtained from all subjects involved in this study.

Data Availability Statement: Data are available upon request from the authors.

Acknowledgments: The authors are grateful to all the volunteer participants, especially to the students of the Haute Ecole Bruxelles-Brabant (Belgium), Motor Sciences Department (Physiotherapy).

Conflicts of Interest: The authors declare no conflict of interest.

Abbreviations

8-iso-PGF2a	8-isoprostane
ATA	Atmosphere absolute
CAT	Catalase
CYSGLY	Cysteinylglycine
EPR	Electron Paramagnetic Resonance
FiO_2	Inspired Fraction of Oxygen
GSH	Glutathione
H_2O_2	Hydrogen peroxide
HBOT	Hyperbaric oxygen therapy
IL-6	Interleukine-6
NO	Nitric oxide
NOx	Nitric oxide metabolites
NRF2	Nuclear Factor Erythroid 2 Related—Factor 2
ROS	Reactive Oxygen Species
SOD	Superoxide dismutase

References

1. Lee, J.S.; Cha, Y.S.; Lim, J. Association between number of hyperbaric oxygen therapy sessions and neurocognitive outcomes of acute carbon monoxide poisoning. *Front. Med.* **2023**, *10*, 1127978. [CrossRef]
2. Biggs, A.T.; Littlejohn, L.F.; Dainer, H.M. Alternative Uses of Hyperbaric Oxygen Therapy in Military Medicine: Current Positions and Future Directions. *Mil. Med.* **2022**, *187*, e40–e46. [CrossRef] [PubMed]
3. Harch, P.G. Systematic Review and Dosage Analysis: Hyperbaric Oxygen Therapy Efficacy in Mild Traumatic Brain Injury Persistent Postconcussion Syndrome. *Front. Neurol.* **2022**, *13*, 815056. [CrossRef]
4. MacLaughlin, K.J.; Barton, G.P.; Braun, R.K.; MacLaughlin, J.E.; Lamers, J.J.; Marcou, M.D.; Eldridge, M.W. Hyperbaric air mobilizes stem cells in humans; a new perspective on the hormetic dose curve. *Front. Neurol.* **2023**, *14*, 1192793. [CrossRef] [PubMed]
5. Perdrizet, G.A. Principles and practice of hyperbaric medicine: A medical practitioner's primer, part I. *Conn. Med.* **2014**, *78*, 325–332. [PubMed]
6. de Wolde, S.D.; Hulskes, R.H.; de Jonge, S.W.; Hollmann, M.W.; van Hulst, R.A.; Weenink, R.P.; Kox, M. The Effect of Hyperbaric Oxygen Therapy on Markers of Oxidative Stress and the Immune Response in Healthy Volunteers. *Front. Physiol.* **2022**, *13*, 826163. [CrossRef]
7. Balestra, C.; Arya, A.K.; Leveque, C.; Virgili, F.; Germonpre, P.; Lambrechts, K.; Lafere, P.; Thom, S.R. Varying Oxygen Partial Pressure Elicits Blood-Borne Microparticles Expressing Different Cell-Specific Proteins-Toward a Targeted Use of Oxygen? *Int. J. Mol. Sci.* **2022**, *23*, 7888. [CrossRef]
8. Fratantonio, D.; Virgili, F.; Zucchi, A.; Lambrechts, K.; Latronico, T.; Lafere, P.; Germonpre, P.; Balestra, C. Increasing Oxygen Partial Pressures Induce a Distinct Transcriptional Response in Human PBMC: A Pilot Study on the "Normobaric Oxygen Paradox". *Int. J. Mol. Sci.* **2021**, *22*, 458. [CrossRef]
9. De Bels, D.; Tillmans, F.; Corazza, F.; Bizzari, M.; Germonpre, P.; Radermacher, P.; Orman, K.G.; Balestra, C. Hyperoxia Alters Ultrastructure and Induces Apoptosis in Leukemia Cell Lines. *Biomolecules* **2020**, *10*, 282. [CrossRef]
10. Cimino, F.; Balestra, C.; Germonpre, P.; De Bels, D.; Tillmans, F.; Saija, A.; Speciale, A.; Virgili, F. Pulsed high oxygen induces a hypoxic-like response in Human Umbilical Endothelial Cells (HUVECs) and in humans. *J. Appl. Physiol.* **2012**, *113*, 1684–1689. [CrossRef]
11. Mrakic-Sposta, S.; Gussoni, M.; Marzorati, M.; Porcelli, S.; Bosco, G.; Balestra, C.; Montorsi, M.; Lafortuna, C.; Vezzoli, A. The "ON-OFF" Switching Response of Reactive Oxygen Species in Acute Normobaric Hypoxia: Preliminary Outcome. *Int. J. Mol. Sci.* **2023**, *24*, 4012. [CrossRef]
12. Leveque, C.; Mrakic Sposta, S.; Theunissen, S.; Germonpré, P.; Lambrechts, K.; Vezzoli, A.; Gussoni, M.; Levenez, M.; Lafère, P.; Guerrero, F.; et al. Oxidative Stress Response Kinetics after 60 Minutes at Different Levels (10% or 15%) of Normobaric Hypoxia Exposure. *Int. J. Mol. Sci.* **2023**, *24*, 10188. [CrossRef] [PubMed]
13. Balestra, C.; Lambrechts, K.; Mrakic-Sposta, S.; Vezzoli, A.; Levenez, M.; Germonpre, P.; Virgili, F.; Bosco, G.; Lafere, P. Hypoxic and Hyperoxic Breathing as a Complement to Low-Intensity Physical Exercise Programs: A Proof-of-Principle Study. *Int. J. Mol. Sci.* **2021**, *22*, 9600. [CrossRef] [PubMed]
14. Theunissen, S.; Balestra, C.; Bolognesi, S.; Borgers, G.; Vissenaeken, D.; Obeid, G.; Germonpre, P.; Honore, P.M.; De Bels, D. Effects of Acute Hypobaric Hypoxia Exposure on Cardiovascular Function in Unacclimatized Healthy Subjects: A "Rapid Ascent" Hypobaric Chamber Study. *Int. J. Environ. Res. Public Health* **2022**, *19*, 5394. [CrossRef]
15. Arya, A.K.; Balestra, C.; Bhopale, V.M.; Tuominen, L.J.; Raisanen-Sokolowski, A.; Dugrenot, E.; L'Her, E.; Bhat, A.R.; Thom, S.R. Elevations of Extracellular Vesicles and Inflammatory Biomarkers in Closed Circuit SCUBA Divers. *Int. J. Mol. Sci.* **2023**, *24*, 5969. [CrossRef]

16. Salvagno, M.; Coppalini, G.; Taccone, F.S.; Strapazzon, G.; Mrakic-Sposta, S.; Rocco, M.; Khalife, M.; Balestra, C. The Normobaric Oxygen Paradox-Hyperoxic Hypoxic Paradox: A Novel Expedient Strategy in Hematopoiesis Clinical Issues. *Int. J. Mol. Sci.* **2022**, *24*, 82. [CrossRef] [PubMed]
17. Leveque, C.; Mrakic-Sposta, S.; Lafere, P.; Vezzoli, A.; Germonpre, P.; Beer, A.; Mievis, S.; Virgili, F.; Lambrechts, K.; Theunissen, S.; et al. Oxidative Stress Response's Kinetics after 60 Minutes at Different (30% or 100%) Normobaric Hyperoxia Exposures. *Int. J. Mol. Sci.* **2022**, *24*, 664. [CrossRef]
18. Louge, P.; Pignel, R.; Serratrice, J.; Stirnemann, J. Validation of sham treatment in hyperbaric medicine: A randomised trial. *Diving Hyperb. Med.* **2023**, *53*, 51–54. [CrossRef]
19. Balestra, C.; Kot, J. Oxygen: A Stimulus, Not "Only" a Drug. *Medicina* **2021**, *57*, 1161. [CrossRef]
20. Franceschi, C.; Bonafè, M.; Valensin, S.; Olivieri, F.; De Luca, M.; Ottaviani, E.; De Benedictis, G. Inflamm-aging. An evolutionary perspective on immunosenescence. *Ann. N. Y. Acad. Sci.* **2000**, *908*, 244–254. [CrossRef]
21. Franceschi, C.; Campisi, J. Chronic inflammation (inflammaging) and its potential contribution to age-associated diseases. *J. Gerontol. A Biol. Sci. Med. Sci.* **2014**, *69* (Suppl. S1), S4–S9. [CrossRef]
22. Akhigbe, R.; Ajayi, A. The impact of reactive oxygen species in the development of cardiometabolic disorders: A review. *Lipids Health Dis.* **2021**, *20*, 23. [CrossRef] [PubMed]
23. Checa, J.; Aran, J.M. Reactive Oxygen Species: Drivers of Physiological and Pathological Processes. *J. Inflamm. Res.* **2020**, *13*, 1057–1073. [CrossRef] [PubMed]
24. Maroon, J.C. The effect of hyperbaric oxygen therapy on cognition, performance, proteomics, and telomere length—The difference between zero and one: A case report. *Front. Neurol.* **2022**, *13*, 949536. [CrossRef]
25. Zhilyaev, S.Y.; Moskvin, A.N.; Platonova, T.F.; Gutsaeva, D.R.; Churilina, I.V.; Demchenko, I.T. Hyperoxic vasoconstriction in the brain is mediated by inactivation of nitric oxide by superoxide anions. *Neurosci. Behav. Physiol.* **2003**, *33*, 783–787. [CrossRef] [PubMed]
26. Schildknecht, S.; Ullrich, V. Peroxynitrite as regulator of vascular prostanoid synthesis. *Arch. Biochem. Biophys.* **2009**, *484*, 183–189. [CrossRef]
27. Muskat, J.C.; Babbs, C.F.; Goergen, C.J.; Rayz, V.L. Transport of nitrite from large arteries modulates regional blood flow during stress and exercise. *Front. Cardiovasc. Med.* **2023**, *10*, 1146717. [CrossRef] [PubMed]
28. Schottlender, N.; Gottfried, I.; Ashery, U. Hyperbaric Oxygen Treatment: Effects on Mitochondrial Function and Oxidative Stress. *Biomolecules* **2021**, *11*, 1827. [CrossRef]
29. Eventoff, W.; Tanaka, N.; Rossmann, M.G. Crystalline bovine liver catalase. *J. Mol. Biol.* **1976**, *103*, 799–801. [CrossRef]
30. Fita, I.; Silva, A.; Murthy, M.; Rossmann, M. The refined structure of beef liver catalase at 2·5 Å resolution. *Acta Crystallogr. Sect. B Struct. Sci.* **1986**, *42*, 497–515. [CrossRef]
31. Benedetti, S.; Lamorgese, A.; Piersantelli, M.; Pagliarani, S.; Benvenuti, F.; Canestrari, F. Oxidative stress and antioxidant status in patients undergoing prolonged exposure to hyperbaric oxygen. *Clin. Biochem.* **2004**, *37*, 312–317. [CrossRef] [PubMed]
32. Eken, A.; Aydin, A.; Sayal, A.; Üstündağ, A.; Duydu, Y.; Dündar, K. The effects of hyperbaric oxygen treatment on oxidative stress and SCE frequencies in humans. *Clin. Biochem.* **2005**, *38*, 1133–1137. [CrossRef] [PubMed]
33. Ballinger, C.A.; Mendis-Handagama, C.; Kalmar, J.R.; Arnold, R.R.; Kinkade, J.M., Jr. Changes in the localization of catalase during differentiation of neutrophilic granulocytes. *Blood* **1994**, *83*, 2654–2668. [CrossRef]
34. Sureda, A.; Ferrer, M.D.; Tauler, P.; Maestre, I.; Aguiló, A.; Córdova, A.; Tur, J.A.; Roche, E.; Pons, A. Intense physical activity enhances neutrophil antioxidant enzyme gene expression. Immunocytochemistry evidence for catalase secretion. *Free. Radic. Res.* **2007**, *41*, 874–883. [CrossRef] [PubMed]
35. Liu, T.; Sun, L.; Zhang, Y.; Wang, Y.; Zheng, J. Imbalanced GSH/ROS and sequential cell death. *J. Biochem. Mol. Toxicol.* **2022**, *36*, e22942. [CrossRef]
36. Han, Y.; Liu, K.; Li, L.; Li, X.; Zhao, P. The effects of hyperbaric oxygen therapy on neuropathic pain via mitophagy in microglia. *Mol. Pain* **2017**, *13*, 1744806917710862. [CrossRef]
37. Gao, W.; Guo, L.; Yang, Y.; Wang, Y.; Xia, S.; Gong, H.; Zhang, B.K.; Yan, M. Dissecting the Crosstalk between Nrf2 and NF-κB Response Pathways in Drug-Induced Toxicity. *Front. Cell Dev. Biol.* **2021**, *9*, 809952. [CrossRef]
38. Burtscher, J.; Mallet, R.T.; Pialoux, V.; Millet, G.P.; Burtscher, M. Adaptive Responses to Hypoxia and/or Hyperoxia in Humans. *Antioxid. Redox Signal.* **2022**, *37*, 887–912. [CrossRef]
39. Michalak, Ł.; Bulska, M.; Strząbała, K.; Szcześniak, P. Neopterin as a marker of cellular immunological response. *Adv. Hyg. Exp. Med.* **2017**, *71*, 727–736. [CrossRef]
40. Huber, C.; Fuchs, D.; Hausen, A.; Margreiter, R.; Reibnegger, G.; Spielberger, M.; Wachter, H. Pteridines as a new marker to detect human T cells activated by allogeneic or modified self major histocompatibility complex (MHC) determinants. *J. Immunol.* **1983**, *130*, 1047–1050. [CrossRef]
41. Huber, C.; Batchelor, J.R.; Fuchs, D.; Hausen, A.; Lang, A.; Niederwieser, D.; Reibnegger, G.; Swetly, P.; Troppmair, J.; Wachter, H. Immune response-associated production of neopterin. Release from macrophages primarily under control of interferon-gamma. *J. Exp. Med.* **1984**, *160*, 310–316. [CrossRef] [PubMed]
42. Ghisoni, K.; Martins Rde, P.; Barbeito, L.; Latini, A. Neopterin as a potential cytoprotective brain molecule. *J. Psychiatr. Res.* **2015**, *71*, 134–139. [CrossRef] [PubMed]

43. Gottfried, I.; Schottlender, N.; Ashery, U. Hyperbaric Oxygen Treatment-From Mechanisms to Cognitive Improvement. *Biomolecules* **2021**, *11*, 1520. [CrossRef] [PubMed]
44. World Medical, A. World Medical Association Declaration of Helsinki: Ethical principles for medical research involving human subjects. *JAMA* **2013**, *310*, 2191–2194. [CrossRef]
45. Bosco, G.; Paganini, M.; Giacon, T.A.; Oppio, A.; Vezzoli, A.; Dellanoce, C.; Moro, T.; Paoli, A.; Zanotti, F.; Zavan, B.; et al. Oxidative Stress and Inflammation, MicroRNA, and Hemoglobin Variations after Administration of Oxygen at Different Pressures and Concentrations: A Randomized Trial. *Int. J. Environ. Res. Public Health* **2021**, *18*, 9755. [CrossRef]
46. Mrakic-Sposta, S.; Vezzoli, A.; D'Alessandro, F.; Paganini, M.; Dellanoce, C.; Cialoni, D.; Bosco, G. Change in Oxidative Stress Biomarkers During 30 Days in Saturation Dive: A Pilot Study. *Int. J. Environ. Res. Public Health* **2020**, *17*, 7118. [CrossRef]
47. Moretti, S.; Mrakic-Sposta, S.; Roncoroni, L.; Vezzoli, A.; Dellanoce, C.; Monguzzi, E.; Branchi, F.; Ferretti, F.; Lombardo, V.; Doneda, L.; et al. Oxidative stress as a biomarker for monitoring treated celiac disease. *Clin. Transl. Gastroenterol.* **2018**, *9*, 157. [CrossRef]
48. Mrakic-Sposta, S.; Vezzoli, A.; Rizzato, A.; Della Noce, C.; Malacrida, S.; Montorsi, M.; Paganini, M.; Cancellara, P.; Bosco, G. Oxidative stress assessment in breath-hold diving. *Eur. J. Appl. Physiol.* **2019**, *119*, 2449–2456. [CrossRef]
49. Bosco, G.; Rizzato, A.; Quartesan, S.; Camporesi, E.; Mrakic-Sposta, S.; Moretti, S.; Balestra, C.; Rubini, A. Spirometry and oxidative stress after rebreather diving in warm water. *Undersea Hyperb. Med.* **2018**, *45*, 191–198. [CrossRef]
50. Mrakic-Sposta, S.; Gussoni, M.; Montorsi, M.; Porcelli, S.; Vezzoli, A. A quantitative method to monitor reactive oxygen species production by electron paramagnetic resonance in physiological and pathological conditions. *Oxidative Med. Cell. Longev.* **2014**, *2014*, 306179. [CrossRef]
51. Mrakic-Sposta, S.; Gussoni, M.; Montorsi, M.; Vezzoli, A. Comment on Menzel et al. Common and Novel Markers for Measuring Inflammation and Oxidative Stress Ex Vivo in Research and Clinical Practice—Which to Use Regarding Disease Outcomes? *Antioxidants* **2021**, *10*, 414. *Antioxidants* **2021**, *10*, 836. [CrossRef]
52. Mrakic-Sposta, S.; Gussoni, M.; Montorsi, M.; Porcelli, S.; Vezzoli, A. Assessment of a standardized ROS production profile in humans by electron paramagnetic resonance. *Oxidative Med. Cell. Longev.* **2012**, *2012*, 973927. [CrossRef]
53. Dellanoce, C.; Cozzi, L.; Zuddas, S.; Pratali, L.; Accinni, R. Determination of different forms of aminothiols in red blood cells without washing erythrocytes. *Biomed. Chromatogr.* **2014**, *28*, 327–331. [CrossRef]
54. Vezzoli, A.; Dellanoce, C.; Mrakic-Sposta, S.; Montorsi, M.; Moretti, S.; Tonini, A.; Pratali, L.; Accinni, R. Oxidative Stress Assessment in Response to Ultraendurance Exercise: Thiols Redox Status and ROS Production according to Duration of a Competitive Race. *Oxidative Med. Cell. Longev.* **2016**, *2016*, 6439037. [CrossRef] [PubMed]
55. Ciccone, M.M.; Bilianou, E.; Balbarini, A.; Gesualdo, M.; Ghiadoni, L.; Metra, M.; Palmiero, P.; Pedrinelli, R.; Salvetti, M.; Scicchitano, P.; et al. Task force on: 'Early markers of atherosclerosis: Influence of age and sex'. *J. Cardiovasc. Med.* **2013**, *14*, 757–766. [CrossRef] [PubMed]

Disclaimer/Publisher's Note: The statements, opinions and data contained in all publications are solely those of the individual author(s) and contributor(s) and not of MDPI and/or the editor(s). MDPI and/or the editor(s) disclaim responsibility for any injury to people or property resulting from any ideas, methods, instructions or products referred to in the content.

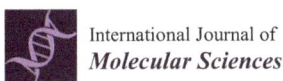

Article

Hyperbaric Oxygenation Prevents Loss of Immature Neurons in the Adult Hippocampal Dentate Gyrus Following Brain Injury

Rada Jeremic [1], Sanja Pekovic [2], Irena Lavrnja [2], Ivana Bjelobaba [2], Marina Djelic [1], Sanja Dacic [3,*,†] and Predrag Brkic [1,*,†]

[1] Institute of Medical Physiology "Richard Burian", Faculty of Medicine, University of Belgrade, 11000 Belgrade, Serbia
[2] Department of Neurobiology, Institute for Biological Research "Sinisa Stankovic", National Institute of the Republic of Serbia, University of Belgrade, 11000 Belgrade, Serbia
[3] Department of General Physiology and Biophysics, Institute of Physiology and Biochemistry, Faculty of Biology, University of Belgrade, 11000 Belgrade, Serbia
* Correspondence: sanjas@bio.bg.ac.rs (S.D.); predrag.brkic@med.bg.ac.rs (P.B.); Tel.: +381-11-2638-500 (S.D.); +381-11-3607-076 (P.B.); Fax: +381-11-3607-093 (P.B.)
† These authors contributed equally to this work.

Abstract: A growing body of evidence suggests that hyperbaric oxygenation (HBO) may affect the activity of adult neural stem cells (NSCs). Since the role of NSCs in recovery from brain injury is still unclear, the purpose of this study was to investigate the effects of sensorimotor cortex ablation (SCA) and HBO treatment (HBOT) on the processes of neurogenesis in the adult dentate gyrus (DG), a region of the hippocampus that is the site of adult neurogenesis. Ten-week-old Wistar rats were divided into groups: Control (C, intact animals), Sham control (S, animals that underwent the surgical procedure without opening the skull), SCA (animals in whom the right sensorimotor cortex was removed via suction ablation), and SCA + HBO (operated animals that passed HBOT). HBOT protocol: pressure applied at 2.5 absolute atmospheres for 60 min, once daily for 10 days. Using immunohistochemistry and double immunofluorescence labeling, we show that SCA causes significant loss of neurons in the DG. Newborn neurons in the subgranular zone (SGZ), inner-third, and partially mid-third of the granule cell layer are predominantly affected by SCA. HBOT decreases the SCA-caused loss of immature neurons, prevents reduction of dendritic arborization, and increases proliferation of progenitor cells. Our results suggest a protective effect of HBO by reducing the vulnerability of immature neurons in the adult DG to SCA injury.

Keywords: traumatic brain injury; hyperbaric oxygenation; adult neurogenesis; dentate gyrus

1. Introduction

After years of debate, it is accepted that adult neurogenesis exists in mammals and new functionally integrated neurons are generated throughout adulthood [1]. Neural stem cells (NSCs) in the adult brain reside in the subventricular zone (SVZ) of the lateral ventricle and the subgranular zone (SGZ) of the dentate gyrus (DG) of the hippocampus [2,3]. Through the lifespan, NSCs in the DG add excitatory granular neurons that can integrate into the neuronal network in the granule cell layer (GCL) [4]. Adult neurogenesis in the DG is thought to significantly increase the neural plasticity of the DG and thereby increasing hippocampal functionality [5].

The characteristics of the neurogenic brain regions that enable the smooth development of adult neurogenesis are unclear. Still, it is known that neurogenesis can be promoted or suppressed by various intrinsic or extrinsic factors [2,6]. Adult neurogenesis increases in response to various brain injuries in both neurogenic regions. A positive correlation has been found between the extent of neurogenesis and recovery after traumatic brain injury (TBI) [5].

It has been extensively reported that TBI is still a global burden on the health care system with its growing age-standardized incidence [7,8]. TBI consists of primary and secondary injuries. Primary injury causes permanent loss of neurons that cannot be repaired. Secondary injury represents neuronal degeneration, which is a consequence of primary injury [9–12]. Our previously published article suggested that secondary injury should be considered as a chronic non-communicable disease [11]. In light of this, and to alleviate symptoms of TBI, the secondary injury should be a potential target for therapeutic procedures. Currently, studies in animal models of TBI are needed to investigate the exact mechanisms of injury and the recovery process [8].

Patients may have post-traumatic amnesia among a wide range of symptoms after TBI [13]. In addition, because damage to the hippocampus has been shown to result in an inability to form new memories [14], cortex lesions can be expected to indirectly affect the morphology and number of neurons in the DG, a part of the hippocampus.

Given the complexity of TBI, a combination of different therapeutic protocols would likely provide the best results. Hyperbaric oxygen therapy (HBOT) has found its place as a preconditioning treatment or adjunctive therapy in treating TBI [8,15]. HBOT is a therapeutic procedure in which the patient intermittently inhales 100% oxygen at a pressure greater than 1 atmosphere absolute (1 ATA) [16]. Many studies have shown that HBOT has positive and negative effects. Interestingly, under hyperbaric conditions, oxygen can deeply penetrate ischemic regions, which may lead to a reduction in lesions caused by TBI [16]. On the other hand, numerous studies have investigated the oxygen toxicity and oxidative stress that may be caused by HBOT [17]. To avoid the side effects of high oxygen concentrations, the treatment parameters of HBOT, such as pressure and duration, must be controlled [18].

As part of neuroplasticity, neurogenesis and synaptogenesis show that the adult brain can adapt even to TBI [19,20]. To our knowledge, we were the first to report that HBOT applied after TBI increases synaptophysin expression, a marker of synaptogenesis. In addition, improvement in locomotor performance and sensorimotor integration was noted after HBOT [21]. Furthermore, a growing number of data suggests that hyperbaric oxygenation can influence the activity of adult NSCs. In addition, recent studies have shown that HBOT stimulates adult neurogenesis [22,23]. Moreover, HBOT promotes the mobilization of neural stem cells to the lesion site to replace presumably damaged neurons [23]. Although the exact mechanisms of HBOT-induced neurogenesis in adults are still unknown, previous studies suggest that various factors, such as hypoxia-inducible factors, are involved [24].

The aim of this study was to investigate the effects of brain injury induced by sensorimotor cortex ablation (SCA) on DG, and the potential therapeutic impact of HBOT on SCA-induced injury by stimulation of adult mammalian neurogenesis. We found that HBOT could prevent SCA-induced loss of newborn immature neurons and impairment of their morphology. In addition, HBOT increased the number of proliferating cells in hippocampal DG after the SCA injury. To our knowledge, this is the first comprehensive immunohistochemical study to visualize the beneficial effects of HBOT on injury-affected neurogenesis in adult hippocampal DG.

2. Results

Notably, there was no statistically significant difference between data obtained for the C and S groups (Figures S2 and S3); therefore, for immunohistochemical and immunofluorescence analysis, all comparisons were made regarding intact controls (data are shown in the Supplemented Material).

2.1. SCA Leads to Layer-Specific Neurodegeneration in the Hippocampal DG

In order to characterize neuronal death in the hippocampal DG and to visualize the location of the cells undergoing degeneration, we used FJB staining (in green, Figure 1A,D) and NeuN to visualize neurons (in red, Figure 1B,E). Given that the GCL of the DG is further divided into an outer-, mid-, and inner-third of granular neurons and the SGZ, where the NSCs are located [25], we wanted to characterize the impact of SCA on the distribution of the FJB-positive neurons in these specific sub-layers. After analysis, no degenerating neurons were seen in any regions of the DG control sections as assessed using FJB staining (Figure 1A,C). In contrast, SCA caused massive neurodegeneration in the DG, as indicated by an increase in the FJB-immunoreactivity (Figure 1D).

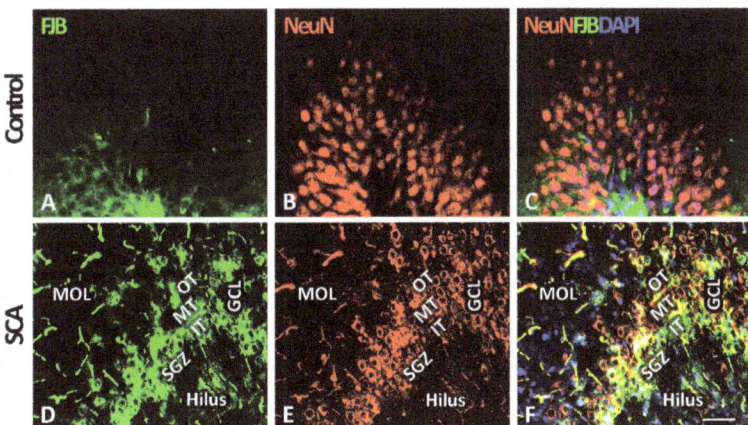

Figure 1. SCA (suction cortical ablation) induces neuronal death predominantly in the inner- and mid-third of the granule cell layer (GCL) and subgranular zone (SGZ) of the dentate gyrus (DG). (**A**–**C**) FJB (green fluorescence) staining in the control sections was weak, and FJB-positive cells were rare. (**D**) After SCA, a substantial increase in FJB-immunoreactivity indicates increased cellular degeneration. (**E**) Reduced NeuN (red) immunoreactivity indicates neuronal loss. (**F**) FJB (green), NeuN (red), and DAPI (blue) fluorescence show strong co-staining, revealing the neuronal identity of degenerating cells. In (**C**,**F**), the sections were counterstained with DAPI (blue) to visualize cell nuclei. Most affected are the inner- and mid-third of the GCL and the SGZ, indicating that neurons are undergoing, degeneration particularly in these compartments. FJB/NeuN-positive neurons were occasionally seen in the molecular layer (MOL) of the DG and the hilus. Outer-third (OT), mid-third (MT), inner-third (IT) of the GCL, and the SGZ of the DG. Scale bar 50 μm.

Importantly, in SCA sections, we found the sub-layer specificity in the distribution of the FJB- and NeuN-positive neurons (Figure 1D–F). Co-labeling of FJB and NeuN (see yellow fluorescence in Figure 1F) allowed us to detect degenerating neurons and revealed that the vast majority of these NeuN/FJB-positive neurons were located in the inner- (IT) and mid-third (MT) of the GCL and partially in the SGZ. On the other hand, FJB/NeuN-positive neurons were rarely detected in the outer-third (OT) of the GCL of the DG. Furthermore, only a few FJB/NeuN-positive neurons were found in the molecular layer (MOL) of the DG and the hilus (Figure 1F). Based on these results, we concluded that SCA has layer-specific effects on the DG, causing cell death of neurons predominantly in the inner GCL and the SGZ.

2.2. HBOT Prevents/Ameliorates SCA-Provoked Loss of Neurons in the GCL of the Hippocampal DG

To determine whether HBOT could prevent or at least ameliorate SCA-induced cellular loss in the hippocampal DG granule neurons, we performed immunofluorescence staining with neuronal marker NeuN. Cortical injury caused a significant loss of granular neurons stained with NeuN (red fluorescence) in the DG (Figure 2B, arrowheads) in comparison to the control sections (Figure 2A). After SCA, 10 successive HBO treatments prevented/ameliorated neuronal death after SCA (Figure 2C).

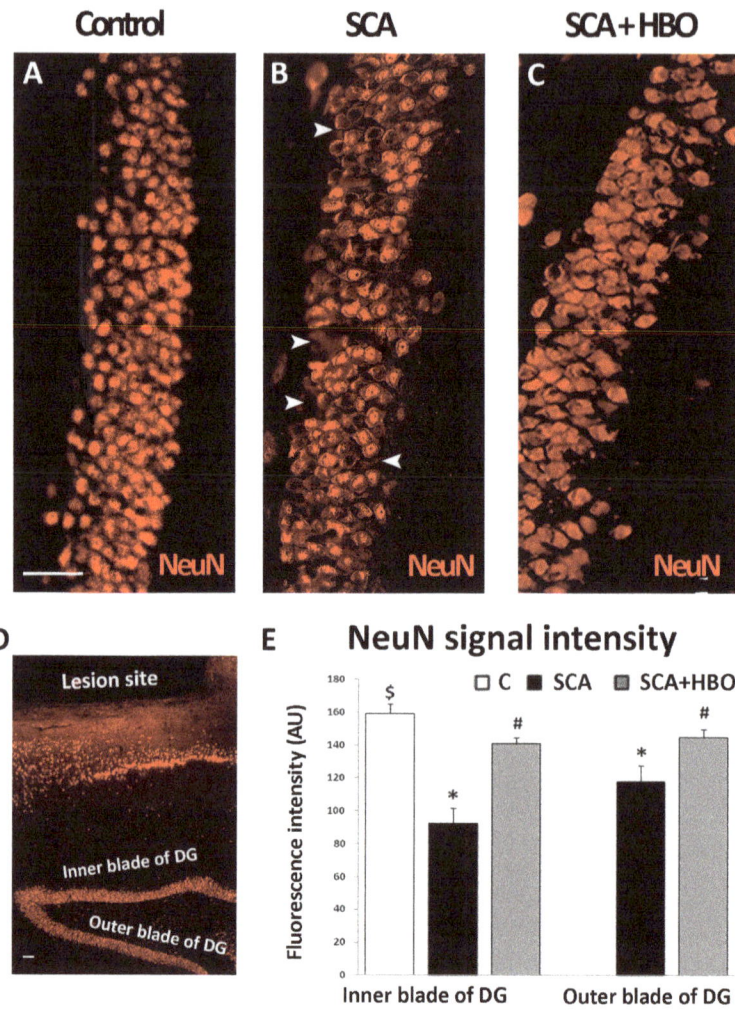

Figure 2. Effect of SCA (suction cortical ablation) and HBOT (hyperbaric oxygen therapy) on NeuN immunoreactivity in the GCL (granule cell layer) of the hippocampal DG (dentate gyrus). Significant loss of granular neurons stained with NeuN (red fluorescence) is seen in the DG after SCA (**B**, arrowheads) in comparison to the control sections (**A**). In contrast, (**C**) HBOT ameliorated neuronal loss. (**D**) NeuN staining in the hippocampus underlying the lesion site. (**E**) NeuN fluorescence signal intensity (in arbitrary units, AU), quantified separately in the inner and outer blades of the DG in controls (**C**, white bar), SCA (black bars), and HBO (hyperbaric oxygenation)-treated animals (SCA + HBO, gray bars). After the SCA, the brain sections show a statistically significant decrease in NeuN signal intensity in the inner blade and, to a less extent, in the outer blade of the DG compared to the controls. Following HBOT, the signal intensity of NeuN was comparable to the control level. C—Control, SCA—Suction cortical ablation, SCA + HBO—SCA animals treated with hyperbaric oxygen. Bars represent mean ± SD. The level of significance was analyzed using One-way ANOVA with Tukey's multiple comparisons post hoc test (* $p < 0.001$ SCA vs. C, $ $p < 0.01$ SCA + HBO vs. C, # $p < 0.001$, SCA + HBO vs. SCA). Scale bar 50 μm (**A–D**).

Since the loss of NeuN immunoreactivity may predict neuronal degeneration in the rodent hippocampus after various brain injuries [26], we quantified separately NeuN labeling in the suprapyramidal (inner) blade and infrapyramidal (outer) blade of the hippocampal DG [27] in coronal sections of the control, SCA, and HBO-treated animals (Figure 2D,E).

In the control sections, there was no significant difference ($p = 0.114$) in the NeuN fluorescence intensity (in arbitrary units, AU) between the inner (159.21 ± 6.18) and outer (153.79 ± 4.56) blades of the DG (Figure S2). Hence, all comparisons were made against the NeuN fluorescence intensity of the inner blade.

SCA caused a significant reduction (41.85%, $p < 0.001$) of NeuN fluorescence intensity (92.59 ± 9.25, black bar) in the inner blade of the DG compared to controls (159.21 ± 6.18, white bar). However, after 10 HBOT, this SCA-induced neurodegeneration was less pronounced (11.49%, $p < 0.01$) (140.93 ± 3.92, gray bar).

In the outer blade of the DG of animals exposed to SCA, the reduction of NeuN fluorescence intensity was lesser but still significant (26.02%, $p < 0.001$) (117.78 ± 9.52, black bar) vs. the signal intensity of the control sections (159.21 ± 6.18, white bar). On the other hand, in the HBOT sections, the effect of SCA was attenuated and no statistically significant (9.04%, $p = 0.227$) difference was observed in the NeuN fluorescence intensity (144.82 ± 5.02) (Figure 2E, gray bar) vs. control. Together, these results suggest that SCA injury induces massive neuronal degeneration in the inner and outer blades of the DG, judging by the significant loss of NeuN immunoreactivity. In contrast, HBOT almost completely prevents/ameliorates this.

2.3. Cell Type of Neurons Undergoing Neurodegeneration in the Hippocampal DG Following SCA Injury and HBOT

Given that a large amount of FJB-positive neurons were detected in the SGZ layer, where the NSCs reside, in this section, we further performed immunofluorescence staining with doublecortin (DCX, green), a marker for early newborn immature neurons [28] and beta-III tubulin (TUJ1, red), which is expressed during hippocampal neurogenesis after DCX and marks newly generated postmitotic neurons [29,30].

2.3.1. HBOT Prevents Loss of DCX-Positive Newborn Immature Neurons in the GCL of the Hippocampal DG Following SCA Injury

First, we performed immunofluorescence staining with doublecortin (DCX, green) to identify the cell layer in which these early newborn immature neurons are localized, as well as to count the number of DCX-positive neurons in the SGZ layer of control, SCA, and HBOT sections separately in the inner and outer blades. As it is apparent from Figure 3, most of the DCX immunoreactivity was found in the SGZ layer. In the control sections (Figure 3A), there was no statistically significant ($p = 0.191$) difference between the number of DCX-positive cells in the inner (114 ± 10.31) and outer (120 ± 5.14) blades of the DG (Figure S3). Therefore, all comparisons were made against the number of DCX-positive cells in the inner blade (Figure 3D, white bar). DCX immunoreactivity is mainly seen in the SGZ in DCX-positive granular neurons with dendrites that elongate from the SGZ until MOL and in the cells located on the hilar border of the granular layer, probably basket cells (Figure 3A, inset).

SCA caused a significant ($p < 0.001$) loss in the number of DCX-positive immature neurons, particularly in the inner blade (50.90%) (56 ± 11.03, black bar) compared to the controls (114 ± 10.31, white bar) (Figure 4B,D), and to a less extent, but still noteworthy (38.90%, $p < 0.001$) in the outer blade (70 ± 10.58, black bar).

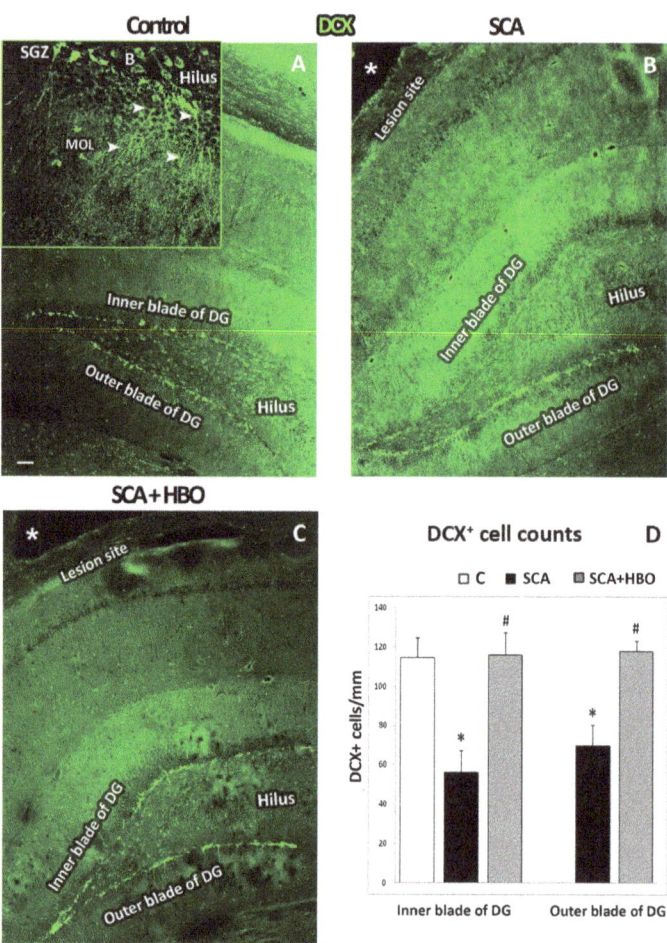

Figure 3. HBOT prevented the loss of doublecortin (DCX)-immunopositive newborn immature neurons after SCA (suction cortical ablation) in the subgranular zone (SGZ) of the hippocampal dentate gyrus (DG). A total of 25 μm thick frozen brain sections of C—Control, SCA—Suction cortical ablation, and SCA + HBO—SCA animals treated with hyperbaric oxygen were stained with DCX (green). (**A**) In the control sections, intensive DCX-immunopositivity was seen in the SGZ of the inner and outer blades of the DG. At higher magnification (inset), intensively DCX-labeled newborn neurons with branched dendrites (arrowheads) extended from the SGZ until the molecular layer (MOL). In addition, DCX immunoreactivity is detected in progenitors and basket cells (**B**) in the hilus. (**B**) SCA reduced DCX-immunofluorescence and was particularly pronounced in the inner blade of the DG beneath the lesion site (asterisk). (**C**) After 10 successive HBOT (hyperbaric oxygen therapy), the level of DCX-immunopositivity was as observed in the control. (**D**) DCX-positive cells were counted separately in the SGZ of the inner and outer blades of the hippocampal DG. Bars represent mean ± SD. Control (C, white bar), SCA (black bars), and HBO (hyperbaric oxygenation)-treated animals (SCA + HBO, gray bars). The significance level was analyzed using One-way ANOVA with Tukey's multiple comparisons post hoc test (* $p < 0.001$ SCA vs. C, # $p < 0.001$ SCA + HBO vs. C). Scale bar: (**A**–**C**)—100 μm.

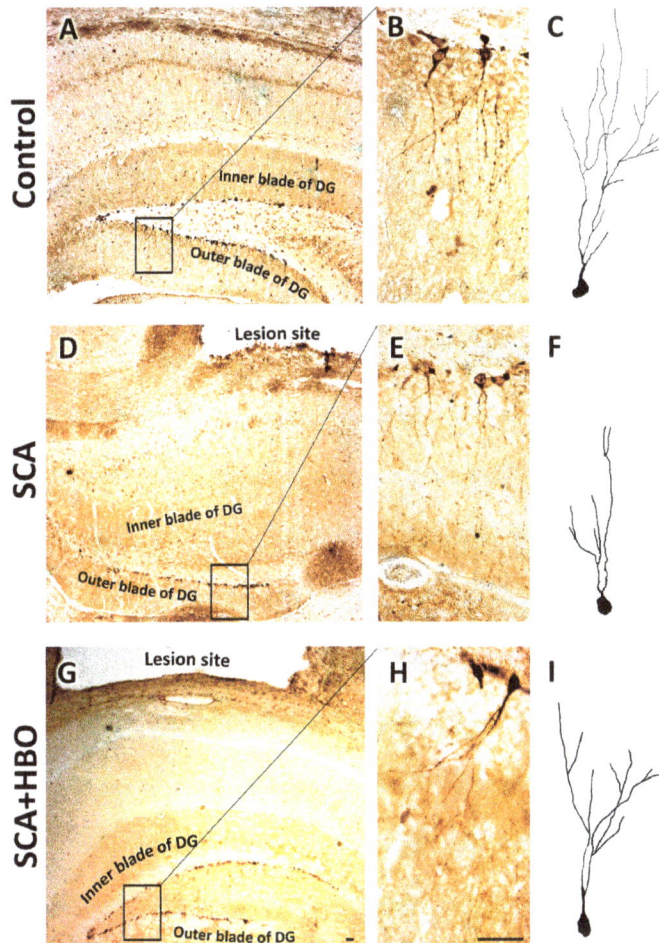

Figure 4. Besides prevention of SCA (suction cortical ablation)—which caused the neuronal loss, HBOT (hyperbaric oxygen therapy) impends dendrite degeneration of immature neurons in the SGZ (subgranular zone) as well. (**A,B**) In the control sections, DCX-stained immature neurons are in the SGZ, with dendrites branching in the inner- and mid-third of the granule cell layer (GCL) until the molecular layer. (**C**) The reconstructed neuron in the control group. (**D,E**) SCA causes the loss of neurons in the inner blade. (**E**) Higher magnification of the outer blade reveals that neurons in the SGZ show significant morphological changes manifested by dendritic shrinkage and reduction of arborization. (**F**) Reconstructed neuron after SCA. (**G,H**) HBOT protects neurons in the SGZ and prevents dendritic degeneration. (**I**) Reconstructed neuron following HBOT. Rectangles indicate where the high-magnification images are taken. Scale bars: (**A,D,G**)—50 μm, and (**B,C,E,F,H,I**)—10 μm.

Ten successive HBOTs prevented the loss of DCX-positive newborn immature neurons in the SGZ (Figure 3C). In addition, the number of DCX-positive cells in both the inner (116 ± 11.48) and outer (118 ± 5.63) blades of the hippocampal DG (Figure 3D, gray bars) was similar to those counted in control animals. These data indicate that newborn neurons are particularly vulnerable to SCA, while HBOT was able to overcome these effects of SCA and protect these newborn neurons from death.

2.3.2. HBOT Prevents SCA-Caused Neuronal Loss and Dendrite Degeneration of Newborn Immature Neurons in the SGZ of the Hippocampal DG

Light microscopic analysis of DCX immunostaining confirmed a significant loss of DCX-stained cells in the inner blade of the DG beneath the site of the lesion (Figure 4D) compared to the control sections (Figure 4A). Moreover, SCA caused morphological alterations of immature neurons in the SGZ layer of the inner and outer blade (Figure 4E,F). Higher-resolution images of the DG revealed that dendrites of spared neurons in the SGZ were damaged and underwent significant morphological changes. Namely, SCA induced an extreme reduction of dendritic complexity of SGZ neurons, which was manifested by the shortening of dendrite length and reduction of dendritic arborization (Figure 4E,F), as compared with controls (Figure 4B,C).

HBOT prevents and ameliorates these SCA-induced morphological alterations of neurons (Figure 4G–I), and these immature neurons resemble those in the control sections.

In order to show the effect of SCA and HBOT on dendrite arborization, we compared the dendrite total length, average segment length, and the number of branching points of the neurons in the outer blade between the groups (Table 1). There were significant decreases in the dendrite total length (by 43.09%, $p < 0.001$) and the number of branching points (by 60.77%, $p < 0.001$) in the SCA group compared to the control and an increase in the average segment length (by 33.18%, $p < 0.01$). According to this, SCA caused a dramatic reduction of dendritic arborization of the immature neurons in SGZ.

Table 1. The number of branching points, dendrite total length, and average segment length in the neurons of control, SCA and HBOT brain sections.

	C	SCA	SCA + HBO	*p* SCA vs. C	SCA + HBO vs. C	SCA + HBO vs. SCA
DTL	261.08 ± 24.39	148.60 ± 21.25	211.51 ± 28.40	<0.001	<0.01	<0.01
ASL	19.08 ± 1.70	25.41 ± 2.84	20.46 ± 3.67	<0.01	0.69	<0.05
BP	6.56 ± 0.96	2.57 ± 0.53	4.83 ± 0.35	<0.001	<0.01	<0.001

All values are shown as mean ± SD. The level of significance was determined using One-way ANOVA with Tukey's multiple comparisons post hoc test. DTL—dendrite total length in μm, ASL—average segment length in μm, BP—branching points. C—Control, SCA—Suction cortical ablation, and SCA + HBO—SCA animals treated with hyperbaric oxygen.

In the SCA + HBO group, the total length of the dendrites was also reduced, but to a lesser extent (by 18.99%, $p < 0.01$), as well as the number of branching points (by 26.3%, $p < 0.01$) compared to the control group. However, values of average segmental length were similar in these two groups ($p > 0.05$).

Altogether, these results suggest that SCA reduces the number of newborn neurons in the DG and causes significant impairment in the development and dendritic arborization. In contrast, HBOT attenuates these changes and protects the morphology of these newborn neurons.

2.3.3. HBOT Prevents Loss of DCX/TUJ1-Positive Newborn Immature Neurons in the GCL of the Hippocampal DG Following SCA Injury

To confirm the results mentioned above, we next performed double immunofluorescence staining with the most accepted markers for early neurons: doublecortin (DCX, green), a marker of early newborn immature neurons in adult DG, and beta-III tubulin (TUJ1, red), which marks newly generated postmitotic neurons (Figure 5). As expected, double staining revealed that in the DG of control sections, DCX/TUJ1-positive immature neurons were mainly located in the SGZ layer of the inner and outer blades (Figure 5A–C). At the higher magnification, DCX/TUJ1-positive cells were also visible in the IT of GCL, with their dendrites extending toward the MT and OT of GCL (Figure 5D–F, arrowheads). Notably, neuronal cell bodies were intensively stained both with DCX and TUJ1 (Figure 5D–F), while dendrites were stained only with DCX (Figure 5D,F, arrowheads). Only a few DCX/TUJ1-positive cells were in the OT of GCL and molecular cell layer (MOL) (Figure 5D–F, white asterisks). In the hilus, a paucity of intensely stained DCX/TUJ1-positive cells with large cell bodies were detected (Figure 5D–F, white arrows), while others with round/oval morphology were mostly TUJ1-positive (Figure 5D–F, yellow arrows).

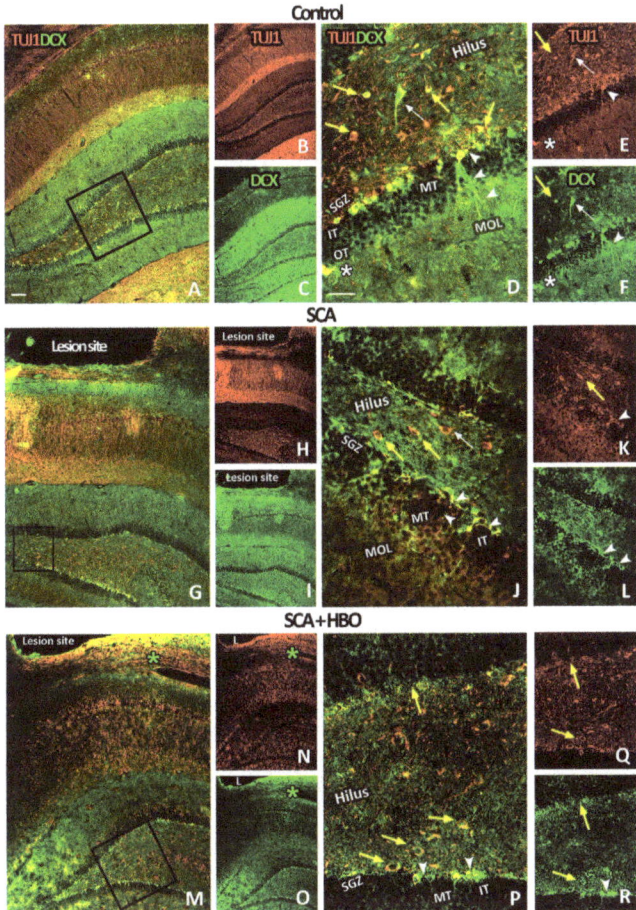

Figure 5. DCX (doublecortin) and TUJ1 (beta-III tubulin) immunoreactivity in the hippocampal DG (dentate gyrus) of control, SCA (suction cortical ablation), and HBO (hyperbaric oxygenation)-treated SCA animals. DCX (green) and TUJ1 (red) staining were used to visualize newborn neurons in the brain sections from controls (**A–F**), animals undergoing SCA (**G–L**), and HBOT (hyperbaric oxygen therapy) (**M–R**). (**D–F**) Higher magnification images of control sections revealed DCX/TUJ1-positive cells in the SGZ (subgranular zone), IT (inner-third) of the GCL (granule cell layer), with dendrites extending toward the MT (mid-) and OT (outer-third) of the GCL (arrowheads). A few DCX/TUJ1-positive cells were located in the OT of the GCL and molecular cell layer (MOL) (white asterisks). In the hilus, we detected some intensely stained DCX/TUJ1-positive cells with large cell bodies (white arrows) and others with round/oval morphology (yellow arrows) that were mostly TUJ1-positive (**J–L**). Higher magnification indicates that SCA reduced the number of DCX/TUJ1-positive immature neurons in the SGZ compared to control sections (**D–F**). (**M–O**) After HBOT, concentrated DCX/TUJ1 immunoreactivity is seen around the lesion site (green asterisks), (**P–R**) in the SGZ (arrowheads) and in the hilus (yellow arrows) as well. Rectangles indicate where the high-magnification images are taken from. C—control; SCA—sensorimotor cortex ablation. SCA + HBO—SCA animals treated with hyperbaric oxygen. Scale bars: (**A,G,M**)—100 µm; (**D,J,P**)—50 µm.

SCA reduced the DCX/TUJ1-immunoreactivity in the SGZ (Figure 5G–I), principally in the inner blade of the DG below the lesion site. The remaining DCX/TUJ1-positive neurons had altered morphology with shortened and less-branched dendrites (Figure 5J–L, arrowheads). In the hilus, TUJ1-positive neurons with round/oval morphology were still predominant (Figure 5J,K, yellow arrows).

Ten repetitive HBOTs prevented the loss of DCX/TUJ1-positive immature neurons mainly located in the SGZ layer of the inner and outer blade (Figure 5M–O). Interestingly, at higher magnification, we detected that besides neurons with round/oval morphology, which were only TUJ1-positive, some of them were also DCX/TUJ1-positive (Figure 5P–R, yellow arrows). Furthermore, these DCX/TUJ1-positive neurons were primarily located at the hilar border of the GCL. Taken together, these data indicate that newborn neurons were especially vulnerable to SCA, particularly in the inner blade facing the lesion site. Moreover, it is noteworthy to mention that after HBOT, a robust increase of DCX/TUJ1-immunoreactivity, which was widely distributed around the lesion site, was seen (Figure 5M–O, green asterisks).

2.4. Proliferation of Ki67-Positive Newborn Immature Neurons Co-Labeled with DCX in the SGZ of the Hippocampal DG Following SCA Injury and HBOT

To evaluate the proliferative cells of the neuronal lineage in the SGZ of the hippocampal DG after the SCA and HBOT, we performed double immunofluorescent staining with Ki67 (a marker of cell division, red fluorescence), and DCX (a marker of immature neurons, green fluorescence). We counted the number of cells with ongoing proliferation along the entire length of the SGZ of the DG in control, SCA, and SCA + HBO brain sections. Counted cells were either Ki67+/DCX+ (yellow fluorescence, Figure 6A,D,G,J), DCX+ (green fluorescence, Figure 6B,E,H,K), or Ki67+ (red fluorescence, Figure 6C,F,I,L). The results revealed that in all the investigated groups, the majority of cells were DCX-positive. Ki67-positive cells were located predominantly in the SGZ and hilus, irrespective of the investigated group. As expected, the Ki67 signal was restricted to the nuclei of cells (red fluorescence, Figure 6A,C, inset). In contrast, the DCX signal was found mainly in the cell cytosol (green fluorescence, Figure 6, inset to A,B) and the cellular processes arising from the SGZ until the MOL (green fluorescence, Figure 6A,B,G,H, arrowheads). It is important to note that HBOT increased the number of neurons with processes protruding until the molecular cell layer (Figure 6G,H) in contrast to SCA sections (Figure 6D,E), where this was only occasionally seen. Moreover, HBOT increased Ki67-stained cells in the SGZ, hilus, and MOL (Figure 6I, asterisk). When quantified, we demonstrated that SCA radically reduced the number of all counted cells. Compared to the control, the number of Ki67+ cells co-expressing DCX+ decreased by 58.7% (yellow fluorescence, Figure 6J), DCX+ cells by 61.47% (green fluorescence, Figure 6K), and Ki67+ cells by 31.11% (red fluorescence, Figure 6L). In contrast to SCA, after HBOT, the number of Ki67-expressing DCX-positive progenitors was slightly (6.52%) increased compared to controls (yellow fluorescence, Figure 6J), while the number of Ki67+ cells was increased by 22.22% (red fluorescence, Figure 6L). The number of DCX+ cells in the SCA + HBO group was slightly decreased (3.67%) vs. the control group. Next, we determined the fraction of dividing Ki67-expressing progenitors in all the investigated groups. In all the investigated groups of animals, control, SCA, and SCA + HBO, almost the same number of DCX-positive cells co-expressed Ki67 (42.2%, 45.2%, and 46.7%, respectively), being the largest in the HBOT group, where around half of all DCX-positive cells were proliferating immature neurons (Ki67+/DCX+). These results suggest that SCA reduced the number of proliferating and total DCX-expressing progenitors and all Ki67-positive cells. In contrast, HBOT increased the number of proliferating cells after the SCA injury.

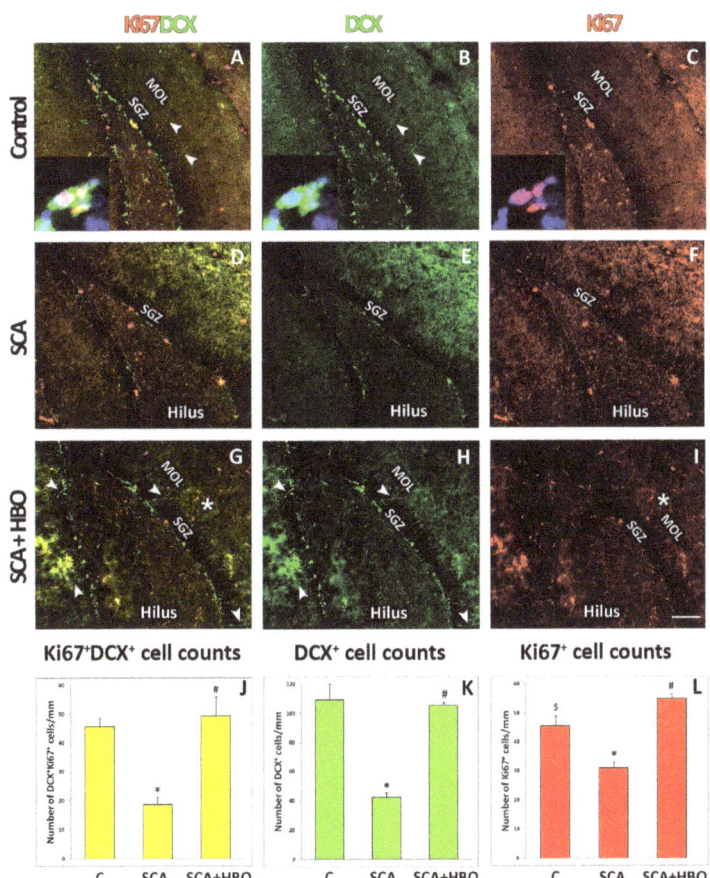

Figure 6. Effect of SCA (suction cortical ablation) and HBOT (hyperbaric oxygen therapy) on cell proliferation in the hippocampal DG (dentate gyrus). The proliferation marker Ki67 was used to quantify the number of dividing cells (red fluorescence), while DCX (a marker of immature neurons, green fluorescence) was used to identify cells of neuronal lineage. The higher magnification images of control sections were counterstained with DAPI (blue) to visualize cell nuclei. (**A–C**, inset) The Ki67 signal was restricted to the nuclei of cells (red fluorescence, **A,C** insert). In contrast, (**A,B**, inset), the DCX signal was mainly located in the cell cytosol (green fluorescence) and the cellular processes arising from the SGZ (subgranular zone) until the MOL (molecular cell layer) (green fluorescence, (**A,B**, arrowheads). SCA reduced Ki67+/DCX+ (**D**, yellow fluorescence), DCX+ (**E**, green fluorescence), and Ki67+ (**F**, red fluorescence) immunoreactivity in SGZ. In contrast, HBOT increased the number of DCX+ neurons with processes extending until the MOL (**G,H** arrowheads) and increased Ki67 cells in SGZ, hilus, and MOL (**I**, red fluorescence, asterisk). C—Control, SCA—Suction cortical ablation, SCA + HBO—SCA animals treated with hyperbaric oxygen. (**J–L**) Cells that were Ki67+/DCX+ (yellow fluorescence), DCX+ (green fluorescence), and Ki67+ (red fluorescence) were counted along the entire SGZ of the DG. While the number of all counted cells was drastically reduced after SCA, following HBOT, the number of proliferating immature neurons was at the same level as observed in the controls. In contrast, the overall proliferation of all Ki67-positive cells increased. Bars represent mean ± SD. The level of significance was analyzed using One-way ANOVA with Tukey's multiple comparisons post hoc test (* $p < 0.001$ SCA vs. C, $ $p < 0.001$ SCA + HBO vs. C, # $p < 0.001$ SCA + HBO vs. SCA). Scale bar 50 μm (**A–I**).

3. Discussion

Considering that adult hippocampal neurogenesis is restricted to only one part of the hippocampal formation, the dentate gyrus—DG [31], in this article, we investigate how hyperbaric oxygenation overcomes the impairments of neurogenesis in the adult DG caused by brain injury. The results show that our model of experimental cortical trauma, ablation of the sensorimotor cortex, causes a loss of DG neurons, mostly in the inner granular neuron layer of the inner blade underlying the lesion site. Analysis with cell-specific markers shows that mostly immature neurons of the subgranular layer of DG degenerate. We also demonstrate that injury leads to a reduction in dendrites branching of spared neurons. The most striking finding of this study is that HBOT prevents SCA-induced neuronal death in both the inner and outer blades of the granular layer of the DG. In addition, HBOT prevents the degeneration of dendrites and significantly reduces the loss of newborn immature neurons. Finally, using the endogenously expressed marker Ki67 to label and detect dividing cells and the marker of neuronal progenitors doublecortin (DCX), we demonstrate that SCA radically reduces the number of proliferating cells in SGZ, particularly those of neuronal lineage. Conversely, HBOT increases overall cell proliferation after SCA.

The experimental results on the effects of TBI on hippocampal neurogenesis are complex and seemingly contradictory [32–36]. An important factor contributing to these discrepancies is that different TBI models have other effects on neurogenesis in the adult hippocampus. To better understand how brain trauma can affect the generation of new neurons, which is a prerequisite for using this process to enhance brain repair, it is essential to examine the effects of different TBI models on hippocampal neurogenesis. For methodological reasons, many studies of the effects of TBI on the hippocampus focus on degenerating cells, changes in neurogenesis, and other morphological alterations that can be visualized by using immunostaining or other standard morphological techniques. The specific TBI lesion model, the suction-ablation of the sensorimotor cortex (SCA), that we use here has been thoroughly characterized previously [21,37,38]. SCA is a well-characterized model of focal traumatic brain injury, which permits highly reproducible lesions in the hindlimb sensorimotor cortex, uniform in size and depth [39]. The advantages of this type of cortex injury are well described in Goldstein's study [37]. Since the lesion is the result of actual removal of brain tissue, pathological events such as inflammatory responses and reactive gliosis are limited [39,40], while secondary processes associated with other types of injuries such as ischemia [41,42], concussive trauma [43], and electrolytic lesions [39] are minimized [37]. This type of injury mimics a clinical condition of immediate brain tissue removal, such as during surgical removal of brain tumors [44].

In our recently published paper, we applied the gray-level co-occurrence matrix algorithm for textural analysis of granular cell bodies to show that SCA resulted in subtle morphological changes in hippocampal DG neurons that could not be detected via classical immunohistochemical analysis [20]. In the present study, we report that SCA causes damage of hippocampal DG neurons, as shown by the reduction of NeuN immunoreactivity, which was used to predict neuronal degeneration in the rodent hippocampus after various brain injuries [26]. The extensive loss of granule cell neurons in this region indicates that the loss of neurons is the most prominent in the part of the granule cell layer below the lesion site. These changes in the GCL probably contribute to the injury-induced impairments of locomotor coordination observed in our previous publications [21,38,45]. Having found that SCA leads to a substantial loss of hippocampal cells, as shown by thinning of the neuronal layers, we want to specify which part of the GCL is most affected. In this way, our results reveal that SCA leads to specific damage of the hippocampus and predominantly affects neurons in the inner-third layer of the inner blade of the GCL. Our findings are consistent with the results of other studies on different animal models of TBI, which also reported that hippocampal neurons are particularly vulnerable to brain injury [32,35,46–48]. On the other hand, Becerra et al. [49] have recently shown that controlled cortical impact (CCI) injury causes the loss of neurons in the CA3 region and relative preserves neurons in the GCL, but they did not quantify NeuN+ cells in this region as we did. Indeed, we quantified NeuN fluorescence intensity in the suprapyramidal (inner) and infrapyramidal (outer) blades of the hippocampal DG of control, SCA, and HBO animals and found massive neuronal loss in both the inner (42%) and outer (26%) blades of the DG after SCA injury. In contrast, after HBOT, this effect of SCA is almost completely attenuated. Our results are consistent with those of Baratz and colleagues, who found that HBOT prevents neuronal loss in the blades of the DG [50].

The distribution and extent of cell death in the hippocampus have been shown to vary depending on the injury model [46,51,52], severity of injury [53,54], and age [55]. Moreover, many studies have shown that neurogenesis increases in a time-dependent manner after brain injury depending on the severity of injury [56,57]. Interestingly, our model eliciting a relatively extensive injury shows a similar specific impairment of adult hippocampal neurogenesis as more moderate CCI injury models [32,58]. By combining FJB-staining and double immunofluorescence staining with specific cell-type markers, we demonstrate that predominantly newborn neurons of the SGZ of the hippocampal DG are affected by SCA. To confirm that these progenitor cells are of neuronal lineage, we use DCX, a marker for putative newborn immature neurons [28]. The quantification of DCX-expressing cells shows that the number of DCX-positive immature neurons is significantly reduced (by more than 50%) in the inner blade compared with the control animals and to a lesser extent, but still remarkably (by about 40%) in the outer blade of the DG after the SCA. Our observations are in line with those of other authors who also reported that DCX-expressing neural progenitors are vulnerable to brain injury and undergo cell death in the ipsilateral DG [32,34,36,58]. Light microscope examination of stained sections revealed that spared DCX-positive immature neurons, despite their survival, exhibit a substantial injury-induced alteration of their morphology, manifested by dendritic shrinkage and a considerable reduction in dendritic arborization. Similarly, Villasana et al. also found abnormal dendritic branching after TBI [59]. This significant dendrite damage, accompanied by a reduction in dendritic spines, may represent a potential anatomical substrate that explains, at least in part, the development of posttraumatic memory deficits [35,48]. In contrast, we have shown that 10 consecutive HBOT prevents the loss of these DCX-expressing neural progenitors, ameliorates the observed SCA-caused changes in the SGZ of DG, and protects their morphology. Taken together, our data suggest that HBOT can overcome the harmful effects of SCA and protect newborn neurons from death and morphological deterioration.

To identify the cell type of neurons undergoing degeneration in the SGZ layer of hippocampal DG, we performed double immunofluorescence staining using DCX as a marker for early newborn immature neurons and beta-III tubulin (TUJ1), which is expressed during hippocampal neurogenesis after DCX and labels newly formed postmitotic neurons [29,30]. After the SCA injury, the reduced DCX/TUJ1-immunoreactivity in the SGZ of the DG inner blade facing the lesion site confirms our observations mentioned above that SCA triggers selective death of immature neurons. We also demonstrate that the development of newborn DCX/TUJ1-positive neurons occurs not only in the SGZ layer of the DG but also in the inner- and outer-thirds of the granule cell layer. Interestingly, in the hilus, we found that in addition to the neurons with round/oval morphology, which were only TUJ1-positive, some of them were also DCX/TUJ1-positive. These DCX/TUJ1-positive neurons are primarily located at the hilar border of the granule cell layer and deep in the hilus and are present in all the groups regardless of the treatment protocol. It is suggested that cells with round/oval shape are neuroblasts that are generated in the hilus and migrate to the SGZ and inner part of the GCL to increase the population of neuronal progenitors [60]. They proposed that a substantial population of these hilar progenitors should differentiate into proliferative neuroblasts and immature neurons within the hilus, probably via transitional intermediate cells expressing both astrocytic and neuronal markers. Ten repetitive HBOTs prevent the loss of DCX/TUJ1-positive immature neurons located in the SGZ layer of the inner and outer blades and increase the appearance of progenitors in the hilus. In addition, it is important to note that, after HBOT, DCX/TUJ1-immunoreactivity is abundantly distributed around the lesion site, suggesting that HBOT also increases the number of neuronal progenitors in the peri-lesioned region. However, it is unclear whether these newly generated neurons proliferate locally at the injury site and/or migrate from neurogenic regions along migratory pathways, extending from the SVZ or SGZ to the lesion site, as suggested by some authors [34,61,62].

Finally, we quantify the number of proliferating cells [4] after SCA and HBOT in the subgranular zone of the DG. Immunostaining analysis reveals radically reduced DCX/Ki67-positivity after SCA, particularly in the inner blade of the DG below the lesion site. These observations confirm the results of cell population quantification, showing that after SCA, the fractions of actively dividing neuronal precursors (Ki67/DCX double-positive) and total DCX-expressing progenitors are significantly reduced (by 60%) in the ipsilateral DG. Interestingly, the number of Ki67-labelled cells is reduced to a lesser extent, indicating that some cell populations are unaffected by SCA. These cells are mainly located in the hilus, and most of them do not co-express DCX, suggesting they probably belong to the glial lineage. Our assumption is consistent with the results of Colicos et al. [47], who found that brain injury does not affect the number of astrocytes and oligodendrocytes. Moreover, Liu et al. [63] suggested that the glial fibrillary acidic protein (GFAP)-positive progenitors in the SGZ of the DG give rise to neuronal progenitors that develop into granule neurons. In contrast to SCA, HBOT administration increases overall cell proliferation in the DG, with the proportion of DCX+/Ki67+ proliferating immature neurons accounting for approximately 50% of all DCX-expressing progenitors. Our results are consistent with the observations of Wei et al. [64], who reported that hyperbaric oxygenation promotes neural stem cell proliferation and protects learning and memory in neonatal hypoxic-ischemic brain damage.

Since our knowledge about the exact mechanisms by which HBOT exerts its beneficial effects still needs to be improved, in our recently published review [16], we summarized up-to-date results of potential cellular and molecular mechanisms underlying the beneficial effects of HBOT. We hypothesize that many of these cellular and molecular mechanisms and signaling pathways work in parallel or together, contributing to the establishment of a stimulating local environment that enhances neurogenesis, thereby allowing tissue repair and the recovery of impaired brain functions.

In conclusion, this study shows that SCA not only causes neuronal loss, but also induces remarkable dendritic degeneration of spared neurons and a reduction in proliferation of progenitor cells. In contrast, treatment with HBO prevents the loss and morphological deterioration of immature neurons, promotes the overall proliferation of progenitors, and thus has the potential to improve neurogenesis in the adult hippocampal DG affected by TBI. According to the literature and our results, adequate rehabilitation of the TBI consequences requires a combination of different therapeutic procedures, among which hyperbaric oxygenation therapy seems promising. However, underlying mechanisms remain to be determined.

4. Materials and Methods

4.1. Animals

The experiment was performed on male Wister albino rats, which were 10 weeks old. Animals were housed in four per cage under standard environmental conditions (23 ± 2 °C, 50–60% relative humidity, 12:12 h light-dark cycle, and food and water ad libitum). Animals were randomly divided into groups: Control group (C; n = 6)—age-matched intact animals; Sham control (S; n = 6)—the rats that underwent the surgical procedure without opening the skull; SCA group (SCA; n = 7)—suction ablation of the right sensorimotor cortex; HBO group (SCA + HBO; n = 6)—the rats that were subjected to the HBO protocol after SCA. There was no significant difference within and between the groups considering the animal body weight (250 ± 30 g). Experimental procedures were approved by the Ethical Committee of the University of Belgrade (No. 61206-2915/2-20). They were carried out in strict accordance with Directive 2010/63/EU on the protection of animals used for scientific purposes. Furthermore, all potential problems were considered to keep animal suffering to a minimum.

4.2. Surgical Procedure

Our previously published work describes the surgical procedure in detail [21]. Before the surgery, the rats were anaesthetized with an intraperitoneal injection of Zoletil®50 (Virbac, Carros, France) at 50 mg/kg body weight. After providing the anesthesia, rats were shaved and placed into the stereotaxic frame. The scalp was cut with a scalpel along the midline to expose the bregma. The craniotomy coordinates were: 2 mm anterior to the bregma, 4 mm posterior to the bregma, and 4 mm lateral from the midline [64]. The suction ablation of the right sensorimotor cortex was carefully carried out through a polypropylene tip to the depth of white matter with the purpose of keeping the white matter layer intact, thus separating the lesion cavity from the underlying hippocampus. Dura and the bone flap were returned to the place, and the skin was sutured. After the surgery, the rats from the SCA + HBO group were left to recover for up to 5 h before the hyperbaric oxygen treatment.

4.3. Hyperbaric Oxygen Treatment

The rats in the SCA + HBO group were placed into experimental HBO chambers (Holywell Neopren, Belgrade, Serbia) and exposed to 100% oxygen according to the following protocol: 10 min compression, 2.5 atmospheres absolute (ATA), for 60 min, and 10 min decompression. In addition, hyperbaric oxygen treatment (HBOT) was performed once daily for 10 successive days. This protocol represents the hyperbaric oxygen treatment that is routinely used in the clinical setting of The Centre for Hyperbaric Medicine, Belgrade, Serbia [21,65].

4.4. Brain Tissue Preparation

After the ending of HBOT, animals from all the groups were overdosed with CO_2 and decapitated. The brains were dissected and fixed at +4 °C in 4% paraformaldehyde overnight. After fixation, the brains were cryoprotected with immersion in graded sucrose solutions (10%, 20%, and 30% in 0.2 M phosphate buffer pH 7.4) at +4 °C followed by freezing in isopentane cooled to −80 °C. Using a cryostat, the brains were cut into 25-μm thick coronal slices. Afterward, sections at 3.12–3.84 mm anteroposterior to the bregma were mounted on glass slides, air-dried at room temperature, and maintained at −20 °C, until following procedures.

4.5. Immunohistochemistry and Immunofluorescence Staining

Single peroxidase immunohistochemistry was performed to visualize DCX as a marker of newborn neurons to determine the effect of SCA on the immature neurons' vulnerability in the hippocampal DG. Heated citrate buffer (pH 6) was used as antigen retrieval. Sections were washed in PBS and then incubated in 0.3% H_2O_2 in methanol for 20 min to block endogenous peroxidase. Normal donkey serum (NDS; 5% solution in PBS; Sigma, Munich, Germany) was used to block unspecific binding. Sections were incubated overnight at 4 °C with an anti-DCX antibody. After using the appropriate primary and peroxidase-linked secondary antibody, the products of immunoreactions were visualized with 3′3-diaminobenzidine (DAB, Dako, Glostrup, Denmark) according to manufacturer instructions. All sections were dehydrated in graded ethanol, cleared in xylene, and mounted in DPX Mounting medium (Sigma-Aldrich, Munich, Germany).

Visualization of TUJ1, a cell marker of neurons from the early stage of neural differentiation, and Ki67, widely accepted as a cell proliferation marker, was performed using double immunofluorescent staining. First, microscopic slides were incubated in 5% NDS with 0.5% Triton X-100 (Sigma-Aldrich, Darmstadt, Germany). After that, sections were incubated overnight with the appropriate primary antibody at +4 °C and with the appropriate secondary for 2 h at room temperature. Immune complexes were visualized after incubation with the secondary antibody.

The double immunofluorescence staining with Fluoro-Jade B (FJB) and Neuronal nuclear antigen (NeuN) was performed as previously described by Parabucki et al. [11]. NeuN was used as a marker of mature neurons. Briefly, sections were first incubated overnight at +4 °C with the primary antibody, and the immune reaction was visualized with a proper secondary antibody. Then, sections were pretreated with a 0.06% potassium permanganate solution for 5 min and incubated with 0.0004% solution of FJB (Chemicon International, Temecula, CA, USA) dissolved in 0.1% acetic acid for 20 min. In addition, sections were counterstained with DAPI (Invitrogen, Grand Island, NY, USA).

The list of the used primary and secondary antibodies is shown in Table 2.

Table 2. The list of the primary and secondary antibodies used for immunohistochemistry and immunofluorescence staining.

Antibody	Source	Dilution	Company
doublecortin	Goat	1:200	Santa Cruz Biotechnology, Santa Cruz, CA, USA
TUJ1	mouse	1:400	Abcam, Cambridge, MA, USA
NeuN	mouse	1:200	Milipore, Burlington, MA, USA
Ki67	rabbit	1:100	Vector Laboratories, Burlingame, CA, USA
anti-goat HRP conjugated IgG	donkey	1:200	Santa Cruz Biotechnology, Santa Cruz, CA, USA
anti-goat Alexa Fluor 488	donkey	1:200	Invitrogen (Eugene, OR, USA)
anti-mouse Alexa Fluor 555	donkey	1:200	Invitrogen (Eugene, OR, USA)
anti-rabbit Alexa Fluor 555	donkey	1:200	Invitrogen (Eugene, OR, USA)

All micrographs of stained sections were made using a Carl Zeiss AxioVert microscope (Zeiss, Gottingen, Germany) at the following magnifications: 5×, 10×, 20×, 40×, and 63×.

4.6. Quantification of Immunoreactive Cells

Quantification of DCX+ cells was done along the length of the SGZ in the inner and separately in the outer blade of the right dentate gyrus [65]. At the micrographs, DCX-positive cells were easily noticeable and were counted manually. The ImageJ open-source platform (National Institutes of Health, USA; http://imagej.nih.gov/ij/download.html, accessed on 30 January 2022) was used to determine the length of the SGZ. The number of marked cells was expressed per 1 mm of the length of the SGZ.

DCX+, Ki67+, and DCX+/Ki67+ cells were quantified along the entire length of the SGZ of the DG in control, SCA, and SCA + HBO brain sections of the DG. Two independent observers manually counted the total number of single and double-positive cells at corresponding channels using Adobe Photoshop Creative Cloud (Version 14.0). The percentage of single- or double-positive cell populations was also calculated and presented.

NeuN immunoreactivity was quantified in an area of interest, which was defined within the inner and outer blades of the right DG (180 × 180 pixels). Raw immunofluorescent micrographs of the DG were taken under the same conditions at a 20× magnification using a Carl Zeiss AxioVert microscope (Zeiss, Gottingen, Germany) and then used to measure integrated fluorescence density (Figure S1). Integrated density was calculated separately for the inner and outer blades of the DG. After conversion into an 8-bit grayscale format, post-image processing was conducted using ImageJ open-source platform. For more details, see the Supplementary Material.

All images of the selected neurons, placed in the outer blade, were taken under 40× magnification for graphic processing. A total of five neurons were studied for each animal in different experimental groups. These images have been processed in the ImageJ open-source platform to analyze the dendritic arborization and total length of the dendrites in the obtained binary images. We counted the number of branching points, dendrite terminals, and segments to quantify dendritic arborization in each neuron. After converting the taken pictures into binary and skeletonized images for measuring the total dendritic length, we used ImageJ macro called measure skeleton length. The average segmental length represents a ratio between the total dendritic length and the number of segments [66].

4.7. Statistical Analysis

Statistical Package for the Social Sciences (SPSS; IBM, version 22.0, Armonk, NY, USA) was used for the data analysis. First, the normal distribution of data was tested using the Shapiro-Wilk test. All values are expressed as mean ± standard deviation (SD). Differences between the groups were estimated using One-way ANOVA with Tukey's multiple comparisons post hoc test. Group differences were assessed using the Independent-Samples T-test. Statistical significance was set at $p < 0.05$, $p < 0.01$, and $p < 0.001$.

Supplementary Materials: The following supporting information can be downloaded at: https://www.mdpi.com/article/10.3390/ijms24054261/s1.

Author Contributions: Conceptualization: R.J., S.P., P.B. and S.D.; animal surgery and HBOT administration: S.P., S.D., P.B. and R.J.; immunohistochemistry and microscopy: S.D. and R.J.; software, R.J., S.D. and S.P.; statistical analysis: R.J.; visualization: S.P.; data analysis and manuscript writing: R.J. and S.P.; manuscript review and editing: P.B., I.L., I.B. and M.D.; supervision/mentoring and funding acquisition: P.B. and S.D.; project administration: R.J. All authors have read and agreed to the published version of the manuscript.

Funding: This research was supported by grants from the Ministry of Science, Technological Development and Innovations of the Republic of Serbia (No. 200110 and No. 451-03-47/2023-01/200007).

Institutional Review Board Statement: The study was conducted in accordance with the Declaration of Helsinki, and experimental procedures were approved by the Ethical Committee of the University of Belgrade (No. 61206-2915/2-20, 22 September 2020), University of Belgrade, and were carried out in strict accordance with recommendations given by the Directive 2010/63/EU on the protection of animals used for scientific purposes.

Informed Consent Statement: Not applicable.

Data Availability Statement: The data presented in this study are available in article and Supplementary Material.

Acknowledgments: The authors are grateful to Center for Hyperbaric Medicine, Belgrade, Serbia.

Conflicts of Interest: The authors declare no conflict of interest.

References

1. Owji, S.; Shoja, M.M. The History of Discovery of Adult Neurogenesis. *Clin. Anat.* **2020**, *33*, 41–55. [CrossRef] [PubMed]
2. Jorgensen, C. Adult mammalian neurogenesis and motivated behaviors. *Integr. Zool.* **2018**, *13*, 655–672. [CrossRef] [PubMed]
3. La Rosa, C.; Parolisi, R.; Bonfanti, L. Brain Structural Plasticity: From Adult Neurogenesis to Immature Neurons. *Front. Neurosci.* **2020**, *14*, 75. [CrossRef] [PubMed]
4. Mensching, L.; Djogo, N.; Keller, C.; Rading, S.; Karsak, M. Stable adult hippocampal neurogenesis in cannabinoid receptor CB2 deficient mice. *Int. J. Mol. Sci.* **2019**, *20*, 3759. [CrossRef]
5. Yu, T.S.; Washington, P.M.; Kernie, S.G. Injury-Induced Neurogenesis: Mechanisms and Relevance. *Neuroscientist* **2016**, *22*, 61–71. [CrossRef]
6. Kempermann, G.; Gage, F.H.; Aigner, L.; Song, H.; Curtis, M.A.; Thuret, S.; Kuhn, H.G.; Jessberger, S.; Frankland, P.W.; Cameron, H.A.; et al. Human Adult Neurogenesis: Evidence and Remaining Questions. *Cell Stem Cell* **2018**, *23*, 25–30. [CrossRef]
7. Rubiano, A.M.; Carney, N.; Chesnut, R.; Puyana, J.C. Global neurotrauma research challenges and opportunities. *Nature* **2015**, *527*, S193–S197. [CrossRef]
8. Feigin, V.L.; Nichols, E.; Alam, T.; Bannick, M.S.; Beghi, E.; Blake, N.; Culpepper, W.J.; Dorsey, E.R.; Elbaz, A.; Ellenbogen, R.G.; et al. Global, regional, and national burden of neurological disorders, 1990–2016: A systematic analysis for the Global Burden of Disease Study 2016. *Lancet Neurol.* **2019**, *18*, 459–480. [CrossRef]
9. Ng, S.Y.; Lee, A.Y.W. Traumatic Brain Injuries: Pathophysiology and Potential Therapeutic Targets. *Front. Cell. Neurosci.* **2019**, *13*, 528. [CrossRef]
10. Brkić, P.; Sanja, P.; Danijela, K.; Jovanović, T. Hyperbaric oxygenation as an adjuvant therapy for traumatic brain injury: A review of literature. *Period. Biol.* **2014**, *116*, 29–36.

11. Parabucki, A.B.; Božić, I.D.; Bjelobaba, I.M.; Lavrnja, I.C.; Brkić, P.D.; Jovanović, T.S.; Savić, D.Z.; Stojiljković, M.B.; Peković, S.M. Hyperbaric oxygenation alters temporal expression pattern of superoxide dismutase 2 after cortical stab injury in rats. *Croat. Med. J.* **2012**, *53*, 586–597. [CrossRef] [PubMed]
12. Pekovic, S.; Subasic, S.; Nedeljkovic, N.; Bjelobaba, I.; Filipovic, R.; Milenkovic, I.; Lavrnja, I.; Stojkov, D.; Jovanovic, S.; Rakic, L.; et al. Molecular basis of brain injury and repair. In *Neurobiological Studies—From Genes to Behavior*; Ruzdijic, S., Rakic, L.J., Eds.; Research Signpost: Kerala, India, 2006; pp. 143–165. ISBN 81-308-0107-8.
13. Capizzi, A.; Woo, J.; Verduzco-Gutierrez, M. Traumatic Brain Injury: An Overview of Epidemiology, Pathophysiology, and Medical Management. *Med. Clin. N. Am.* **2020**, *104*, 213–238. [CrossRef] [PubMed]
14. Terranova, J.I.; Ogawa, S.K.; Kitamura, T. Adult hippocampal neurogenesis for systems consolidation of memory. *Behav. Brain Res.* **2019**, *372*, 112035. [CrossRef] [PubMed]
15. Margulies, S.; Hicks, R. Combination therapies for traumatic brain injury: Prospective considerations. *J. Neurotrauma* **2009**, *26*, 925–939. [CrossRef]
16. Pekovic, S.; Dacic, S.; Krstic, D.; Jeremic, R.; Djelic, M.; Brkic, P. Hyperbaric oxygen therapy in traumatic brain injury: Cellular and molecular mechanisms. In *Hyperbaric Oxygen Treatment in Research and Clinical Practice—Mechanisms of Action in Focus*; Drenjančević, I., Ed.; InTechOpen: Rijeka, Croatia, 2018; pp. 25–46. ISBN 978-953-51-5916-2. [CrossRef]
17. De Wolde, S.D.; Hulskes, R.H.; Weenink, R.P.; Hollmann, M.W.; Van Hulst, R.A. The effects of hyperbaric oxygenation on oxidative stress, inflammation and angiogenesis. *Biomolecules* **2021**, *11*, 1210. [CrossRef]
18. Daly, S.; Thorpe, M.; Rockswold, S.; Hubbard, M.; Bergman, T.; Samadani, U.; Rockswold, G. Hyperbaric Oxygen Therapy in the Treatment of Acute Severe Traumatic Brain Injury: A Systematic Review. *J. Neurotrauma* **2018**, *35*, 623–629. [CrossRef]
19. Manivannan, S.; Marei, O.; Elalfy, O.; Zaben, M. Neurogenesis after traumatic brain injury—The complex role of HMGB1 and neuroinflammation. *Neuropharmacology* **2021**, *183*, 108400. [CrossRef]
20. Pantic, I.; Jeremic, R.; Dacic, S.; Pekovic, S.; Pantic, S.; Djelic, M.; Vitic, Z.; Brkic, P.; Brodski, C. Gray-Level Co-Occurrence Matrix Analysis of Granule Neurons of the Hippocampal Dentate Gyrus Following Cortical Injury. *Microsc. Microanal.* **2020**, *26*, 166–172. [CrossRef]
21. Brkic, P.; Stojiljkovic, M.; Jovanovic, T.; Dacic, S.; Lavrnja, I.; Savic, D.; Parabucki, A.; Bjelobaba, I.; Rakic, L.; Pekovic, S. Hyperbaric oxygenation improves locomotor ability by enhancing neuroplastic responses after cortical ablation in rats. *Brain Inj.* **2012**, *26*, 1273–1284. [CrossRef]
22. Hu, Q.; Manaenko, A.; Xu, T.; Guo, Z.; Tang, J.; Zhang, J.H. Hyperbaric oxygen therapy for traumatic brain injury: Bench-to-bedside. *Med. Gas Res.* **2016**, *6*, 102–110. [CrossRef]
23. Shandley, S.; Wolf, E.G.; Schubert-Kabban, C.M.; Baugh, L.M.; Richards, M.F.; Prye, J.; Arizpe, H.M.; Kalns, J. Increased circulating stem cells and better cognitive performance in traumatic brain injury subjects following hyperbaric oxygen therapy. *Undersea Hyperb. Med.* **2017**, *44*, 257–269. [CrossRef] [PubMed]
24. Mu, J.; Krafft, P.R.; Zhang, J.H. Hyperbaric oxygen therapy promotes neurogenesis: Where do we stand? *Med. Gas Res.* **2011**, *1*, 14. [CrossRef] [PubMed]
25. Kempermann, G.; Gast, D.; Kronenberg, G.; Yamaguchi, M.; Gage, F.H. Early determination and long-term persistence of adult-generated new neurons in the hippocampus of mice. *Development* **2003**, *130*, 391–399. [CrossRef] [PubMed]
26. Collombet, J.M.; Masqueliez, C.; Four, E.; Burckhart, M.F.; Bernabé, D.; Baubichon, D.; Lallement, G. Early reduction of NeuN antigenicity induced by soman poisoning in mice can be used to predict delayed neuronal degeneration in the hippocampus. *Neurosci. Lett.* **2006**, *398*, 337–342. [CrossRef]
27. Amaral, D.G.; Scharfman, H.E.; Lavenex, P. The dentate gyrus: Fundamental neuroanatomical organization (dentate gyrus for dummies). *Prog. Brain Res.* **2007**, *163*, 3–22. [CrossRef]
28. Couillard-Despres, S.; Winner, B.; Schaubeck, S.; Aigner, R.; Vroemen, M.; Weidner, N.; Bogdahn, U.; Winkler, J.; Kuhn, H.G.; Aigner, L. Doublecortin expression levels in adult brain reflect neurogenesis. *Eur. J. Neurosci.* **2005**, *21*, 1–14. [CrossRef]
29. Von Bohlen Und Halbach, O. Immunohistological markers for staging neurogenesis in adult hippocampus. *Cell Tissue Res.* **2007**, *329*, 409–420. [CrossRef]
30. Korzhevskii, D.E.; Karpenko, M.N.; Kirik, O.V. Microtubule-Associated Proteins as Indicators of Differentiation and the Functional State of Nerve Cells. *Neurosci. Behav. Physiol.* **2012**, *42*, 215–222. [CrossRef]
31. Kempermann, G. What Is Adult Hippocampal Neurogenesis Good for? *Front. Neurosci.* **2022**, *16*, 852680. [CrossRef]
32. Chen, J. Selective Death of Newborn Neurons in Hippocampal Dentate Gyrus Following Moderate Experimental Traumatic Brain Injury. *J. Neurosci. Res.* **2008**, *86*, 2258–2270. [CrossRef]
33. Gao, X.; Enikolopov, G.; Chen, J. Moderate traumatic brain injury promotes proliferation of quiescent neural progenitors in the adult hippocampus. *Exp. Neurol.* **2009**, *219*, 516–523. [CrossRef] [PubMed]
34. Coates, D.R.; Chin, J.M.; Chung, S.T.L. Forebrain Neurogenesis after Focal Ischemic and Traumatic Brain. *Bone* **2011**, *23*, 1–7. [CrossRef]
35. Gao, X.; Deng, P.; Xu, Z.C.; Chen, J. Moderate traumatic brain injury causes acute dendritic and synaptic degeneration in the hippocampal dentate gyrus. *PLoS ONE* **2011**, *6*, e24566. [CrossRef] [PubMed]
36. Wang, X.; Gao, X.; Michalski, S.; Zhao, S.; Chen, J. Traumatic Brain Injury Severity Affects Neurogenesis in Adult Mouse Hippocampus. *J. Neurotrauma* **2016**, *33*, 721–733. [CrossRef] [PubMed]
37. Goldstein, L.B. Model of recovery of locomotor ability after sensorimotor cortex injury in rats. *ILAR J.* **2003**, *44*, 125–129. [CrossRef]

38. Lavrnja, I.; Trifunovic, S.; Ajdzanovic, V.; Pekovic, S.; Bjelobaba, I.; Stojiljkovic, M.; Milosevic, V. Sensorimotor cortex ablation induces time-dependent response of ACTH cells in adult rats: Behavioral, immunohistomorphometric and hormonal study. *Physiol. Behav.* **2014**, *125*, 30–37. [CrossRef]
39. Szele, F.G.; Alexander, C.; Chesselet, M.F. Expression of molecules associated with neuronal plasticity in the striatum after aspiration and thermocoagulatory lesions of the cerebral cortex in adult rats. *J. Neurosci.* **1995**, *15*, 4429–4448. [CrossRef]
40. Pearlson, G.D.; Robinson, R.G. Suction lesions of the frontal cerebral cortex in the rat induce assymetrical behavioral and catecholaminergic responses. *Brain Res.* **1981**, *218*, 233–242. [CrossRef]
41. Pulsinelli, W.A.; Brierley, J.B.; Plum, F. Temporal profile of neuronal damage in a model of transient forebrain ischemia. *Ann. Neurol.* **1982**, *11*, 491–498. [CrossRef]
42. Saunders, D.E.; Howe, F.A.; Van den Boogaart, A.; McLean, M.A.; Griffiths, J.R.; Brown, M.M. Continuing ischemic damage after acute middle cerebral artery infarction in humans demonstrated by short-echo proton spectroscopy. *Stroke* **1995**, *26*, 1007–1013. [CrossRef] [PubMed]
43. Povlishock, J.T.; Erb, D.E.; Arstruc, J. Axonal response to traumatic brain injury: Reactive axonal change, deafferentation, and neuroplasticity. *J. Neurotrauma* **1992**, *9*, S189–S200.
44. de Freitas, H.T.; da Silva, V.G.; Giraldi-Guimarães, A. Comparative study between bone marrowmononuclear fraction andmesenchymal stemcells treatment in sensorimotor recovery after focal cortical ablation in rats. *Behav. Brain Funct.* **2012**, *8*, 58. [CrossRef] [PubMed]
45. Lavrnja, I.; Ajdzanovic, V.; Trifunovic, S.; Savic, D.; Milosevic, V.; Stojiljkovic, M.; Pekovic, S. Cortical ablation induces time-dependent changes in rat pituitary somatotrophs and upregulates growth hormone receptor expression in the injured cortex. *J. Neurosci. Res.* **2014**, *92*, 1338–1349. [CrossRef] [PubMed]
46. Colicos, M.A.; Dash, P.K. Apoptotic morphology of dentate gyrus granule cells following experimental cortical impact injury in rats: Possible role in spatial memory deficits. *Brain Res.* **1996**, *739*, 120–131. [CrossRef] [PubMed]
47. Grady, M.S.; Charleston, J.S.; Maris, D.; Witgen, B.M.; Lifshitz, J. Neuronal and Glial Cell Number in the Hippocampus after Experimental Traumatic Brain Injury: Analysis by Stereological Estimation. *J. Neurotrauma* **2003**, *20*, 929–941. [CrossRef] [PubMed]
48. Winston, C.N.; Chellappa, D.; Wilkins, T.; Barton, D.J.; Washington, P.M.; Loane, D.J.; Zapple, D.N.; Burns, M.P. Controlled cortical impact results in an extensive loss of dendritic spines that is not mediated by injury-induced amyloid-beta accumulation. *J. Neurotrauma* **2013**, *30*, 1966–1972. [CrossRef] [PubMed]
49. Becerra, A.P.; Logsdon, A.F.; Banks, W.A.; Ransom, C.B. Traumatic brain injury broadly affects GABAergic signaling in dentate gyrus granule cells. *eNeuro* **2021**, *8*, 1–15. [CrossRef]
50. Baratz-Goldstein, R.; Toussia-Cohen, S.; Elpaz, A.; Rubovitch, V.; Pick, C.G. Immediate and delayed hyperbaric oxygen therapy as a neuroprotective treatment for traumatic brain injury in mice. *Mol. Cell. Neurosci.* **2017**, *83*, 74–82. [CrossRef]
51. Kelly, K.M. Modeling traumatic brain injury and posttraumatic epilepsy. *Epilepsy Curr.* **2004**, *4*, 160–161. [CrossRef]
52. Witgen, B.M.; Lifshitz, J.; Smith, M.L.; Schwarzbach, E.; Liang, S.L.; Grady, M.S.; Cohen, A.S. Regional hippocampal alteration associated with cognitive deficit following experimental brain injury: A systems, network and cellular evaluation. *Neuroscience* **2005**, *133*, 1–15. [CrossRef]
53. Markgraf, C.G.; Clifton, G.L.; Aguirre, M.; Chaney, S.F.; Bois, C.K.D.; Kennon, K.; Verma, N. Injury severity and sensitivity to treatment after controlled cortical impact in rats. *J. Neurotrauma* **2001**, *18*, 175–186. [CrossRef] [PubMed]
54. Hellmich, H.L.; Capra, B.; Eidson, K.; Garcia, J.; Kennedy, D.; Uchida, T.; Parsley, M.; Cowart, J.; DeWitt, D.S.; Prough, D.S. Dose-dependent neuronal injury after traumatic brain injury. *Brain Res.* **2005**, *1044*, 144–154. [CrossRef] [PubMed]
55. Tong, W.; Igarashi, T.; Ferriero, D.M.; Noble, L.J. Traumatic brain injury in the immature mouse brain: Characterization of regional vulnerability. *Exp. Neurol.* **2002**, *176*, 105–116. [CrossRef] [PubMed]
56. Ton, S.T.; Adamczyk, N.S.; Gerling, J.P.; Vaagenes, I.C.; Wu, J.Y.; Hsu, K.; O'Brien, T.E.; Tsai, S.Y.; Kartje, G.L. Dentate Gyrus Proliferative Responses After Traumatic Brain Injury and Binge Alcohol in Adult Rats. *Neurosci. Insights* **2020**, *15*, 1–13. [CrossRef] [PubMed]
57. Ngwenya, L.B.; Danzer, S.C. Impact of traumatic brain injury on neurogenesis. *Front. Neurosci.* **2019**, *13*, 1014. [CrossRef]
58. Yu, T.S.; Zhang, G.; Liebl, D.J.; Kernie, S.G. Traumatic brain injury-induced hippocampal neurogenesis requires activation of early nestin-expressing progenitors. *J. Neurosci.* **2008**, *28*, 12901–12912. [CrossRef] [PubMed]
59. Villasana, L.E.; Kim, K.N.; Westbrook, G.L.; Schnell, E. Functional integration of adult-born hippocampal neurons after traumatic brain injury. *eNeuro* **2015**, *2*, 1–17. [CrossRef]
60. Namba, T.; Mochizuki, H.; Onodera, M.; Mizuno, Y.; Namiki, H.; Seki, T. The fate of neural progenitor cells expressing astrocytic and radial glial markers in the postnatal rat dentate gyrus. *Eur. J. Neurosci.* **2005**, *22*, 1928–1941. [CrossRef]
61. Masuda, T.; Isobe, Y.; Aihara, N.; Furuyama, F.; Misumi, S.; Kim, T.S.; Nishino, H.; Hida, H. Increase in neurogenesis and neuroblast migration after a small intracerebral hemorrhage in rats. *Neurosci. Lett.* **2007**, *425*, 114–119. [CrossRef]
62. Zheng, W.; Zhuge, Q.; Zhong, M.; Chen, G.; Shao, B.; Wang, H.; Mao, X.; Xie, L.; Jin, K. Neurogenesis in adult human brain after traumatic brain injury. *J. Neurotrauma* **2013**, *30*, 1872–1880. [CrossRef]
63. Liu, Y.; Namba, T.; Liu, J.; Suzuki, R.; Shioda, S.; Seki, T. Glial fibrillary acidic protein-expressing neural progenitors give rise to immature neurons via early intermediate progenitors expressing both glial fibrillary acidic protein and neuronal markers in the adult hippocampus. *Neuroscience* **2010**, *166*, 241–251. [CrossRef]

64. Wei, L.; Wang, J.; Cao, Y.; Ren, Q.; Zhao, L.; Li, X.; Wang, J. Hyperbaric oxygenation promotes neural stem cell proliferation and protects the learning and memory ability in neonatal hypoxic-ischemic brain damage. *Int. J. Clin. Exp. Pathol.* **2015**, *8*, 1752–1759.
65. Brkic, P.; Mitrovic, A.; Rakic, M.; Grajic, M.; Jovanovic, T. Hyperbaric oxygen therapy of angiopathic changes in patients with inherited gene imbalance. *Srpski Arhiv za Celokupno Lekarstvo* **2007**, *135*, 669–671. [CrossRef]
66. Puškaš, N.; Zaletel, I.; Stefanović, B.D.; Ristanović, D. Fractal dimension of apical dendritic arborization differs in the superficial and the deep pyramidal neurons of the rat cerebral neocortex. *Neurosci. Lett.* **2015**, *589*, 88–91. [CrossRef]

Disclaimer/Publisher's Note: The statements, opinions and data contained in all publications are solely those of the individual author(s) and contributor(s) and not of MDPI and/or the editor(s). MDPI and/or the editor(s) disclaim responsibility for any injury to people or property resulting from any ideas, methods, instructions or products referred to in the content.

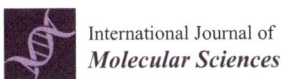

Article

Elevations of Extracellular Vesicles and Inflammatory Biomarkers in Closed Circuit SCUBA Divers

Awadhesh K. Arya [1], Costantino Balestra [2,3], Veena M. Bhopale [1], Laura J. Tuominen [3], Anne Räisänen-Sokolowski [3], Emmanuel Dugrenot [4,5], Erwan L'Her [6], Abid R. Bhat [1] and Stephen R. Thom [1,*]

[1] Department of Emergency Medicine, University of Maryland School of Medicine, Baltimore, MD 21201, USA
[2] Environmental, Occupational, Aging (Integrative) Physiology Laboratory, Haute Ecole Bruxelles-Brabant (HE2B), 1090 Brussels, Belgium
[3] DAN Europe Research Division, DAN Europe Foundation, 64026 Roseto degli Abruzzi, Italy
[4] Divers Alert Network, Durham, NC 27707, USA
[5] Laboratoire ORPHY, EA 4324, Université de Bretagne Occidentale UFR Science, 29238 Brest, France
[6] LaTIM INSERM UMR 1101, Université de Bretagne Occidentale UFR Science, 29238 Brest, France
* Correspondence: sthom@som.umaryland.edu

Abstract: Blood-borne extracellular vesicles and inflammatory mediators were evaluated in divers using a closed circuit rebreathing apparatus and custom-mixed gases to diminish some diving risks. "Deep" divers ($n = 8$) dove once to mean ($\pm$SD) 102.5 ± 1.2 m of sea water (msw) for 167.3 ± 11.5 min. "Shallow" divers ($n = 6$) dove 3 times on day 1, and then repetitively over 7 days to 16.4 ± 3.7 msw, for 49.9 ± 11.9 min. There were statistically significant elevations of microparticles (MPs) in deep divers (day 1) and shallow divers at day 7 that expressed proteins specific to microglia, neutrophils, platelets, and endothelial cells, as well as thrombospondin (TSP)-1 and filamentous (F-) actin. Intra-MP IL-1β increased by 7.5-fold ($p < 0.001$) after day 1 and 41-fold ($p = 0.003$) at day 7. Intra-MP nitric oxide synthase-2 (NOS2) increased 17-fold ($p < 0.001$) after day 1 and 19-fold ($p = 0.002$) at day 7. Plasma gelsolin (pGSN) levels decreased by 73% ($p < 0.001$) in deep divers (day 1) and 37% in shallow divers by day 7. Plasma samples containing exosomes and other lipophilic particles increased from 186% to 490% among the divers but contained no IL-1β or NOS2. We conclude that diving triggers inflammatory events, even when controlling for hyperoxia, and many are not proportional to the depth of diving.

Keywords: extracellular vesicles; exosomes; filamentous actin; decompression sickness; diving; hyperoxia; interleukin-1β; microglia; microparticles; nitric oxide synthase; plasma gelsolin

1. Introduction

The goal of this work was to improve the understanding of decompression sickness (DCS) pathophysiology. DCS is traditionally viewed as related to gas bubble formation from insoluble gas on decompression. However, the inconsistent presence of bubbles in human studies has prompted investigations that are focused instead on inflammatory pathways [1–3]. A body of work implicates a subset of extracellular vesicles (EVs), 0.1 to 1 μm microparticles (MPs), that are elevated in humans and rodent models exposed to high gas pressure and rise further after decompression [4–15]. MPs initiate a systemic inflammatory response related to neutrophil activation [13,16–18].

EVs are lipid bilayer-enclosed sub-cellular structures present in all bodily fluids that increase in association with inflammation [19]. EVs include exosomes (20–120 nm diameter particles generated by the endosomal pathway), 0.1–1 μm microparticles (MPs) generated by an outward budding of plasma membrane, and ~0.5–5 μm apoptotic bodies generated during cell self-destruction. Exosomes and MPs play roles in cell-to-cell communication due to their contents, which include nucleic acids, inflammatory mediators, and enzymes or organelles that generate free radicals [16,19–21].

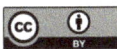

This study evaluated inflammatory biomarkers in response to open water diving conducted by human subjects using closed circuit rebreathing (CCR) apparatus. This differs from typical self-contained underwater breathing apparatus (SCUBA) gear because exhaled gases are recycled after carbon dioxide removal and oxygen supplementation. Oxygen partial pressure is kept within narrow limits through the operation of intrinsic sensors. Breathing air at a high pressure involves exposure to elevated partial pressures of oxygen, nitrogen, and other respired gases. CCR is often used with custom-mixed gases rather than air to diminish the risks of oxygen toxicity and nitrogen narcosis. Thus, our rationale was to evaluate EVs production and other manifestations of inflammation in a cadre of open-water divers, where some of the confounding variables posed by breathing air were diminished due to CCR utilization.

High pressures of nitrogen and noble gases such as helium and argon activate leukocytes via an oxidative stress process that triggers MPs production [22]. Exposure to high gas pressure and subsequent decompression pose a dual insult. Studies with human volunteers have demonstrated that while under pressure and before decompression, there are elevations in MPs number and those expressing filamentous (F-) actin on the membrane surface [5,23]. Similar responses occur in a murine DCS model, and when these MPs are purified and injected into naïve mice, they cause the same spectrum of injuries as seen in decompressed mice [13,15,23]. The second insult occurs because some MPs generated due to high gas pressure are enriched with inflammatory nitric oxide synthase (NOS)2. Enzyme activity within the MPs is responsible for generating a gas phase which provides a nucleation site for inert gas uptake on decompression. This causes MPs to enlarge, and they then cause vascular damage and neutrophil activation that can be abrogated by reversing particle enlargement [16–18].

The mechanism for the dual risk of MPs is related to neutrophil responses. As mentioned, some MPs formed in response to high gas pressures have F-actin on the surface. These particles will exacerbate MPs production because they trigger neutrophil auto-activation [24]. The rigidity caused by the MPs F-actin shell allows phosphatidylserine that is ubiquitously present in the MPs membrane to be recognized by a complex of receptors, including CD36, Toll-like receptor (TLR)4, and the receptor for advanced glycation end-products (RAGE). These proteins are linked to a scaffold protein called NOS1 adaptor protein. When the receptors bind to a MP, an increase in membrane colocalization occurs and NOS2 binds to the complex [24,25]. NOS2 facilitates S-nitrosylation of Src kinases and the cytoskeleton, resulting in formation of the nucleotide-binding domain leucine rich repeat (NOD)-like receptor, pyrin containing 3 (NLRP3) inflammasome. The NLRP3 inflammasome is responsible for producing mature interleukin (IL)-1β [15,22,25]. Inflammasome assembly correlates with MP production, and the MPs that contain high amounts of IL-1β are a factor in diffuse vascular damage in a murine DCS model [15,26]. It is unclear whether the MPs expressing F-actin are the same as those containing NOS2.

2. Results

2.1. Study Subjects and Protocol

This investigation involved two groups of CCR divers. One group of 8 deep divers performed a single dive to a mean depth of 102.5 ± 1.2 (SD) meters of sea water (msw) for 167.3 ± 11.5 min. The diluent gas in the CCR apparatus was a mixture of 10% oxygen, 20% nitrogen, and 70% helium (used to diminish the risk of nitrogen narcosis). A second group of 6 divers performed a series of 9 to 12 dives at lesser depths over a span of 7 days (termed shallow group) using a CCR apparatus with 18% nitrogen, 50% helium, and the balanced oxygen. All divers in this group did three dives on day one, to allow for comparisons with the deep divers, and repetitive dives for the subsequent week. The daily activity in this group is illustrated in Figure 1. The mean diving depth for the shallow group was 16.4 ± 3.7 msw, with a mean time of 49.9 ± 11.9 min. For both groups of divers, the CCR apparatus was set to maintain constant oxygen partial pressure at 120 kPa, and a built-in safety threshold kept the level greater than 140 kPa during the shallow return phase of dives (to accelerate inert gas removal). There were no diving mishaps and none of the 14 divers sustained signs or symptoms of DCS.

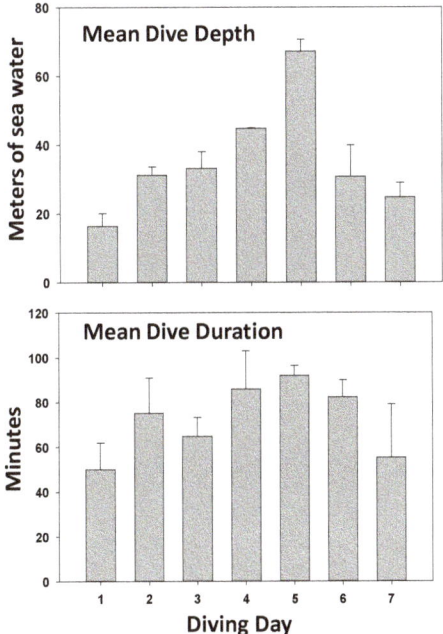

Figure 1. Diving activity in the shallow diver group. Data show diving depth and duration (mean ± SD) for the 6 individuals in the shallow diver group. On day 1, all performed 3 dives; on days 2 and 3, all performed 2 dives; on day 4, only 5 of 6 each performed one dive; on day 5, all 6 performed 1 dive; on day 6, three divers each performed 2 dives; and on day 7, four divers performed 2 dives.

2.2. Blood-Borne EVs Elicited by Diving

Blood counts are shown for MPs in Table 1. MPs were identified based on the size (0.1–1 μm) and surface expression of annexin V (which binds to phosphatidylserine, Table 1). In addition to the total number of particles, the expression of surface proteins on MPs originated from neutrophils (CD66b), platelets (CD41), endothelial cells (CD146), and microglia (TMEM119) were analyzed. To gain further insight into MPs, surface expression of thrombospondin-1 (TSP) and staining with phalloidin were also assessed. Phalloidin binding is an index of F-actin expression, and recent work in the murine model has indicated an inflammatory role for TSP-expressing MPs [27]. Both dive profiles caused significant elevations in total MPs, whereas only the deep divers also showed significant elevations in the various MPs subgroups, expressing cell-specific proteins after the first day of diving. However, after the 7-day course of repetitive diving, the shallow group divers exhibited significant elevations in subgroups versus pre-dive values (Table 1).

Exosomes were enumerated (Table 2), as described more extensively in Methods, as particles with diameters between 20 and 120 nm that were stained with lipophilic PKH67 dye, and subsets were analyzed for the expression of several tetraspanin proteins. The analysis involves an initial evaluation based on particle size, and additional steps are necessary to separate bilayer-enclosed particles from random debris. We used the PKH67 dye as our prime stain, which has been used by others [28]. In preliminary studies, we found PKH stained 52.1 ± 11.4% (n = 9) of all 20–120 nm diameter structures, whereas an alternative lipid stain, Laurdan, only detected 22.2 ± 6.9% in pre-diving samples. Laurdan detects changes in lipid phase properties through its sensitivity to bilayer polarity.

After diving, PKH stained 51.7 ± 19.2% (NS, versus pre-dive), whereas Laurdan stained 75.5 ± 5.2% ($p < 0.001$ versus pre-dive, t-test) of all 20 to 120 nm diameter particles. The Laurdan emission spectrum maximum is centered at 490 nm in a disordered (gel) phase and 430 nm in a packed (liquid crystalline phase) [29]. When selecting 20 to 120 nm PKH-staining particles, prior to diving 41.3 ± 26.0% also stain with Laurdan, but after diving all stained positive (the bandpass filter allowed passage of 457 ± 45 nm light).

Table 1. Microparticles in blood. Flow cytometry was used to evaluate MPs. Total MPs/μL plasma is shown in the first column, and other columns show the percent of each that expressed proteins specific to different cells, including neutrophils (CD66b), endothelial cells (CD146), platelets (CD41a), and microglia (transmembrane protein 119, TMEM). As discussed in the text, proteins expressing TSP-1 and F-actin, evaluated as those binding phalloidin, were also assessed. Rows show values for divers in the deep group prior to their dive and after the ~100 m dive. The next three rows show results for divers in the shallow group prior to their first dive, after the first day of 3 dives, and after the last of 7 days diving. Data are mean ± SD (n = number of diver's samples; + $p < 0.001$, t-test; * $p < 0.001$ vs. control, RM-ANOVA). Bold numbers are to indicate statistically significant values.

	MPs/μL	% CD66b	%CD146	%TSP	%CD41	%TMEM	%Phalloidin
Deep-Pre (8)	900 ± 68	11.0 ± 0.5	25.1 ± 0.5	12.7 ± 0.4	3.5 ± 0.4	31.3 ± 0.9	17.3 ± 0.2
Deep-Post (8)	**1089 ± 68 +**	**14.3 ± 2.0 +**	**28.4 ± 1.8 +**	**15.9 ± 2.3 +**	**5.7 ± 1.6 +**	**34.4 ± 2.1 +**	**20.0 ± 1.9 +**
Shallow-pre (6)	799 ± 68	11.4 ± 2.6	23.0 ± 2.5	13.6 ± 2.5	3.1 ± 1.1	29.2 ± 2.0	18.4 ± 1.5
Shallow-1 day post (6)	**947 ± 31 ***	12.8 ± 1.5	23.6 ± 1.5	14.5 ± 1.4	4.8 ± 1.9	29.9 ± 0.8	19.4 ± 1.3
Shallow-7 day post (6)	**1016 ± 48 ***	**18.7 ± 1.5 ***	**27.4 ± 1.5 ***	16.2 ± 1.8	**7.1 ± 1.8 ***	**33.2 ± 1.7 ***	20.7 ± 1.5

Table 2. Exosomes/lipophilic particles in blood. Imaging flow cytometry was used to evaluate exosomes and lipophilic particles as total number/μL (mean ± SD, n = number of samples) pre- and post-deep and shallow dives. Note that due to insufficient plasma volume, analysis could only be conducted on 4 of the 8 participants in the deep diver group (+ $p < 0.001$, t-test; * $p < 0.001$ vs. control, RM-ANOVA). Bold numbers indicate statistically significant values.

	Pre-Dive (#/μL)	Post-Day 1 (#/μL)	Post Day 7 (#/μL)
Deep divers (n = 4)	$9.3 \pm 0.9 \times 10^7$	$\mathbf{16.5 \pm 5.2 \times 10^7}$ **+**	
Shallow divers (n = 6)	$6.1 \pm 2.6 \times 10^7$	$\mathbf{14.7 \pm 3.6 \times 10^7}$ *****	$\mathbf{17.3 \pm 3.8 \times 10^7}$ *****

Exosome membranes are rich in tetraspanins, endosomal proteins that organize membrane microdomains. Several were evaluated in the shallow diver group (inadequate sample volumes precluded assays from the deep divers) among PKH-positive particles between 20 and 120 nm in diameter. CD63 expression pre-dive occurred on 74.7 ± 2.4%, and 94.7 ± 0.6% after day 1, and 94.6 ± 3.5 % after day 7 ($p < 0.001$ versus pre-diving, RM-ANOVA). CD81 expression pre-dive occurred on 67.7 ± 2.4%, 93.3 ± 0.4% after day 1, and 94.5 ± 4.1% after day 7 ($p < 0.001$ versus pre-diving, RM-ANOVA).

2.3. Neutrophil Activation Elicited by Diving

The activation of neutrophils, which express the CD66b protein, was assessed by flow cytometry as the surface expression of the CD18 protein component of the β_2 integrin, or myeloperoxidase (MPO) above background on CD66b-positive cells. Neither diver group exhibited activation after day 1. Only after the 7th day of diving was there a statistically significant increase in cells expressing MPO in the shallow diver group (Table 3).

Table 3. Activation of neutrophils from all divers in both groups. Data are the mean ± SD (n = sample number) % of neutrophils (identified in the flow cytometer based on CD66b expression) expressing myeloperoxidase (MPO) and CD18 above a threshold value as an index of cell activation. Pre- and post-day 1 are values from the deep and shallow groups, and those in the third column reflect values from the shallow group, and the statistical analysis compared against the values only takes this group into account (pre- and post-day 1 as repeated measures ANOVA. (* $p < 0.001$ vs. pre-dive, RM-ANOVA).

	Pre-Dive	Post-Day 1	Post Day 7
% MPO	8.7 ± 4.0 (13)	8.7 ± 6.1 (13)	10.7 ± 5.4 (6) *
% CD18	2.1 ± 1.9 (13)	4.5 ± 3.4 (13)	3.7 ± 4.7 (6)

2.4. IL-1β in MPs Increased by Diving

IL-1β secretion requires unconventional pathways, involving packaging into either MPs or exosomes, to be liberated to the extracellular milieu [30]. To assess cargo differences in MPs versus exosomes, the plasma preparation used for enumerating EVs were centrifuged at 21,000× g for 30 min. Afterwards, 67.6 ± 17.8 (n = 13) % of all MPs and only 15.5 ± 5.2 (n = 13) % of the exosomes/lipophilic particles were found in the pellet. There was no detectable IL-1β in 21,000× g supernatants, indicating the absence of this cytokine in exosomes. Contents in pellets are shown in Table 4. There was a statistically significant difference between the pre-dive IL-1β levels in the deep versus the shallow divers, which suggests some pre-diving differences between groups. Within each group, there were significant differences in values on day 1 diving in the deep divers, and at day 7 in the shallow diver group (Table 4).

Table 4. Intra-MPs IL-1β as pg/million MPs. Data are the mean ± SD (n = sample number) pre- and post-diving for both diver groups (+ $p < 0.02$, t-test; * $p < 0.001$ RM-ANOVA; [1] $p < 0.01$ t-test within columns).

	Pre-Dive	Post-Day 1	Post-Day 7
Deep divers (8)	10.0 ± 9.5 [1]	65.6 ± 23.1 + [1]	
Shallow divers (6)	3.1 ± 1.5	21.6 ± 16.5	104.9 ± 14.0 *

2.5. NOS2 in MPs Increased by Diving

Animal studies suggest there is a role for NOS2 generating a gas phase in MPs [16]. Others have reported NOS activity and presence of NOS2 in exosomes [31,32]. There was no detectable NOS2 in the 21,000× g supernatant preparation (exosomes exosomes/lipophilic particles and few MPs), but there were significant elevations versus pre-dive values in the pellets, as shown in Table 5.

Table 5. Intra-MPs NOS2 as pg/million MPs. Data are the mean ±SD (n = sample number) pre- and post-diving for both diver groups (+ $p \leq 0.02$, t-test; * $p < 0.001$ RM-ANOVA.

	Pre-Dive	Post-Day 1	Post-Day 7
Deep divers (8)	0.03 ± 0.06	0.17 ± 0.12 +	
Shallow divers (6)	0.04 ± 0.06	0.16 ± 0.11 *	0.17 ± 0.06 *

2.6. Plasma Gelsolin (pGSN) Decreased by Diving

Plasma gelsolin is a highly conserved, cytoplasmic actin-binding protein that has been reported to decrease in post-diving samples in a murine DCS model and in human subjects exposed to pressure in a hyperbaric chamber [23]. The open-water diver data shown in Table 6 demonstrate significant reductions in pGSN post-dive in the deep divers at day 1, and among the shallow divers at day 7.

Table 6. Plasma gelsolin (µg/mL). Data are the mean ± SD (*n* = sample number) pre- and post-diving for both diver groups (+ *p* < 0.001, *t*-test; * *p* < 0.001 RM-ANOVA; There is not a statistically significant difference in pre-dive values between the two groups).

	Pre-Dive (µg/mL)	Post-Day 1	Post-Day 7
Deep divers (8)	121.3 ± 33.1	34.8 ± 20.4 +	
Shallow divers (6)	168.5 ± 21.5	151.9 ± 13.7	106.7 ± 30.9 *

3. Discussion

This study demonstrates that MPs elevations and neutrophil activation in CCR divers mirror changes previously reported in air-breathing divers, where oxygen partial pressures were variable and often higher [4,5,7–9,11,12,14]. Changes in MPs subgroups expressing different cell-specific proteins and concurrent changes in IL-1β, NOS2, and pGSN provide additional insight. Based on the mechanisms of MPs production by high pressure gases, one would anticipate that exposure to higher pressures will trigger more MPs to be formed than in lower gas pressures, as was observed. However, helium triggers less oxidative stress than an equal pressure of nitrogen, so one cannot directly compare responses between the diver groups [22]. It is notable that elevations in MPs expressing microglial-specific TMEM were found after the single ~100 msw dive, whereas a similar elevation in shallow divers was only observed after 7 days of repetitive diving. We recently reported that TMEM-expressing MPs that also expressed TSP generated in the brain are released via the brain glymphatic system to the systemic circulation, where they activate neutrophils to generate a second array of MPs, some of which express F-actin (29). This cascade of MPs responses could explain differences between the diver groups. MPs-bearing proteins specific to neutrophils (CD66b), endothelial cells (CD146), and platelets (CD41a) support activation of these cells from diving. We cannot rule out a role for platelet-derived TSP in the elevation of MPs expressing this protein in the deep diver group.

We also report, for the first time, exosome/lipophilic particle elevations in response to diving. We assessed these particles based on their 20 to 120 nm diameter and staining with the lipophilic PKH67 dye. There is a complex interplay between exosomes, the NLRP3 inflammasome, and IL-1β. Inflammatory stimuli can enhance exosome formation and exosomes can either enhance or inhibit inflammasome formation and IL-1β production [33]. Mechanism (s) for exosome formation with diving will require further investigation, but could be linked to MPs, given their IL-1β cargo. We found that there were higher percentages of sub-micron particles expressing CD63 and CD81 post-diving, supporting the presence of exosomes versus merely non-specific lipophilic particles. We also utilized Laurdan staining in the protocol. The changes in CD63 and 81 and Laurdan staining are indicative of new exosome populations with differing protein and lipid content. The higher percentage of particles detected by Laurdan in the post-dive samples is likely due to the emission spectrum of the dye (490 nm in a disordered lipid [gel] phase versus 430 nm in an ordered [liquid crystalline] phase), and because the detection channel bandpass filter in the flow cytometer was 475 ± 45 nm. This is not the same as providing direct information about lipid packing domains (so-called lipid rafts) which requires more precise dual wavelength measurements to assess the generalized polarization [34].

Plasma gelsolin (pGSN) blood levels fall in numerous acute and chronic inflammatory states. Among studies, the magnitude of pGSN reduction parallels the extent of tissue damage, and depletion precedes and predicts adverse clinical outcomes [35–41]. In the present study, we observed significantly lower pGSN concentrations in post-dive plasma. Prior work suggests that the decrease occurs due to pGSN consumption from binding and lysis of F-actin-expressing MPs. In the murine DCS model, and numerous animal studies of infection, injury, and inflammation, pGSN supplementation can abrogate organ damage [23,42]. Our study is the first to show reductions of pGSN in open-water divers.

Elevations of IL-1β following high gas pressure exposure have been described in the murine model and in humans after simulated diving [5,15,26]. Here, we show IL-1β elevations in CCR divers, and that it is present in MPs but not in exosomes. This is consistent with NLRP3 inflammasome assembly occurring concurrently with MPs formation in response to high gas pressure exposures. We also demonstrate NOS2 presence in human MPs and an increased content post-diving. When neutrophils are stimulated by binding MPs, synthesis of many proteins associated with NLRP3 inflammasome formation are increased, including NOS2 [24,25]. This has important implications for diving physiology because NOS2 is a high-output Ca^{++}-independent NOS isoform. After expressional induction, it continuously produces nitric oxide until the enzyme is degraded. This alone (separate from other changes post-diving) can impair normal vascular tone and endothelial integrity [31,32]. Moreover, murine studies indicate that MPs NOS2 is responsible for generating a gas phase of NO_2 (from oxidized nitric oxide) within MPs [16]. As these MPs enlarge on decompression, the data suggest that enzyme activity provides a nucleation site for bubble formation. The findings in this project–that MPs are more numerous and possess higher NOS2 concentrations post-dive, somewhat proportional to dive depth–imply greater potential for bubble nucleation and greater risk for bubble-induced vascular damage. It should be noted that, given the micro-dimensions of MPs, bubbles related to MPs (that would be expected to lyse with sufficient growth) would still be below the detection limits of current ultrasound technology.

This project reconfirms the pro-inflammatory effects of diving in humans. It also, for the first time, documents elevations in exosomes/lipophilic particles, although their pathophysiological role in diving remains unclear. It should be emphasized that divers in this study exhibited no adverse health effects. Oxidative stress and inflammatory responses are not necessarily manifestations of toxicity and organ damage. However, all changes seen in these research subjects are directly linked to tissue damage in the murine DCS model. Clearly, therefore, additional events are necessary for symptom development and overt DCS. An attractive hypothesis is that some individuals may exhibit lower pGSN at baseline and/or more exuberant NOS2 production and activity, such that nucleation-site-carrying MPs generate more intravascular bubbles or carry more IL-1β in response to diving. These issues are currently under investigation.

4. Materials and Methods

4.1. Experimental Protocol

All subjects gave their informed consent for inclusion before they participated in the study. The study was conducted in accordance with the Declaration of Helsinki, and the protocol was approved by the Bio-Ethical Committee for Research and Higher Education, Brussels (N° B200-2020-088). Analyses of deidentified blood samples were approved by the University of Maryland Institutional Review Board (N° HP-00059996). After written, informed consent, 13 male, healthy, non-smoking divers (Minimum certification "Autonomous Divers" according to European norm EN 14153-2 or ISO 24801-2 with at least 50 logged dives) volunteered for this study. None of them had a history of previous cardiac abnormalities or were under any cardio- or vaso-active medication. They were selected from a large population of divers in order to have a homogenous sample: aged 44.7 ± 12.4 years old (mean ± SD); height 173 cm ± 6.6; weight 75.2 ± 13.7 kg.

4.2. Reagents

Chemicals were purchased from Sigma–Aldrich (St. Louis, MO, USA) unless otherwise noted. Annexin-binding buffer and the following agents were purchased from BD Pharmingen (San Jose, CA, USA): fluorescein isothiocyanate (FITC) conjugated Annexin V (cat # 556419), R-PE conjugated anti-human CD18 (cat # 555924), and PerCP/Cy5.5 conjugated anti-human CD41a (cat # 340931). APC-conjugated anti-human CD146 (cat # 340931) was purchased from BioScience (San Diego, CA, USA), AlexaFluor488-conjugated anti-human TMEM119 (cat # FAB103131G) was from R & D Systems (Minneapolis, MN, USA), anti-thrombospondin (TSP)-1 (cat # sc-393504) was from Santa Cruz Biotechnology (Dallas, TX, USA), and FITC-conjugated anti-human myeloperoxidase (MPO, cat # HM1051PE-100) was from Hycult Biotech (Plymouth Meeting, PA, USA). Antibodies purchased from Biolegend (San Diego, CA, USA) included: AlexaFluor647-conjugated anti-human CD63 (cat # 353016), PercpCy5.5-conjugated anti-human CD81 (cat # 349520), and BV421-conjugated anti-human CD66b (cat # 347201).

4.3. Blood Sampling and Laboratory Procedure

Blood samples were obtained before and 120 min after the last dive on the first day from both diver groups (deep and shallow), and after the last dive on the 7th day for the shallow group. Blood (~5 mL) was drawn into Cyto-Chex BCT test tubes that contained a proprietary preservative (Streck, Inc., Omaha, NE, USA). Samples were sent by express mail to the University of Maryland (Dr. Thom) laboratory, where all analyses were performed following published techniques described in previous publications [25,43]. In brief, total MPs and subtypes were assayed in an 8-color, triple-laser MACSQuant (Version 2.13.3, Miltenyi Biotec Corp., Auburn, CA, USA) flow cytometer with the manufacturers' acquisition software using standard methods, including a "fluorescence minus one control test" [44]. This analysis provides a way to define the boundary between positive and negative particles in an unbiased manner by defining the maximum fluorescence expected for a given subset after outlining the area in a two-dimensional scatter diagram when a fluorophore-tagged antibody is omitted from the stain set. The analysis allows for a simple decision as to where to place the upper boundary for non-staining particles in a fluorescence channel. All supplies, reagents, and manufacturer sources have been described in previous publications [8,9,11,12].

The blood was centrifuged for 5 min at $1500\times g$, the supernatant was made to 12.5 mmol/L EDTA to impede MP aggregation, and then centrifuged at $15,000\times g$ for 30 min. Aliquots of the $15,000\times g$ supernatant were stained with antibodies for MP analysis by flow cytometry, and a portion was used for exosome analysis. Plasma stored at $-80\ °C$ after a $15,000\times g$ centrifugation step preceding MP analysis was used for IL-1β, NOS2, and pGSN assays.

4.4. Neutrophil Activation Analysis

Whole fixed blood from the Cyto-Chex tubes (100 μL) was stained for 30 min at room temperature in the dark with optimized concentrations of antibodies as listed above. After staining, 2 mL phosphate buffered saline (PBS) was added to dilute each sample tube prior to analysis, with the cytometer acquisition set to use anti-human CD66b as the fluorescence trigger to recognize neutrophils.

4.5. IL-1β and NOS2 Measurements

Human-specific ELISA Kits (eBioscience, San Diego, CA, USA) that detect pro- and mature forms of IL-1β or NOS2 were used following the manufacturer's instructions. Measurements were made using plasma supernatant after blood was centrifuged at $15,000\times g$, as described for flow cytometry studies, and also in supernatant and pellet fractions separated by a second centrifugation at $21,000\times g$ for 30 min. The MPs in pellets were placed in a 0.3 mL lysis buffer, the protein content of the sample was measured, diluted to 5 mg/mL, and 20 μg protein was used for analysis.

4.6. Gelsolin Assay

A human-specific commercial pGSN ELISA kit (LSBio, Inc. Seattle, WA, USA) was used following the manufacturer's instructions. Serial dilutions in PBS were prepared using the supernatant after $15,000\times g$ centrifugation of plasma, as described above, and analyzed concurrent with a range of known pGSN standards.

4.7. Exosome/Lipophilic Particles Assay

Using 15,000 g supernatants from plasma as described above, 5 μL samples were diluted in 100 μL PBS and incubated with dyes [2.5 μmol PKH67 (Sigma Cat#SIG-MINI67),

2.5 μmol Laurdan (1-[6-(Dimethylamino)-2-naphthalenyl]-1-dodecanone, Tocris Biotech Cat#7275)], and antibodies for 30 min prior to analysis using an ImageStream®X Mk II: Imaging Flow cytometer. FluoSphere™ carboxylate-modified microspheres (Thermofisher, 20 and 100 nm in diameter) were used to provide size bracketing, and initial standardization of methods was conducted with 120 nm (range 80–140 nm) synthetic lipid vesicles from Cellarcus Biosciences (San Diego, CA, USA) that were made with a lipid composition comparable to mammalian cells. For initialization, the instrument bright field and lasers were set to maximum power, side scatter (SSC) set to 70 mW, and the 60× imager magnification set to high gain. Channel 1 was used for bright field and Ch.6 for SSC. After setting the compensation matrix with bright field off and all channels enabled, single-color compensations were set for each color, with gates set to detect particles between 20 and 100 nm in diameter.

4.8. Statistical Analysis

Results are expressed as the mean ± SD. Data were analyzed using SigmaStat (Version 12.5, Jandel Scientific, San Jose, CA, USA). The normality of the data was assessed with the Shapiro–Wilk tests, and if passed, data was analyzed with a Student's t-test between groups and repeated measures analysis of variance (RM-ANOVA) with the post-hoc Tukey test, where appropriate. A small number of data sets for the deep diver group failed the normality test, and comparisons within the group were performed by means of the non-parametric Mann–Whitney test. For all studies, we deemed a result to be statistically significant if $p < 0.05$.

Author Contributions: All authors listed have made a substantial, direct and intellectual contribution to the work, and approved it for publication: Conceptualization: C.B. and S.R.T.; Investigation: A.K.A., V.M.B., A.R.B., L.J.T., A.R.-S., C.B., S.R.T., E.L. and E.D.; Writing: A.K.A., S.R.T. and C.B.; Funding: S.R.T. and C.B. All authors have read and agreed to the published version of the manuscript.

Funding: This work was supported in part by grants from the US Office of Naval Research N00014-20-1-2641 (Thom), the National Institutes for Health (NINDS) R01-NS122855 (Thom), and internal funding from the Environmental, Occupational, Ageing (Integrative) Physiology Laboratory, Haute Ecole Bruxelles-Brabant (HE2B), Belgium). The sponsors had no role in the design and conduct of the study; collection, management, analysis, and interpretation of the data; preparation, review or approval of the manuscript; and the decision to submit the manuscript for publication.

Institutional Review Board Statement: All experimental procedures were conducted in accordance with the Declaration of Helsinki [45]. Ethics Committee approval from the Bio-Ethical Committee for Research and Higher Education, Brussels (N° B 200-2020-088) and University of Maryland Institutional Review Board (N° HP-00059996).

Informed Consent Statement: Informed consent was obtained from all subjects involved in the study.

Data Availability Statement: Data are available at request from the authors.

Acknowledgments: Authors are grateful to all volunteer participants.

Conflicts of Interest: The authors declare no conflict of interest.

Abbreviations

CCR	Closed circuit rebreather
DCS	Decompression sickness
EVs	Extracellular vesicles
IL-1β	Interleukin-1β
MPO	Myeloperoxidase
MPs	Blood Borne Microparticles
NLRP3	Nucleotide-binding domain leucine rich repeat (NOD)-like receptor, pyrin containing 3 inflammasome
NOS2	Nitric oxide synthase-2

pGSN	Plasma gelsolin
PO$_2$	Oxygen Partial Pressure
RAGE	Receptor for advanced glycation end products
TMEM	Transmembrane protein 119
TLR4	Toll-like receptor 4
TSP	Thrombospondin 1

References

1. Francis, T.J.; Pearson, R.R.; Robertson, A.G.; Hodgson, M.; Dutka, A.J.; Flynn, E.T. Central nervous system decompression sickness: Latency of 1070 human cases. *Undersea Hyperb. Med.* **1988**, *15*, 404–417.
2. Bigley, N.J.; Perymon, H.; Bowman, G.C.; Hull, B.E.; Stills, H.F.; Henderson, R.A. Inflammatory cytokines and cell adhesion molecules in a rat model of decompression sickness. *J. Interferon Cytokine Res.* **2008**, *28*, 55–63. [CrossRef]
3. Martin, J.D.; Thom, S.R. Vascular leukocyte sequestration in decompression sickness and prophylactic hyperbaric oxygen therapy in rats. *Aviat. Space Environ. Med.* **2002**, *73*, 565–569. [PubMed]
4. Barak, O.F.; Janjic, N.; Drvis, I.; Mijacika, T.; Mudnic, I.; Coombs, G.B.; Thom, S.R.; Madic, D.; Dujic, Z. Vascular dysfunction following breath-hold diving. *Can. J. Physiol. Pharmacol.* **2020**, *98*, 124–130. [CrossRef] [PubMed]
5. Brett, K.D.; Nugent, N.Z.; Fraser, N.K.; Bhopale, V.M.; Yang, M.; Thom, S.R. Microparticle and interleukin-1ß production with human simulated compressed air diving. *Sci. Rep.* **2019**, *87*, 13320. [CrossRef] [PubMed]
6. Vince, R.V.; McNaughton, L.R.; Taylor, L.; Midgley, A.W.; Laden, G.; Madden, L.A. Release of VCAM-1 associated endothelial microparticles following simulated SCUBA dives. *Eur. J. Appl. Physiol.* **2009**, *105*, 507–513. [CrossRef]
7. Madden, L.A.; Chrismas, B.C.; Mellor, D.; Vince, R.V.; Midgley, A.W.; McNaughton, L.R.; Atkins, S.L.; Laden, G. Endothelial function and stress response after simulated dives to 18 msw breathing air or oxygen. *Aviat. Space Environ. Med.* **2010**, *81*, 41–51. [CrossRef]
8. Thom, S.R.; Milovanova, T.N.; Bogush, M.; Bhopale, V.M.; Yang, M.; Bushmann, K.; Pollock, N.W.; Ljubkovic, M.; Denoble, P.; Dujic, Z. Microparticle production, neutrophil activation and intravascular bubbles following open-water SCUBA diving. *J. Appl. Physiol.* **2012**, *112*, 1268–1278. [CrossRef]
9. Thom, S.R.; Milovanova, T.N.; Bogush, M.; Yang, M.; Bhopale, V.M.; Pollock, N.W.; Ljubkovic, M.; Denoble, P.; Madden, D.; Lozo, M.; et al. Bubbles, microparticles and neutrophil activation: Changes with exercise level and breathing gas during open-water SCUBA diving. *J. Appl. Physiol.* **2013**, *114*, 1396–1405. [CrossRef]
10. Pontier, J.M.; Gempp, E.; Ignatescu, M. Blood platelet-derived microparticles release and bubble formation after an open-sea dive. *Appl. Physiol. Nutr. Metab.* **2012**, *37*, 888–892. [CrossRef]
11. Madden, D.; Thom, S.R.; Milovanova, T.N.; Yang, M.; Bhopale, V.M.; Ljubkovic, M.; Dujic, Z. Exercise before SCUBA diving ameliorates decompression-induced neutrophil activation. *Med. Sci. Sports Exerc.* **2014**, *46*, 1928–1935. [CrossRef] [PubMed]
12. Madden, D.; Thom, S.R.; Yang, M.; Bhopale, V.M.; Milovanova, T.N.; Ljubkovic, M.; Dujic, Z. High intensity cycling before SCUBA diving reduces post-decompression microparticle production and neutrophil activation. *Eur. J. Appl. Physiol.* **2014**, *114*, 1955–1961. [CrossRef] [PubMed]
13. Thom, S.R.; Yang, M.; Bhopale, V.M.; Huang, S.; Milovanova, T.N. Microparticles initiate decompression-induced neutrophil activation and subsequent vascular injuries. *J. Appl. Physiol.* **2011**, *110*, 340–351. [CrossRef]
14. Thom, S.R.; Bennett, M.; Banham, N.D.; Chin, W.; Blake, D.F.; Rosen, A.; Pollock, N.W.; Madden, D.; Barak, O.; Marroni, A.; et al. Association of microparticles and neutrophil activation with decompression sickness. *J. Appl. Physiol.* **2015**, *119*, 427–434. [CrossRef] [PubMed]
15. Thom, S.R.; Bhopale, V.M.; Yu, K.; Yang, M. Provocative decompression causes diffuse vascular injury in mice mediated by microparticles containing interleukin-1beta. *J. Appl. Physiol.* **2018**, *125*, 1339–1348. [CrossRef]
16. Thom, S.R.; Yang, M.; Bhopale, V.M.; Milovanova, T.N.; Bogush, M.; Buerk, D.G. Intra-microparticle nitrogen dioxide is a bubble nucleation site leading to decompression-induced neutrophil activation and vascular injury. *J. Appl. Physiol.* **2013**, *114*, 550–558. [CrossRef] [PubMed]
17. Yang, M.; Milovanova, T.N.; Bogush, M.; Uzan, G.; Bhopale, V.M.; Thom, S.R. Microparticle enlargement and altered surface proteins after air decompression are associated with inflammatory vascular injuries. *J. Appl. Physiol.* **2012**, *112*, 204–211. [CrossRef] [PubMed]
18. Yang, M.; Kosterin, P.; Salzberg, B.M.; Milovanova, T.N.; Bhopale, V.M.; Thom, S.R. Microparticles generated by decompression stress cause central nervous system injury manifested as neurohypophiseal terminal action potential broadening. *J. Appl. Physiol.* **2013**, *115*, 1481–1486. [CrossRef]
19. Mause, S.F.; Weber, C. Microparticles: Protagonists of a novel communication network for intercellular information exchange. *Circ. Res.* **2010**, *107*, 1047–1057. [CrossRef]
20. Cabral, J.; Ryan, A.E.; Griffin, M.D.; Riter, T. Extracellular vesicles as modulators of wound healing. *Adv. Drug. Deliv. Rev.* **2018**, *129*, 394–406. [CrossRef]
21. Slater, T.W.; Finkilesztein, A.; Mascarenhas, L.A.; Mehl, L.C.; Butin-Israeli, V.; Sumagin, R. Neutrophil microparticles deliver active myeloperoxidase to injured mucosa to inhibit epithelial wound healing. *J. Immunol.* **2017**, *198*, 2886–2897. [CrossRef] [PubMed]

22. Thom, S.R.; Bhopale, V.M.; Yang, M. Neutrophils generate microparticles during exposure to inert gases due to cytoskeletal oxidative stress. *J. Biol. Chem.* **2014**, *289*, 18831–18845. [CrossRef]
23. Bhopale, V.M.; Ruhela, D.; Brett, K.D.; Nugent, N.Z.; Fraser, N.K.; Levinson, S.L.; DiNubile, M.J.; Thom, S.R. Plasma gelsolin modulates the production and fate of IL-1β-containing microparticles following high-pressure exposure and decompression. *J. Appl. Physiol.* **2021**, *130*, 1604–1613. [CrossRef] [PubMed]
24. Thom, S.R.; Bhopale, V.M.; Arya, A.K.; Ruhela, D.; Bhat, A.R.; Mitra, N.; Hoffstad, O.; Malay, D.S.; Mirza, Z.K.; Lantis, J.C.; et al. Blood-borne microparticles are an inflammatory stimulus in type-2 diabetes mellitus. *ImmunoHorizons* **2023**, *1*, 71–80. [CrossRef]
25. Thom, S.R.; Bhopale, V.M.; Yu, K.; Huang, W.; Kane, M.A.; Margolis, D.J. Neutrophil microparticle production and inflammasome activation by hyperglycemia due to cytoskeletal instability. *J. Biol. Chem.* **2017**, *292*, 18312–18324. [CrossRef] [PubMed]
26. Thom, S.R.; Bhopale, V.M.; Yang, M. Microparticle-induced vascular injury in mice following decompression is inhibited by hyperbaric oxygen: Effects on microparticles and interleukin-1beta. *J. Appl. Physiol.* **2019**, *126*, 1006–1014. [CrossRef] [PubMed]
27. Thom, S.R.; Bhopale, V.M.; Bhat, A.R.; Arya, A.K.; Ruhela, D.; Qiao, G.; Li, X.; Tang, S.; Xu, S. Neuroinflammation with increased glymphatic flow in a murine model of decompression sickness. *J. Neurophysiol.* **2023**, *129*, 662–671. [CrossRef]
28. Pospichalova, V.; Svoboda, J.; Dave, Z.; Kotrbova, A.; Kaiser, K.; Klemova, D.; Ilkovics, L.; Hampl, A.; Crha, I.; Jandakova, E.; et al. Simplified protocol for flow cytometry analysis of fluorescently labeled exosomes and microvesicles using dedicated flow cytometer. *J. Extracell. Vesicles* **2015**, *4*, 25530. [CrossRef]
29. Harris, F.M.; Best, K.B.; Bell, J.D. Use of laurdan fluorescence intensity and polarization to distinguish between changes in membrane fluidity and phospholipid order. *Biochem. Biophys. Acta* **2002**, *1565*, 123–128. [CrossRef]
30. Cypryk, W.; Nyman, T.A.; Matikainen, S. From inflammasome to exosome-does extracellular vesicle secretion constitute an inflammasome-dependent immune response? *Front. Immunol.* **2018**, *9*, 2188. [CrossRef]
31. Gambim, M.H.; do Carmo, A.O.; Marti, L.; Verrissimo-Filho, S.; Lopes, L.R.; Janiszewski, M. Platelet-derived exosomes induce endothelial cell apoptosis through peroxynitrite generation: Experimental evidence for a novel mechanism of septic vascular dysfunction. *Crit. Care* **2007**, *11*, R107. [CrossRef] [PubMed]
32. Webber, R.J.; Sweet, R.M.; Webber, D.S. Inducible nitric oxide synthase in circulating microvesicles: Discovery, evolution, and evidence as a novel biomarker and the probable causative agent for sepsis. *J. Appl. Lab. Med.* **2019**, *3*, 698–711. [CrossRef] [PubMed]
33. Noonin, C.; Thongboonkerd, V. Exosome-inflammasome crosstalk and their roles in inflammatory responses. *Theranostics* **2021**, *11*, 4436–4451. [CrossRef] [PubMed]
34. Sanchex, S.S.; Tricerri, M.A.; Gratton, E. Laurdan generalized polarization fluctuations measures membrane packing micro-heterogeneity in vivo. *PNAS* **2012**, *109*, 7314–7319. [CrossRef] [PubMed]
35. Khatri, N.; Sagar, A.; Peddada, N.; Choudhary, V.; Singh Chopra, B.; Garg, V. Ashish, Plasma gelsolin levels decrease in diabetic state and increase upon treatment with F-actin depolymerizing versions of gelsolin. *J. Diab. Res.* **2014**, *2014*, 152075.
36. Lu, C.-H.; Lin, S.-T.; Chou, H.-C.; Lee, Y.-R.; Chan, H.-L. Proteomic analysis of retinopathy-related plasma biomarkers in diabetic patients. *Arch. Biochem. Biophys.* **2013**, *529*, 146–156. [CrossRef]
37. Lee, P.S.; Patel, S.R.; Christiani, D.C.; Bajwa, E.; Stossel, T.P.; Waxman, A.B. Plasma gelsolin depletion and circulating actin in sepsis: A pilot study. *PLoS ONE* **2008**, *3*, e3712. [CrossRef]
38. Lee, P.S.; Sampath, K.; Karumanchi, S.A.; Tamez, H.; Bhan, I.; Isakova, T.; Gutierrez, O.M.; Wolf, M.; Chang, Y.; Stossel, T.P.; et al. Plasma gelsolin and circulating actin correlate with hemodialysis mortality. *Am. Soc. Nephrol.* **2009**, *20*, 1140–1148. [CrossRef]
39. Osborn, T.M.; Verdrengh, M.; Stossel, T.P.; Tarkowski, A.; Bokarewa, M. Decreased levels of the gelsolin plasma isoform in patients with rheumatoid arthritis. *Arthritis Res. Ther.* **2008**, *10*, R117. [CrossRef]
40. Peddada, N.; Sagar, A.; Ashish; Garg, R. Plasma gelsolin: A general prognostic marker of health. *Med. Hypotheses.* **2012**, *778*, 203–210. [CrossRef]
41. Overmyer, K.A.; Shishkova, E.; Miller, I.J.; Balnis, J.; Bernstein, M.N.; Peters-Clarke, T.M.; Meyer, J.G.; Quan, Q.; Muehlbauer, L.K.; Trujillo, E.A.; et al. Large-scale multi-omic analysis of COVID-19 severity. *medRxiv* **2020**. [CrossRef] [PubMed]
42. Piktel, E.; Levental, I.; Durnás, B.; Janmey, P.; Bucki, R. Plasma gelsolin: Indicator of inflammation and its potential as a diagnostic tool and therapeutic target. *Int. J. Mol. Sci.* **2018**, *19*, 2516. [CrossRef] [PubMed]
43. Balestra, C.; Arya, A.K.; Leveque, C.; Virgili, F.; Germonpre, P.; Lambrechts, K.; Lafere, P.; Thom, S.R. Varying oxygen partial pressure elicits blood-borne microparticles expressing different cell-specific proteins—Toward a targeted use of oxygen? *Int. J. Mol. Sci.* **2022**, *23*, 7888. [CrossRef] [PubMed]
44. Tung, J.W.; Parks, D.R.; Moore, W.A.; Herzenberg, L.A.; Herzenberg, L.A. New approaches to fluorescence compensation and visualization of FACS data. *Clin. Immunol.* **2004**, *110*, 277–283. [CrossRef] [PubMed]
45. World Medical, A. World Medical Association Declaration of Helsinki: Ethical principles for medical research involving human subjects. *JAMA* **2013**, *310*, 2191–2194.

Disclaimer/Publisher's Note: The statements, opinions and data contained in all publications are solely those of the individual author(s) and contributor(s) and not of MDPI and/or the editor(s). MDPI and/or the editor(s) disclaim responsibility for any injury to people or property resulting from any ideas, methods, instructions or products referred to in the content.

MDPI
St. Alban-Anlage 66
4052 Basel
Switzerland
www.mdpi.com

International Journal of Molecular Sciences Editorial Office
E-mail: ijms@mdpi.com
www.mdpi.com/journal/ijms

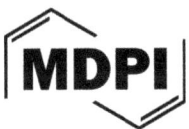

Disclaimer/Publisher's Note: The statements, opinions and data contained in all publications are solely those of the individual author(s) and contributor(s) and not of MDPI and/or the editor(s). MDPI and/or the editor(s) disclaim responsibility for any injury to people or property resulting from any ideas, methods, instructions or products referred to in the content.

www.ingramcontent.com/pod-product-compliance
Lightning Source LLC
LaVergne TN
LVHW070635100526
838202LV00012B/811

9 7 8 3 0 3 6 5 8 8 9 2 6